Hallucinations

Hallucinations
The Science of Idiosyncratic Perception

André Aleman and **Frank Larøi**

American Psychological Association
Washington, DC

Published by
American Psychological Association
750 First Street, NE
Washington, DC 20002
www.apa.org

To order
APA Order Department
P.O. Box 92984
Washington, DC 20090-2984
Tel: (800) 374-2721; Direct: (202) 336-5510
Fax: (202) 336-5502; TDD/TTY: (202) 336-6123
Online: www.apa.org/books/
E-mail: order@apa.org

In the U.K., Europe, Africa, and the Midde East, copies may be ordered from
American Psychological Association
3 Henrietta Street
Covent Garden, London
WC2E 8LU England

Typeset in Goudy by Stephen McDougal, Mechanicsville, MD

Printer: McNaughton & Gunn, Ann Arbor, MI
Cover Designer: Naylor Design, Washington, DC
Technical/Production Editor: Harriet Kaplan

The opinions and statements published are the responsibility of the authors, and such opinions and statements do not necessarily represent the policies of the American Psychological Association.

Library of Congress Cataloging-in-Publication Data

Aleman, André.
    Hallucinations : the science of idiosyncratic perception / André Aleman and Frank Larøi. — 1st ed.
        p. ; cm.
    Includes bibliographical references and index.
    ISBN-13: 978-1-4338-0311-6
    ISBN-10: 1-4338-0311-9
    1. Hallucinations and illusions. I. Larøi, Frank. II. American Psychological Association. III. Title.
        [DNLM: 1. Hallucinations. 2. Cognition. WM 204 A367h 2008]

    RC553.H3A44 2008
    616.8—dc22   2007033125

British Library Cataloguing-in-Publication Data
A CIP record is available from the British Library.

Printed in the United States of America
First Edition

Til Jørgen og Johann. Hva i all verden skulle jeg giort uten dere!
To Jørgen and Johann. What in the world would I have done without you!

CONTENTS

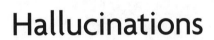

Hallucinations

INTRODUCTION

Hallucinations are an intriguing psychological phenomenon. A person perceives something: a sound, a voice, an image. However, there is no corresponding source in the outside world. How can a person who took LSD see vivid objects when no corresponding photons hit the eye? Or how can a patient with schizophrenia hear people conversing about him loudly and clearly when no sound waves are registered by his ears? Hallucinations can occur in several medical conditions, including psychiatric disorders, but they can also arise because of the intake of a variety of substances, such as LSD or PCP (Brasić, 1998; Slade & Bentall, 1988). Further, hallucinations have also been reported in healthy people from the nonpatient population (Johns & van Os, 2001). The riddle of how hallucinations come about has puzzled clinicians, researchers, and laypeople alike.

Hallucinations are not only an intellectual mystery but also frequently a clinical problem. They can be severely distressing and disruptive of normal functioning. This is vividly illustrated by an excerpt from a first-person account by a woman who was hospitalized several times with severe psychosis. After describing some initial delusional and hallucinatory experiences, she wrote the following:

> The next day I am listening to the soundtrack of the film *The Hurricane*, as I clean my apartment. Suddenly there is an excruciating pain in my

head. It is as if sandpaper were being pulled across the surface of my brain. I hear nasty voices: "You little dumb *** bitch think you can hang out with your special friends. We are here to teach you otherwise. You New World people we can't stand your guts you're all such a bunch of phonies. We're the white lighting [sic] people the Tellurian Hounds and once we're finished with you, you won't recognize the world you live in." I can't stand these voices, the bemoaning belittling laughs. What is going on? I am devastated. . . . "We're going to do some work on your brain Yvonne. You like the *Hurricane* huh? We can't stand these good black people. You think you've accomplished something getting white lightning out of your toilet bowl, try getting it out of your head." The most brutish roaring laughter follows. I am distraught. I run up and down the hallway of my apartment. I can't believe what is happening. I pull my hair. It can't be true what these voices are saying. I try to hide my head, between cushions, between objects, tables, chairs, inside a chest of drawers, anywhere, any place in the apartment, to make the voices stop. But they don't. (*Writing: Hallucinations*, n.d.)

WHO IS THIS BOOK FOR?

This book is written for researchers, clinicians, and students with a background in psychology, psychiatry, cognitive neuroscience, neurology, social work, or philosophy. In fact, it may appeal to any reader interested in hallucinations and how these originate in the mind and brain. For clinicians, the discussion of novel approaches to treatment will extend their "tool kit." Researchers and students will find not only a comprehensive, empirically based review of hallucinogenic phenomena but also proposals for integration of current theory and findings and directions for future research.

WHAT IS IN THIS BOOK?

The purpose of this book is to bring together current knowledge from psychological and neuroscience research into hallucinations and thereby provide a state-of-the-art overview. To this end, we review and integrate all major findings regarding epidemiology, phenomenology, cognitive processing, emotional factors, neurochemistry, brain imaging, and treatment of hallucinations. We intend to cover hallucinations in different sensory modalities and in different clinical and nonclinical groups. Besides discussing conceptual issues, we also review the epidemiology and phenomenology of hallucinations in different sensory modalities. In addition, studies investigating cognitive processes such as attention, perception, and memory in relation to hallucinations are discussed, and we outline the neural basis of hallucinations, drawing on evidence from neurology and brain imaging. Detailed attention is paid to hallucination characteristics in the psychoses, although hallucinations associated with other clinical groups and conditions (e.g., brain damage, Charles Bonnet syndrome, drugs) are also discussed. The book not only summarizes recent progress in understanding the cognitive and neural basis of hallucinations but also describes novel treatments and future research avenues. Finally, the book moves beyond a critical overview of current research and findings and proposes an integrative framework that may help in the understanding of hallucinations and may guide future research.

The approach we have adopted in writing this book can broadly be defined as being multidisciplinary. More specifically, we start from a psychological approach, with emphasis on single symptoms as the unit of analysis and consistent with the cognitive neuropsychiatry approach. We discuss these interrelated and complementary approaches in turn.

PSYCHOLOGICAL APPROACH

The psychological approach emphasizes mechanisms common to both "normal" perception and hallucinations but at the same time specifies what factors lead to the emergence of the latter. Thus, in our view, hallucinations are not by definition discontinuous with normal perception. The approach takes into account cognitive factors underlying perception and also acknowledges the role of emotion and motivation. In our view, that part of contemporary psychology that is concerned with the science of the mind–brain and behavior can be seen as part of the cognitive neurosciences. In this area of enquiry, psychologists strongly cooperate with researchers and clinicians from disciplines such as neurophysiology, neurology, and psychiatry. We have therefore also integrated findings from these fields into our book.

In our psychological approach, we focus on a single symptom. In psychiatry and neurology, researchers frequently focus their investigations on *syndromes*, that is, particular collections of symptoms that have been described under a clinical category, such as Alzheimer's disease, epilepsy, or schizophrenia. There are some disadvantages to this approach, however, which are especially apparent in psychiatry. The main problem is the heterogeneity of syndromes. For example, although hallucinations feature as a prominent symptom of schizophrenia in the widely used classification manual, *Diagnostic and Statistical Manual of Mental Disorders* (4th ed.; American Psychiatric Association, 1994), not every patient with schizophrenia experiences hallucinations. The diagnosis can also be made on the basis of delusions and negative symptoms (apathy, emotional blunting, and social withdrawal). It is hard to imagine that an explanation involving one mechanism will suffice to help one understand emotional blunting and social withdrawal on one hand and also account for hallucinations and delusions on the other.

The symptom-oriented approach argues that to understand the nature of the psychological processes underlying phenomena or symptoms, research should concentrate directly on these individual phenomena (e.g., hallucinations) and not on diagnostic categories (e.g., schizophrenia). There are a number of advantages associated with this approach, but there are also disadvantages. Some of these are presented and discussed in this volume; however, for more detailed information concerning this (interminable) debate, the reader may refer to the specific references.

Persons (1986) provided six important advantages of the symptom approach. First, it avoids misclassification and confounding, which can occur with the diagnostic-category design (e.g., not all schizophrenia patients have hallucinations, and nonschizophrenic patients may also experience hallucinations). Second, it enables the study of important phenomena that are ignored by the diagnostic-category design. Third, there is a greater facilitation of theoretical development (e.g., symptom-specific theories are clearer and easier to test). Fourth, it permits the isolation of single elements of pathology for study. Fifth, it recognizes the continuity of clinical phenomena with normal phenomena and mechanisms. Sixth, it is less vulnerable to the lack of adequate reliability and validity of diagnostic categories. In addition to these arguments, C. G. Costello (1992) added two more arguments in favor of a single-symptom approach: Useful animal models of symptoms are more likely to be developed, and symptoms may be better phenotypes than syndromes and thus more amenable to genetic research.

Mojtabai and Rieder (1998) critically reviewed the arguments in favor of a symptom-oriented approach compared with a syndrome and/or diagnostic category–oriented approach, arguing that there is little or no evidence supporting some of the major assumptions of a symptom-oriented approach. For example, they presented evidence showing that symptoms do not necessarily have higher reliability and validity than syndromes or diagnostic categories. They also argued that some underlying pathological processes are not exclusively symptom specific (e.g., mechanisms underlying hallucinations in schizophrenia may be different from those in hallucinations observed in neurological disorders). Finally, they provided examples in which an understanding of the etiology of diagnostic categories or syndromes did not precede an understanding of symptoms. They concluded that each approach has different aims and answers different questions and, therefore, should be seen as complementary.

COGNITIVE NEUROPSYCHIATRIC APPROACH

A cognitive neuropsychiatric approach is also adopted in this book (David, 1993; Halligan & David, 2001). This approach also takes single symptoms as its unit of analysis, but in particular, it aims to uncover abnormalities or dysfunctions in cognitive mechanisms that may account for the clinical phenomena. Furthermore, the neural basis of such cognitive alterations is investigated. Thus, three levels of explanation are distinguished and related to each other (see Mortimer & McKenna, 1994): phenomenology (the symptom to be understood), cognition (mental processes), and neurophysiology (the brain correlates). This approach assumes that the cognitive level is intermediate between symptoms and neurophysiology and that the neuropsychology of hallucinations may thus have the potential to connect neuroscience with phenomenology. In this book, we take a cognitive neuropsychiatry approach by focusing on one single phenomenon, hallucinations, and by investigating cognitive processes that might be involved together with their corresponding neural basis.

TOWARD A UNIFYING ACCOUNT

Hallucinations can take myriad appearances, as we review in the chapter on phenomenology (chap. 2). For example, whereas visual hallucinations predominate in neurological conditions, auditory hallucinations predominate in a number of psychiatric conditions. Drug-induced hallucinations tend to be visual but might also be auditory or somatosensory. With regard to underlying mechanisms of all these different types of hallucinations, we adopt the stance taken by David (2004) that in each case, hallucinations of different classes have their unique pathophysiologies but additionally involve generic mechanisms that render the individual vulnerable to hallucinations per se. David suggested that such generic mechanisms may operate in a dose-related manner. Such mechanisms could be of a physiological nature (e.g., arousal), of a more psychological nature (e.g., top-down perceptual factors), or an interaction of these.

OUTLINE OF A COGNITIVE MODEL

To give a preliminary impression of the key components involved, we provide a brief outline of our cognitive model here. Chapters 1 through 6 provide extensive background information in addition to a thorough discussion of different cognitive approaches in the literature. After presenting evidence from dozens of empirical studies, we describe our model, which integrates a number of ideas and suggestions put forward by other investigators (whose work is cited accordingly), in more detail in chapter 7.

In short, our model presumes that a sensory experience (either perception due to external input or hallucination due to internal input) can be induced by activation of sensory cortical areas (either primary or secondary). In normal perception, signals emanating from the sensory organs play a decisive role, whereas in imagery and hallucinations, internally generated signals (emanating from cortical centers) play a decisive role in determining the final "percept." Interactions between sensory signals and top-down signals abound, and it is thus very well possible that external perception triggers hallucination in certain individuals (e.g., some patients with schizophrenia have reported hearing voices when the vacuum cleaner was switched on).

The activation in primary and/or secondary sensory brain areas can be due to input from the senses, lesions to perceptual areas, or input from higher brain centers. The model posits key roles for (a) attention, (b) emotion and motivation, (c) top-down perceptual factors, and (d) monitoring mechanisms. *Attention* refers to the selective focusing on particular inputs, thoughts, or actions while ignoring irrelevant or distracting ones (Gazzaniga, Ivry, & Mangun, 2002). *Emotion and motivation* refers to internal desires and goals. *Top-down perceptual factors* refers to prior knowledge and expectations that affect perception and may involve the mental recreation of a sensory experience (mental imagery). *Monitoring mechanisms* refers to the involvement of a number of processes such as distinguishing between whether an event was internally generated by the individual or externally presented and perceived by the individual.

For all types of hallucinations, attention and monitoring (e.g., external attribution bias) are considered to be of importance. However, in neurological and pharmacological hallucinations, monitoring errors might be more a consequence than a cause of the experience of hallucinations, whereas in psychiatric hallucinations, metacognitive factors may play an important role in the emergence of the hallucinations. Whereas in neurological hallucinations, physiological hyperreactivity of sensory and attentional processes may be the main alterations leading to hallucinatory experiences, in psychiatric hallucinations, the complex interplay of emotion and motivation, top-down factors, and monitoring mechanisms may play a more decisive role.

1

DEFINITION AND
CONCEPTUAL ISSUES

In this chapter, we explore the history of the investigation of hallucinations and the conceptual issues that have arisen from there. We then define hallucination and discuss the various definitions used in the literature.

HISTORICAL DESCRIPTIONS

As was noted by Leudar and Thomas (2000), it is not possible to provide a continuous history of the phenomenon of hallucination. The information is simply not available. However, we do know that hallucinations are as old as humankind. It is curious that the possibility of perception seems to imply the possibility of misperception. Ancient texts described the phenomenon of hallucinations, showing that their authors regarded hallucinations as a culturally integrated aspect of human experience that conveyed a meaningful message.

Socrates (4th century BC) heard voices and was guided by them in making decisions. Such hallucinations may not be attributed solely to sociocultural factors, however, because the experience of a "demon" that spoke to

9

Socrates was controversial in Athenian culture at that time (Leudar & Thomas, 2000; Smith, 2007). Thanks to writers and philosophers such as Plato, Plutarch, and Xenophon, relatively detailed (although perhaps not entirely objective) accounts of Socrates' life are available to us. This is not always the case for other important historical figures, but although not always documented in sufficient detail, evidence does suggest that other important historical figures may also have had hallucinatory experiences, including scientists and philosophers (e.g., Galileo, Freud, Jung, Pascal, Pythagoras, Swedenborg) and artists (e.g., Schumann, Blake, Munch, Milton, Artaud; see Leudar & Thomas, 2000; D. B. Smith, 2007; Watkins, 1998). That Joan of Arc was guided by hallucinations has been well documented (D. B. Smith, 2007; Spence, 2004). We can also read in the literature that Galileo heard the voice of his dead daughter (Leudar & Thomas, 2000), and Freud (1901/1966) himself wrote,

> During the days when I was living alone in a foreign city . . . I quite often heard my name suddenly called by an unmistakable and beloved voice; I then noted down the exact moment of the hallucination and made anxious enquiries of those at home about what had happened at that time. (p. 261)

Of course, in religious experience, be it in the past or in the present, idiosyncratic perceptions (i.e., an individual perceives something others in the immediate vicinity do not perceive) abound.

Drug-induced hallucinations have been mentioned in ancient Chinese texts. The Pên-ts'ao Ching, the oldest pharmacopoeia known, stated that the fruits (flowering tops) of hemp, "if taken in excess will produce hallucinations" (literally "seeing devils"; Li, 1974). The ancient medical work also stated, "If taken over a long term, it makes one communicate with spirits and lightens one's body" (Li, 1974). Not until the 18th century, however, were hallucinations systematically described as a separate entity and considered to be "fallacies of the senses" (Dufour, cited in Berrios, 1996) or even as a "disease" (Berrios, 1996). Before the 19th century, hallucinations were termed *apparitions* and were generally not seen as erroneous perceptions but as mystical and spiritual experiences.

In *De genesi ad litteram*, Augustine (354–430 AD) outlined three types of apparitions or visions: *intellectual*, *imaginative*, and *corporeal*. An example of the first type is the experience alluded to by St. Paul as a vision of the "third heaven." The second is exemplified in the vision of St. Peter at Joppa, and the third is exemplified in the vision of Belshazzar in the book of Daniel. Paul described a vision of the third heaven as follows in his letter to the Corinthians:

> Although there is nothing to be gained, I will go on to visions and revelations from the Lord. I know a man in Christ who fourteen years ago was caught up to the third heaven. Whether it was in the body or out of

the body I do not know—God knows. And I know that this man—whether in the body or apart from the body I do not know, but God knows—was caught up to paradise. He heard inexpressible things, things that man is not permitted to tell. (2 Cor. 12:1–4)

The vision of Peter was described as follows in the book of Acts:

I was in the city of Joppa praying, and in a trance I saw a vision. I saw something like a large sheet being let down from heaven by its four corners, and it came down to where I was. I looked into it and saw four-footed animals of the earth, wild beasts, reptiles, and birds of the air. Then I heard a voice telling me, "Get up, Peter. Kill and eat." (Acts 11: 5–7)

The Bible also contains a vivid description of the vision of Belshazzar:

King Belshazzar gave a great banquet for a thousand of his nobles and drank wine with them. . . . Suddenly the fingers of a human hand appeared and wrote on the plaster of the wall, near the lampstand in the royal palace. The king watched the hand as it wrote. His face turned pale and he was so frightened that his knees knocked together and his legs gave way. (Daniel 5:1, 5–6)

According to Augustine, the intellectual vision is an essentially mystic experience without the presence of a visual object. The object of an intellectual vision usually concerns higher theological concepts, such as the Holy Trinity, the essence of the soul, the nature of heaven, and the like. The imaginative vision, in contrast, is somewhat more concrete than the intellectual and may accompany mystical experiences but is not limited to believers. Although it also lacks a visual object, the human imagination is touched to create a visual representation. Often the visionary is aware that it is a purely reproduced or composite image that exists only in the imagination. This kind of vision occurs most frequently during sleep.

The difference between an imaginative and a corporeal vision, according to Augustine, is that the imaginative vision, although having a visual component, is not seen by the eyes and leaves no physical evidence of its effects. The corporeal vision, on the other hand, is registered by the human eye and at times leaves physical effects. The corporeal vision can either be a figure really present or a supernatural power that directly modifies the visual organ and produces in the composite a sensation equivalent to that which an external object would. The presence of an external figure may be seen in two ways. Sometimes the very substance of the being or the person will be present; sometimes it will be merely an appearance consisting of a certain arrangement of luminous rays. Although Augustine mainly limited his discussion of apparitions to visual phenomena, mystics in his tradition also recognized auditory apparitions, usually as an inner voice. This phenomenon was called *locution*.

French and German Psychiatry

Although visions and locutions were widely reported earlier, it was not until the 19th century that more systematic and scientific study was made of the phenomenon. It was at that time that the concept of hallucination was introduced, with a major contribution by French psychiatrists, for example, Jean-Etienne Esquirol in 1832, Alfred Maury in 1855, and Brierre de Boismont in 1856. Overviews of their conceptual thinking have been given by Sarbin and Juhasz (1967), Berrios (1996), and Leudar and Thomas (2000), among others.

The word *hallucination* has its roots in the Latin *hallucinere* or *allucinere*, meaning "to wander in mind" or "idle talk." The first usage of the word *hallucination* in the English language was in the 1572 translation of a work by Lewes Lavater, to refer to "ghostes and spirites walking by nyght" (quoted in Sarbin & Juhasz, 1975). However, it was Esquirol (1817) who introduced the concept of hallucination, as currently understood, into psychiatry. Before the 19th century, there was no generic class to include all hallucinatory experiences (Berrios, 1996). Esquirol proposed that *hallucination* be used as the generic name.

> Hallucinations of eyesight have been called visions but this term is appropriate only for that sensory modality. One cannot talk about "auditory visions", "taste visions", or "olfactory visions". The latter phenomena, however, share with visions the same mechanisms and are seen in the same diseases. A generic term is needed for all. I propose the word hallucination. (quoted in Berrios, 2005, p. 242)

In his book *Mental Maladies: A Treatise on Insanity*, Esquirol (1845/1965) described a person experiencing hallucinations to have a "thorough conviction of the perception of a sensation, when no external object, suited to excite this sensation, has impressed the senses." Shorter (2005) noted that Esquirol thus used the term in its modern sense of perceptions without a real external stimulus. That is not to say, however, that the phenomena of hallucinations as such (without using the word *hallucination*) had not been described earlier in psychiatric literature, as is evident from the writings of William Cullen (who lived from 1710 to 1790), the Scottish systematizer of illnesses, among others (see Shorter, 2005). Esquirol also wrote about possible mechanisms underlying hallucinations. He started from the assumption that "seeing" is the capture of a public stimulus, applied this to visions (which only differ in the fact that no external object is present), and generalized this to other sense modalities (Berrios, 1996). Furthermore, Esquirol (1832) regarded hallucinations as arising from neural hyperactivity during memory retrieval: "The activity of the brain is so energetic that the visionary, the person hallucinating, ascribes a body and an actuality to images that the memory recalls without the intervention of the senses." Lelut, in 1846, and

Tanzi, in 1909 (cited in Berrios, 1996) voiced similar beliefs by suggesting that hallucinations were transformations of thoughts into sensations, or ideas stored in memory that go back to perceptual centers and thus become hallucinations. A number of current cognitive theories can be considered elaborations of this position (see chap. 4, this volume).

Whereas early French psychiatrists such as Louis François Lelut and Jules Baillarger considered hallucinations always to be pathological (i.e., signs of mental illness), Brierre de Boismont in 1861 maintained that not all hallucinations should be tied to madness (see Leudar & Thomas, 2000). Instead, he distinguished between *physiological* and *pathological* hallucinations. Physiological hallucinations can occur in healthy people: They are compatible with reason and can be voluntary (as was the case with Goëthe, according to Brierre). Thus, hallucinations of thinkers like Socrates or religious visionaries like Joan of Arc would be regarded as physiological hallucinations by Brierre. Pathological hallucinations, on the other hand, are almost always associated with "delirious conceptions" and "childish terrors." This approach is radically different from the medicalization of hallucinations by other French psychiatrists of the time. Leudar and Thomas (2000) summarized Brierre's position as follows: "The madness of hallucinations was in their involuntariness, delirious content, its falsity, childish terror of the hallucinator; in other words, nothing specific to hallucinating" (p. 12). We will see in chapter 3 of this volume that current researchers distinguish between pathological and nonpathological hallucinations in a similar way.

According to Berrios (2005), it was the French psychiatrists in the first 30 years of the 19th century who decided that hallucinations were (a) primary disorders of perception; (b) the same class of phenomena, regardless of the sense modality in which they occurred; (c) generated by stimulation of brain regions related to perception and hence mechanical responses with no semantic or informational import; and (d) medical problems. It could be added that the focus was not on the content of the hallucinations but rather on the formal occurrence per se (i.e., that one perceived something that was not objectively present). The content or meaning of the hallucination was considered to be of little relevance.

Berrios (2005) noted that the German contribution to the development of the concept of hallucination has received less attention than the French one. He drew attention to a German book published in 1826 by Johannes Müller (1801–1858), *Ueber die phantastischen Gesichtserscheinungen* (Fantastic Phenomena of Vision). Berrios argued that Müller's book, also written during the first half of the 19th century, offers insight into the early stage of the process of naturalization of hallucinations. Apparently, the development of conceptualizing hallucinations as homogeneous phenomena that form a "natural kind" (i.e., analogous to everyday objects around us rather than being abstract entities) was not an exclusively French pursuit.

Berrios (2005) cited a paper by Brierre that made reference to Müller. This way of viewing hallucinations profoundly affected the way hallucinatory experiences were interpreted. Increasingly, mystical visions and similar experiences were no longer seen as the communication of supernatural origin. Instead, natural explanations were advanced. Müller, for example, claimed that visions are "fantastic," by which he meant that they are the result of overactivity of a putative faculty of fantasy or imagination (Berrios, 2005). Others maintained that hallucinations involve processes similar to dreaming. Brewer (1898/2005) made this point using examples from literature ranging from Shakespere to Descartes to Sir Walter Scott.

Medical Versus Psychological Viewpoints

Berrios (1985) and Slade and Bentall (1988) pointed out that from the very beginning of conceptual thinking about hallucinations, two different approaches can be distinguished: the psychological and the medical. In general, the former considers the hallucinatory experience as continuous with normal experience, whereas the latter regards it as discontinuous with normal experience. For instance, taking a psychological approach, Hibberts (1825) considered imaginations and hallucinations ("apparitions") to be part of a continuum of completely natural and ordinary mental experiences. In a similar vein, Sir Francis Galton (1883/1943), one of the pioneers of scientific psychology, argued that there is a continuity between all forms of visual imagination, from an almost absence of pictorial thought to images so vivid that they are indistinguishable from full percepts, thereby ending in complete hallucination. In contrast, Arnold (1806) and Esquirol (1832) considered hallucinations to be pathological and categorically distinct from normal mental events. Thus, there is a discontinuity between hallucination and normal perception. According to Arnold, hallucinations only arise after a defect to bodily organs whereby incorrect information is transmitted to the brain.

Although the medical model has been dominant over the past centuries, the controversy about pathology versus normality of hallucinations continues up to the present day. During the second part of the 20th century, hallucinations were widely regarded to be signs of mental illness by psychiatrists, presumably due to the strong influence of Schneider's (1957) classification of hallucinations as a "first rank" symptom of schizophrenia. However, large population-based studies have established that people from the normal population, without psychiatric illnesses, experience hallucinations (see chap. 2, this volume). A consensus seems to emerge that pathological and nonpathological forms of hallucination exist, whereby aspects such as attributions (e.g., of omnipotence of the "voices"), loudness, frequency, degree of distress that they elicit, and negative and emotionally threatening content seem to be decisive factors (Chadwick & Birchwood, 1994; Choong,

Hunter, & Woodruff, 2007; Johns & van Os, 2001). Chapters 2 and 3 (this volume) further discuss the phenomenology of hallucinatory experiences and different groups of hallucinators, respectively.

It is interesting that Freud (1900/1938) regarded hallucinations as regressions—that is, to thoughts transformed into images. He suggested that "only such thoughts undergo this transformation as are in intimate connection with suppressed memories, or with memories which have remained unconscious" (p. 462). Freud proposed this explanation as the basis for "the hallucinations of hysteria and paranoia, as well as the visions of mentally normal persons" (p. 462), suggesting that he recognized a continuum between hallucinatory experiences in the normal population and in psychiatric disorders. As noted before, Freud had even experienced hallucinations himself.

DEFINING HALLUCINATION

In more contemporary accounts of hallucination, it has been difficult to find an unambiguous definition. Nonetheless, it is important to agree on a suitable working definition that will guide theory and research, and in describing efforts at reaching such a definition, we will be able to demarcate hallucinations from other phenomena that might share some phenomenological features. The APA *Dictionary of Psychology* defined hallucinations as "a false sensory perception that has the compelling sense of reality despite the absence of an external stimulus" (VandenBos, 2007, p. 427; see Exhibit 1.1 for the complete definition). This certainly captures the essence of a hallucinatory experience, although a more precise description should be possible. For example, the statement "despite the absence of an external stimulus" might not be entirely accurate, because some hallucinations are triggered by (irrelevant) external stimuli—for example, patients who start hearing voices when the vacuum cleaner is switched on. Hallucinations have been defined in different ways (see Exhibit 1.1 for a list), although they have a number of elements in common.

We favor the definition provided recently by David (2004):

> A sensory experience which occurs in the absence of corresponding external stimulation of the relevant sensory organ, has a sufficient sense of reality to resemble a veridical perception, over which the subject does not feel s/he has direct and voluntary control, and which occurs in the awake state. (p. 108)

Veridical perception here refers to the accurate perception of what is real. This definition by David (2004) is a revision and extension of previous definitions proposed by Slade and Bentall (1988) and Aleman and de Haan (1998). Slade and Bentall defined hallucinations as "any percept-like experi-

EXHIBIT 1.1
Definitions of Hallucinations

- Hallucination is a false perception characterized by externalization and a continued belief that the experience is a perception of something outside the self rather than an internal thought or image. (Campbell, 2004, p. 312)
- A true hallucination will be perceived as being in external space, distinct from imagined images, outside conscious control, and as possessing relative permanence. (*Oxford Handbook of Psychiatry*; Semple, Smyth, Burns, Darjee, & McIntosh, 2005)
- A false sensory perception that has a compelling sense of reality despite the absence of an external stimulus. It may affect any of the senses, but auditory hallucinations and visual hallucinations are most common. Hallucination is typically a symptom of psychosis, although it may result from substance abuse or a medical condition, such as epilepsy, brain tumor, or syphilis. (*APA Dictionary of Psychology*; VandenBos, 2007, p. 427)
- Hallucinations are images based on immediately internal sources of information, which are appraised as if they came from immediately external sources of information. (Horowitz, 1975, p. 165)
- Any percept-like experience which (a) occurs in the absence of the appropriate stimulus, (b) has the full force or impact of the corresponding actual (real) perception, and (c) is not amenable to direct and voluntary control by the experiencer. (Slade & Bentall, 1988, p. 23)
- A sensory experience which occurs in the absence of external stimulation of the relevant sensory organ, but has the compelling sense of reality of a true perception, is not amenable to direct and voluntary control by the experiencer, and occurs in the awake state. (Aleman & de Haan, 1998, p. 657)
- A sensory experience which occurs in the absence of corresponding external stimulation of the relevant sensory organ, has a sufficient sense of reality to resemble a veridical perception, over which the subject does not feel s/he has direct and voluntary control, and which occurs in the awake state. (David, 2004, p. 108)

---

ence which (a) occurs in the absence of the appropriate stimulus, (b) has the full force or impact of the corresponding actual (real) perception, and (c) is not amenable to direct and voluntary control by the experiencer" (p. 23). The definition demarcates hallucinations from illusions by indicating that the hallucination arises in the absence of the appropriate stimulus and emphasizes the sensory quality of hallucinations by specifying that a hallucination has "the full force or impact of the corresponding actual (real) perception." Furthermore, this definition distinguishes hallucinations from mental imagery by adding that the hallucination "is not amenable to direct and voluntary control by the experiencer." After all, mental imagery, in contrast to hallucination, is generally under the control of the experiencer (Kosslyn, 1994).

Despite its merits, however, this definition runs into a number of problems. First, the meaning of "percept-like" remains vague. Is mental imagery also percept-like? In addition, the phrase "in the absence of the appropriate stimulus" may need specification. Hallucinations can be triggered in some patients by certain stimuli, such as background noise. In some patients a sensory stimulus is required in the sensory organ corresponding to the modality in which the hallucination is occurring (i.e., hearing church bells when the telephone is ringing). Here "hearing church bells" is a hallucination and "the telephone ringing" is the stimulus in the sensory organ (ear in this case) corresponding to the modality in which hallucination is occurring. Thus, the hallucination is precipitated by a specific function of the corresponding sensory organ.

In other cases, the hallucination can be triggered by certain thoughts, fears, or events. David's (2004) definition circumvents this by stating that a hallucination is "a sensory experience which occurs in the absence of corresponding external stimulation of the relevant sensory organ" (p. 108). In the second part of their definition, Slade and Bentall (1988) required the hallucination to have "the full force or impact of the corresponding actual (real) perception" (p. 23). This might be a rather stringent condition because some patients may hear soft, mumbling voices or see fleeting silhouettes on the neighbors' roof. The phrase proposed by David may capture the intention of this part of the definition better: "has a sufficient sense of reality to resemble a veridical perception" (p. 108).

The final part of Slade and Bentall's (1988) definition concerns voluntary control of the experience, when they stated that a hallucination "is not amenable to direct and voluntary control by the experiencer." This may again be too stringent, because a number of patients do have a certain amount of control. For example, some patients apply coping techniques, such as turning on the television, to diminish their hallucinations. Conversely, other patients are able to induce hallucinations by certain thoughts or actions. The crucial point is that patients generally do not feel they are in control of the experience. Hence, David's (2004) revised definition states that hallucinations are states "over which the subject does not feel s/he has direct and voluntary control" (p. 108).

Finally, Aleman and de Haan (1998) pointed out that vivid dreams can be considered hallucinations by most current definitions but argued that dream imagery should be excluded from the definition. Although dreams certainly share important characteristics of hallucinations, they only occur in the context of sleeping (i.e., REM sleep), which is a fundamental alteration of consciousness. A defining aspect of hallucinations, and a major reason to distinguish them as a separate category, is that they concern false perceptions that occur in an awake state. During a dream, people are usually not aware of their actual surroundings, whereas most hallucinating people are (with the exception of some extreme conditions such as severe psychosis). During a dream, people usually do not interact with other people or actively participate in society, whereas hallucinations may frequently occur in such circumstances and have a stronger impact on everyday functioning. For completeness, it is therefore appropriate to include in any definition of hallucination that the experience should occur in the awake state. At the same time, this implies that daydreaming might be a phenomenon related to hallucinations. There is empirical evidence to bolster this claim (Launay & Slade, 1981).

REALITY CHARACTERISTICS OF HALLUCINATIONS

Some authors have maintained that when a person experiences a hallucination but knows it to be such, then it is no longer a hallucination but a *pseudohallucination* (we discuss this concept later). This raises the question whether awareness of a direct correspondence of a hallucinatory experience to an objective external reality—that is, absence of the insight that the hallucination is a perception without external foundation—is a defining characteristic of hallucination. We emphasize that what defines the experience as a hallucination is not so much the conviction that the hallucinated object exists independent of the hallucinator but the conviction that one perceives an object through the senses even though one can be aware that the object does not exist independent of the observer. This conviction, in the absence of corresponding sensory stimulation, is a crucial component of a hallucination.

Hallucination Versus Illusion

Although psychiatrists and psychologists have distinguished between hallucinations and illusions from the time Jaspers (1923/1962) wrote *General Psychopathology*, the boundary between the two phenomena is not always easy to establish. An illusion is a misperception that is based on an existing stimulus, for example, misinterpreting a coat and hat on a coat rack for a man standing in the hall. In contrast, a hallucination is entirely based on internal representations with no corresponding stimulus coming through the senses. The fact that in a large number of individuals hallucinations can be triggered by certain environmental stimuli already makes this distinction problematic. McManus (1996) argued that the significance of the difference between mistaking an X for a Y (illusion) and mistaking nothing at all for a Y (hallucination) may be overstated. Or, as he put it, where does the major difference lie between cases of hearing the sound of a drill as a scream and seeing a shadow as an animal or an oasis in heat haze? Even if there is "nothing there," that may not make a hallucination qualitatively different from some more familiar kinds of sensory error. Berrios (2005) maintained that there is a problem of circularity in defining hallucinations and illusions as distinct phenomena.

Nevertheless, hallucinations can generally be regarded as a different type of misperception, compared with illusions in the sense that the lack of a direct relationship between trigger and percept for independent observers is much more pronounced in the case of hallucinations. Thus, there is a difference in the degree that the sense experience is transformed as a perception relative to the sensory input received at the moment. So if one mistakes the sound of a drill for a scream, this may be considered an illusion under certain circumstances because the sounds are highly similar. If one hears voices and screams when the toilet is flushed, this may more readily be considered a hallucination because other people will not generally report this type of perceptual mistake. In other words, compared with illusions, hallucinations are more idiosyncratic perceptions.

The Concept of Pseudohallucination

The concept of pseudohallucination first appeared in 19th-century French writings on hallucination (e.g., Baillarger, 1886), but the word as such was introduced into psychiatry by Victor Kandinsky in 1881 and Karl Jaspers in 1911. According to Jaspers, *pseudohallucinations* are vivid images with far more sensory content than normal images and ideas. As such, they come close to normal sense perception. However, they have a character of subjectivity and occur in an inner subjective space. In contrast, "true hallucinations" are experienced as objective and located in external space. Berrios (1996) noted that historical accounts are confusing because authors have used the concept in rather different ways. There is no consensus as to whether pseudohallucinations are a form of perception or a form of imagery, whether they are continuous or discontinuous with true hallucinations or with normality, and whether subjects have insight or not (i.e., whether they experience pseudohallucinations as "real").

More recently, pseudohallucinations have been defined mainly in two different ways (Kraupl Taylor, 1981): (a) as hallucinatory experiences that lack strong realistic qualities (i.e., they are not considered a true perception at the time by the percipient) and (b) as subjectively experienced images of great vividness and clarity. Both types of definitions can be traced to work by earlier writers, as noted above. Slade and Bentall (1988) diplomatically concluded that although many observers have acknowledged the validity of distinguishing among true hallucinations, illusions, pseudohallucinations, and various forms of vivid mental experience, many authors have also tended to view them as points on a continuum, with mental imagery at one end and true hallucinations at the other. This idea can be found in the writings of Galton (1883/1943) and Jaspers (1923/1962), among others. In recent years, because of the lack of agreement on a definition of pseudohallucination and uncertainty regarding its conceptual and diagnostic value, the usefulness of the distinction between true hallucinations and pseudohallucinations has been disputed (Bentall, 2003), and several authors have suggested that the concept of pseudohallucination be abandoned altogether (Berrios, 1996).

A question that is closely related to the issue of pseudohallucinations is whether the perceived location of hallucinations is of clinical and etiological importance. More specifically, according to Jaspers (1923/1962), it matters whether hallucinations (especially hearing voices) are perceived as being inside or outside one's head, and clinicians often attach diagnostic significance to this distinction. Although there is some psychiatric evidence that the latter is associated with more severe psychopathology than the former, and distinct neural correlates have been suggested for voices located inside versus outside the head (Hunter et al., 2003), we do not think there is a need for conceptualizing these as two different kinds of experiences. For example, Junginger and Frame (1985) argued that the important characteristic of voices perceived as outside the head is not their location per se but rather the person's delusional attribution that they are alien. Thus, an internal voice can be as disturbing as an external voice—for example, in terms of the degree of distortion of reality (Larøi & Woodward, 2007). There is no evidence for different cognitive processes, and they share the defining feature of hallucination, that is, a conviction of perceiving a stimulus through the senses in the absence of the corresponding stimulation.

PHILOSOPHICAL NOTES

The phenomenon that people can, under certain circumstances, apparently perceive something "out there" when there is no corresponding stimulus in the external physical world raises several philosophical questions. The fact that people can perceive nonexistent objects or events even questions a fundamental human assumption: the reliability of sense perception. Sense perception is generally regarded as an accurate source of information about the physical environment and is the source of beliefs in which people place most confidence. A classic example concerns the apostle Thomas, who could not believe that the crucified Jesus had risen from the dead and exclaimed, "Unless I see the nail marks in his hands and put my finger where the nails were, and put my hand into his side, I will not believe it" (John 20:25).

Hallucinations not only incite epistemological questions, but they also touch on the problem of consciousness and its neural basis. Daniel Dennett (1991), in his book *Consciousness Explained*, opened the very first chapter with an intriguing discussion of the problem of hallucination, which he described as "an illusion without an illusionist." Dennett persuasively argued against a model of consciousness that posits a controlling self that directs traffic and "decides" what to think and what to image. Instead, he argued for a pandemonium model, with different thoughts and images competing for conscious realization. The "winner" will be that which achieves most coherence with other representations that are unfolding. This is consistent with Hoffman's (1986) proposal that one makes automatic inferences about the intentionality of thoughts and images that depend on how these fit into one's overall frame of mind. According to Hoffman, a breakdown in the subject's normal discourse-planning processes could result in some inner speech utterances being experienced as unintended, with the result that they are attributed to an external source.

In cognitive neuroscience and psychiatry, three approaches can be distinguished in research on hallucinations: a phenomenological–hermeneutic approach, idealism, and realism. A phenomenological–hermeneutic approach has been advocated by Leudar and Thomas (2000). It is not primarily concerned with proposing and testing neurocognitive models of hallucinations that will for once and ever explain how hallucinations come about. Rather, their aim has been to document what hallucinatory experiences mean to people. Making reference to Martin Heidegger and Maurice Merleau-Ponty, Thomas, Bracken, and Leudar (2004) discussed the case of a woman experiencing bereavement hallucinations. From a phenomenological theory of embodiment, Thomas et al. then considered the totality of human experience to understand the meaning of hallucinations. They proposed that such an approach can be a valuable clinical tool.

Realism is presumably most widely endorsed, albeit implicitly, by researchers. Idealism takes an inferential approach to perception and holds that perceptions are ideas formed by the perceiving mind about the physical world. In contrast, realism holds that perceptions directly correspond to what is in the world. However, in hallucinations, subjects perceive things that in fact do not directly correspond to objects in the world around them, which has led some philosophers to conclude that the mere fact that hallucinations are possible is at odds with direct realism. This objection has been termed "the problem from hallucination" in the philosophical literature (McManus, 1996). A more moderate version of realism holds that representations in the mind are directly related to external objects. For example, representations of visual objects may even maintain the spatial relationships of the features of the real-world object (Kosslyn, 1994). This approach will not be affected by the problem from hallucination as it will maintain that hallucinations arise from the activation of these "proto-objects" (Collerton, Perry, & McKeith, 2005).

Behrendt and Young (2004) advocated a philosophical approach to hallucination that they called *transcendental idealism* (with reference to Kant). According to this position, "the world that we see around us is internally created and a fundamentally subjective experience that in the state of normal wakefulness is merely constrained by external physical reality" (p. 771). Or, put another way, "What we perceive as being around us is not the external physical world; instead, it is a part of our mind that is projected outside" (p. 772). This approach has been criticized for assuming that the experienced world emerges from autonomous neural activity, without providing any explanation for how autonomous neural activity could ever give rise to the experience of a real world in all its infinite variety (Myin-Germeys & Myin, 2004). Myin-Germeys and Myin (2004) even questioned the logical consistency of the transcendental idealism in the context of scientific research: "How would we know about the constraining role of external reality if all of experience were subjective?" (p. 802). Along the same lines, Foss (2004) argued that modern scientific methodology is only compatible with the philosophical position of realism.

Another philosophical issue that comes to mind when considering several contemporaneous explanations of hallucinations concerns sense of subjectivity and sense of agency of one's own thoughts and actions. Stephens and Graham (2000) pointed to the distinction made by William James between my awareness that a thought exists or occurs and my awareness that I think the thought. The first event concerns my mere introspective awareness of a thought, whereas the latter concerns my experience of my thought as mine. Stephens and Graham proposed that in hallucinations, self-consciousness is disturbed and unravels in such a way that I retain my sense that I am the subject in whom a thought occurs but no longer have the sense that I am the agent who thinks or carries out the thought. This is an interesting suggestion because it may account for what Fernyhough (2004) called the "alien-yet-self" paradox in hallucinations. This paradox is particularly apparent in auditory–verbal hallucinations of schizophrenia. A majority of patients report their experience of a hallucination as a perception (e.g., a voice) that is internal to themselves but is not their own (inner) voice. This forms a problem for any account of hallucinations that is based on a confusion between self and other. If it is simply an error of differentiating between self and other, it is difficult to see how the patients can at the same time accept the hallucinations as being of themselves.

CONCLUSION

In summary, the scientific study of hallucinations as a conceptual entity can be traced back to 19th-century French and German psychiatry. Many of the notions that were then raised are still relevant in contemporary theory and research. However, the distinction between pseudohallucinations (recognized as coming from within the boundaries of the self) and true hallucinations (with an entirely external attribution) is of little theoretical and clinical importance. The study of hallucinations may be of relevance to the philosophy of mind (and vice versa) as it bears on epistemological questions (how reliable is sense perception?), the nature of mental representation, and issues of consciousness and agency.

In the following chapters, we do not elaborate on philosophical issues and implications but rather try to offer more insight into how such disturbances of self-consciousness or errors of perception can emerge in terms of neurocognitive processes in the mind and brain by reviewing empirical studies. First, however, in the next chapter, we describe the phenomenological landscape of hallucinations.

CHAPTER HIGHLIGHTS

- Over the 20th century, hallucinations have been mostly regarded as discontinuous with normal experience and as signs of mental illness (medical viewpoint). Others, however, have regarded hallucinations as continuous with normal experience (psychological viewpoint).
- A hallucination can be defined as a conscious sensory experience that occurs in the absence of corresponding external stimulation of the relevant sensory organ and has a sufficient sense of reality to resemble a veridical perception. In addition, the subject does not feel he or she has direct and voluntary control over the experience.
- A distinction has been made between pseudohallucinations, which have a character of subjectivity and occur in an inner subjective space, and true hallucinations, which are experienced as objective and located in external space. The validity and utility of this concept remain uncertain, however.

2

THE PHENOMENOLOGY
OF HALLUCINATIONS

As shown in chapter 1, defining hallucinations has been no easy task in the past and will probably continue to generate debate in the future. As Lowe (1973) pointed out,

> the variety in the manners in which hallucinations have been defined does not imply that any given definition is invalid, but it does confirm that hallucinations are complex phenomena, whose investigation almost certainly requires multi-dimensional research designs and multiple initial criteria. (p. 626)

A large number of studies suggest that hallucinations are phenomenologically heterogeneous experiences (Carter, Mackinnon, Howard, Zeegers, & Copolov, 1995; Copolov, Trauer, & MacKinnon, 2004; Ey, 1973; Hunter et al., 2003; Junginger & Frame, 1985; Miller, O'Connor, & DePasquale, 1993; Nayani & David, 1996; Oulis, Mavreas, Mamounas, & Stefanis, 1995; Stephane, Thuras, Nasrallah, & Georgopoulos, 2003). For instance, hallucinations may involve a wide variety of modalities and types, including auditory, verbal (i.e., only involving voices), visual, olfactory, kinesthetic, gustatory, tactile, musical, hypnagogic (occurring at sleep onset), hypnopompic (occurring upon awakening), or multimodal (occurring simultaneously in more than one modality). Important to note, however, is that although auditory hallucinations are often reported as being the most prevalent (especially in schizophrenia), findings from a number of studies suggest that other, nonauditory hallucinations are underreported in the literature and are probably more common than traditionally thought (Baba & Hamada, 1999; Bracha, Wolkowitz, Lohr, Karson, & Bigelow, 1989; Delespaul, deVries, & van Os, 2002; Evers & Ellger, 2004; Gauntlett-Gilbert & Kuipers, 2003; D. W. Goodwin, Alderton, & Rosenthal, 1971; Jansson, 1968; A. R. Larkin, 1979; Lowe, 1973; Miller, 1996; Miller et al., 1993; Mueser, Bellack, & Brady, 1990; Phillipson & Harris, 1985; Small, Small, & Andersen, 1966).

Neuroimaging studies suggest that hallucinations in a given modality involve areas that normally process sensory information in that modality (for a detailed review of neuroimaging studies, see chap. 6, this volume). For instance, studies have shown the involvement of the primary and auditory association areas in auditory hallucinations. In visual hallucinations, among the areas that seem to be involved are the primary and visual association areas. Likewise, for somatic hallucinations, studies have observed somatosensory cortical involvement. In an interesting case study, Izumi, Terao, Ishino, and Nakamura (2002) found evidence of differing patterns of regional cerebral blood flow during musical hallucinations versus verbal hallucinations. In a similar study, Shergill et al. (2001) studied a patient with both auditory and somatic hallucinations and used functional magnetic resonance imaging to identify differences in brain activation underlying both. This analysis revealed that somatic hallucinations were primarily associated with activation in areas classically associated with tactile processing (e.g., primary somatosensory cortex, posterior parietal cortex, thalamus), whereas auditory hallucinations were primarily associated with activation in a distinct set of brain areas, particularly the right temporal cortex.

The phenomenological characteristics of hallucinations may vary across clinical populations. (For a detailed review of hallucinations in these clinical groups, in addition to a more detailed comparison of phenomenological characteristics across these clinical groups, see chap. 3, this volume.) For instance, auditory hallucinations may be congruent with the person's mood (e.g., in psychotic depression, mania), or its content may be similar to past (traumatic) events (e.g., in those with posttraumatic stress disorder). In the case of the dementias, in Lewy body dementia and Parkinson's disease, hallucinations are often rich and detailed, whereas in Alzheimer's disease they are commonly simple or isolated. Furthermore, whereas hallucinations in Alzheimer's disease are more frequently visual than auditory, the reverse is true in older patients with schizophrenia (e.g., with late onset schizophrenia-like psychosis) who fall in approximately the same age group. Whereas hallucinations often reflect the concerns of schizophrenic patients and are highly personally salient and emotionally charged, hallucinations in some nonpsychiatric patients (e.g., those suffering from tumors, epilepsy, drug or alcohol withdrawal) usually give rise to contentless or arbitrary perceptual phenomena such as noises or flashes of light or color. Because these populations differ in terms of the presence of sensory deficits, brain anomalies, environmental factors, traumatic events, genetic factors, and so on, this may at least in part explain how the phenomenological characteristics of hallucinations vary across clinical populations.

CULTURE

Culture may modulate the phenomenological characteristics of hallucinations. Bourguignon (1970), who surveyed anthropological data collected from 488 societies worldwide, was one of the first to report on this relation. He found evidence that hallucinations play a role in ritual practices in 62% of the cultures studied. Furthermore, the presence of hallucinations was not associated with the intake of psychoactive chemicals, hallucinations were positively valued, and they could be understood in the context of local beliefs and practices. Al-Issa (1995) suggested that the positive attitude that many developing societies have toward hallucinations mostly reflects general metaphysical attitudes that are often quite different from those held by people in the West. In particular, Western rational–scientific societies strive to clarify and distinguish whether a given experience is real or imaginary, and when individuals are not able to make such a distinction between percepts and images, they are likely to be labeled as out of contact with reality and therefore pathological (i.e., are having hallucinations).[1] In contrast, many non-Western (or less rational–scientific) societies do not make such a rigid distinction between reality and fantasy even tending to encourage individuals to fantasize, and therefore the possibility of misclassifying an imaginary event as real is less important. Al-Issa went on to show how these contrasting attitudes may affect the emotional reaction to hallucinatory experiences, with a predominance of negative reactions and negative attitudes toward hallucinations in Western societies, in contrast to more open and positive attitudes to such experiences in non-Western societies.

There is evidence of cultural variation in the frequency of different kinds of hallucinations between cultures. Auditory hallucinations seem to be the most frequently reported by schizophrenic patients in the West, with visual hallucinations only appearing in the more deteriorated patients (Mueser et al., 1990; E. W. Strauss, 1962). In 15 published studies, Slade and Bentall (1988) found that on average, auditory hallucinations were reported by about 60% of patients with schizophrenia (range 25%–94%) and visual hallucina-

---

[1]The exception to this in Western culture may be children, for whom confusion of percepts and images may be developmental in nature and therefore not necessarily a sign of pathology (Cangas et al., 2003).

tions by 29% (range 4%–72%). In contrast, a number of studies have found that visual hallucinations are a more common type of hallucination in African and Asian countries compared with the West (Al-Issa, 1977, 1978; Murphy, Wittkower, Fried, & Ellenberger, 1963; Ndetei & Singh, 1983; Ndetei & Vadher, 1984; Okulate & Jones, 2003; Sartorius et al., 1986; Suhail & Cochrane, 2002; Zarroug, 1975).[2] For instance, in a study of schizophrenic symptoms in selected regions of the world, Murphy et al. (1963) found that whereas visual hallucinations are the least frequently reported complaint in Europeans and in Americans, they are the most frequently reported by people in Africa and the Near East. Similarly, Al-Issa (1977, 1978) found visual hallucinations to be more common in developing countries than in the developed world. This finding was replicated later in the World Health Organization's multinational study of new cases of psychosis (Sartorius et al., 1986). More recently, Okulate and Jones (2003) reported that the frequency of auditory hallucinations that were commanding, abusive, cursing, arguing, and frightening was generally lower among their Nigerian patients with schizophrenia than among patients in the United Kingdom, on the basis of the study by Nayani and David (1996). Furthermore, in this study, voices discussing the patient in the third person were not as frequent among the Nigerian schizophrenic patients as in the U.K. study.

Kent and Wahass (1996) investigated the content and characteristics of auditory hallucinations in a group of schizophrenic patients in Saudi Arabia and the United Kingdom and found that characteristics of the voices (e.g., frequency, loudness, degree of intrusiveness, source, perceived reality) did not differ between the two cultures. In terms of hallucination content, there were similarities between the two cultures (e.g., involving animosity and friendliness of voices), but there was also evidence of clear differences: A religious and superstitious content was more likely to be reported by patients from Saudi Arabia, whereas instruction and running commentary were more commonly reported by the U.K. patients. The authors interpreted these latter differences in terms of the greater emphasis placed on religion in Saudi Arabian culture (resulting in the fact that religious and supernatural ideation is more salient there than in the West) in contrast to Western societies, which emphasize other aspects of social life (resulting in instructional and running commentary content being more prominent).

Finally, findings from Suhail and Cochrane (2002) suggest that immediate influences (immediate environment and life experiences) may be more important in determining the content of hallucinations than cultural background. They compared the modalities and themes of hallucinations in three different groups of psychotic patients: (a) White, British patients; (b) Paki-

---

[2]Note that one recent, large-scale study comparing patients from the United States with patients from India did not reveal such a trend (Thomas et al., 2007). In this study, auditory hallucinations were more prevalent in U.S. patients (83%) compared with Indian patients (64%), and visual hallucinations were more prevalent in the U.S. patients (57%) than in the Indian patients (37%).

stani patients living in Britain; and (c) Pakistani patients living in Pakistan. They found that whereas the hallucinations in Pakistani patients clearly differed from those reported in the group of White, British patients (i.e., more visual hallucinations in the former group compared with the latter group, and the two groups differed clearly in terms of the themes of their hallucinations), Pakistani patients residing in Britain more closely resembled the White, British group (i.e., more auditory and fewer visual hallucinations, and they differed much less in terms of themes of the hallucinations).

There is also evidence of cultural variations in the frequency of different kinds of hallucinations within (multiethnic) cultures. Johns, Nazroo, Bebbington, and Kuipers (2002) showed that reports of hallucinations varied significantly across different ethnic groups living in the United Kingdom. In this study, 5,196 subjects from ethnic minorities (Caribbean, Indian, African, Asian, Pakistani, Bangladeshi, and Chinese) and 2,867 White U.K. respondents were screened for mental health problems and asked about hallucinations. Results revealed that reports of hallucinations were 2.5 times higher in the Caribbean sample (9.4%) compared with the White sample (4%). Furthermore, rates of hallucinations in the Caribbean sample did not vary by migration (i.e., those who moved to the United Kingdom before the age of 11, compared with those who moved after the age of 11).

Some evidence suggests that a decline in the prevalence of visual hallucinations in the West has been matched by an increase in auditory hallucinations. Kroll and Bachrach (1982) found as many as 134 descriptions of visionary experiences (i.e., visual hallucinations) contained in texts from the Middle Ages. Important to note is that although medieval society did have a notion of mental illness, only 4 of the 134 descriptions (3%) could be associated with probable mental illness or alcohol intoxication. The authors provided two possible explanations for this: Either the symptomatology of mental illness in the Middle Ages did not include reports of hallucinations (and delusions) or, alternatively, people during this time (including the chroniclers) did not confuse the mentally ill with visionaries (suggesting that many of these visionary experiences were attributed to a religious or transcendental experience and therefore were not considered as being necessarily pathological). Furthermore, the visions were not always accepted unquestioningly. Six examples of this type were found, by and large in cases in which the visionary was a person of low status (e.g., a child or an unknown cleric). In contrast, Lenz (1964) examined psychiatric records from Vienna and found that reports of visual hallucinations decreased over a 100-year period, whereas reports of auditory hallucinations rose. Although these studies suggest a decline in the prevalence of visual hallucinations and an increase in auditory hallucinations over time, it is undeniable that far too little work has been done in this important, yet methodologically challenging area. Also, it is important to add that Kroll and Bachrach did not report the number of descriptions of auditory hallucinations, so that we do not know how many visual compared with auditory hallucination descriptions were contained in these texts from the Middle Ages.

Finally, the content of hallucinations also appears to be influenced by culture over time. For example, whereas hallucinatory experiences reported in the Middle Ages were almost universally religious in content (consisting either of messages from God and the saints or of interactions with demons and angels; Kroll & Bachrach, 1982), those recorded by psychologists and psychiatrists today have persecutory or technological themes (Bentall, 2000). This observation is somewhat analogous to the finding (described above) that visual hallucinations may have predominated in the past (e.g., in medieval Europe) compared with modern-day societies, in which auditory hallucinations seem to dominate. If we consider hallucinations to be personal experiences or the expressions of personal concerns and ideas, then it is not difficult to suggest that these experiences (i.e., hallucinations) will be shaped by the person's immediate environment. Religious ideas and practices had a great influence on medieval people's (psychological, social, political) lives, and it is therefore unsurprising that hallucinations were principally religious in content and thus could be perfectly adapted to the cultural norms of that period (Cangas, García-Montes, de Lemus, & Olivencia, 2003). The fact that the hallucinations might have been predominantly visual may simply reflect the fact that it is more fitting or apt to hallucinate religious themes in the visual modality than in auditory, tactile, or olfactory modalities. Similarly, technology has an undeniably important (psychological, social, political) influence on people's lives today, and the fact that many hallucinations have a technological content may therefore not be surprising. Again, perhaps such themes are more readily expressed in the auditory modality.

Mitchell and Vierkant (1989) compared hallucinations in patients admitted in an East Texas hospital during the 1930s with those reported in patients in the same hospital in the 1980s (patients were matched for age, race, and gender distribution). They found that the primary sources of the hallucinations in the 1930s were religious in nature (God, the Holy Ghost, spirits), whereas the primary sources of the hallucinations in the 1980s included not only God, devils, and demons but also doctor, scanner, television, and radio. The content of hallucinations also differed between the two periods. This difference was particularly dramatic for command hallucinations, in which the commands of the 1930s were primarily benign and religious (e.g., "be a better person," "live right," "be good and go to heaven," "lean on the Lord"), compared with the negative and destructive nature of the command hallucinations from the 1980s (e.g., kill oneself or others, "do perverse things," "set fire to the lawn"). Similar differences in the affective content of hallucinations between the two periods were also observed for auditory hallucinations (e.g., a voice saying "we want to go to heaven" vs. a voice saying "you will be crucified for your sins") and visual hallucinations.

These findings that reveal that hallucinations may be influenced by the culture have important clinical implications. Simply put, the clinician, in addition to providing a detailed account of the hallucinations, must also take into account a person's cultural background when assessing and treating hallucinations (Al-Issa, 1995; Wahass & Kent, 1997a, 1997b, 1997c). For instance, in chapter 8, this volume, we present evidence showing that patients in Saudi Arabia tend to use coping strategies for their hallucinations that are associated with their religion, whereas patients in the United Kingdom are more likely to use distraction or physiologically based approaches (Wahass & Kent, 1997b).

As is described in more detail in chapter 3, this volume, studies reveal that it is common for people to see, hear, or feel the presence of the deceased person during bereavement and that there are cultural differences in terms of the rates of hallucinatory experiences in the context of bereavement. Although a series of studies including a group of Swedish widows found that 36% had experienced at least one type of hallucination (Grimby, 1993, 1998), nearly 90% of Japanese widows in another study were found to have hallucinatory experiences involving their dead husband (Yamamoto, Okonogi, Iwasaki, & Yosimura, 1969). Furthermore, a cross-cultural study (Wahass & Kent, 1997a) found that whereas patients from the United Kingdom were more likely to use biological and psychological approaches to explain the apparition of their hallucinations, patients from Saudi Arabia were more likely to evoke religious and superstitious causes.[3] Thus, the treatment strategies that clinicians propose should attempt to take into account the etiological beliefs of their patients. For instance, on the basis of results from this study, a clinician who proposes typically Western interventional approaches (e.g., biological and/or psychological interventions) for hallucinations to patients from Saudi Arabia (or to patients with a Saudi Arabian background but who live in a Western country) will probably be met with skepticism and noncompliance.[4] As Bentall (2003) pointed out, failure to appreciate the cultural context may prevent clinicians from responding appropriately to the distress experienced by their patients. On the other hand, where hallucinatory experiences are culturally accepted reactions to various life events (and therefore might be quite common), the clinician may consider not intervening at all. Thus, awareness of people's attitudes toward hallucinations may help the clinician distinguish between pathological and culturally sanctioned hallucinations (Al-Issa, 1995).

---

[3] It is interesting that in this study, patients in both cultures agreed that stress is one of the important causes of auditory hallucinations.

[4] It is important to note, however, that Wahass and Kent (1997c) have shown that psychological methods for hallucinations as developed in the West can be effective for hallucinations in patients from non-Western backgrounds, that is, if they are modified appropriately (i.e., when the patient's cultural beliefs are taken into account).

TYPES OF HALLUCINATIONS

Numerous reports have suggested that hallucinations are not restricted to any specific sensory modality. Hallucinations may in fact involve a wide variety of modalities, including auditory, visual, olfactory, kinesthetic, gustatory, tactile, musical, hypnagogic, hypnopompic, or multimodal hallucinations. Some of these types are described below.

Auditory Hallucinations

Auditory hallucinations (also referred to as *verbal hallucinations* when only involving voices) represent a particularly rich and varied phenomenology. They may vary both in form and in content. They may involve *acousmas* (primitive sounds, such as blowing, rustling, rattling, shooting, or thundering) or other types of sounds such as humming, crying, laughing, whispering, and talking (Nayani & David, 1996a; Watkins, 1998). More specifically, verbal hallucinations may consist of a voice speaking the individual's thoughts aloud, a voice carrying out a running commentary on the person's behavior, a collection of voices speaking about the individual in the third person, or voices issuing commands and instructions.

In terms of localization, subjects may attribute auditory hallucinations as coming from inside or outside their head (Nayani & David, 1996a). There are also some cases in which patients find it difficult to say whether the voice is inside or outside of their head (Nayani & David, 1996a) or report them as occurring both internally and externally (Copolov, Trauer, & Mackinnon, 2004). Voices heard in external auditory hallucinations may come from behind walls; within air ducts or ventilators; or from animals, plants, and inanimate objects. Hallucinators may hear these voices as coming from either side of them, from above or below them, or from behind. Rarely, however, do auditory hallucinations seem to come from directly in front (Watkins, 1998). Finally, in some cases, there is no specific external source of the voices, in which case they may be said to emanate from the sky or even from some distant part of the universe (Watkins, 1998).

When auditory hallucinations are not localized in the external physical environment, they may be localized within the subject's own head or body. Some subjects describe voices as coming from their mind or as coming from their head, whereas others describe hearing voices with their ears. Similarly, people who are aware of the inner subjective origin of the voices sometimes believe that they are somehow connected to their own thoughts. Voices can be located in one side of the body only or may be divided between the two sides of the hearer's body (e.g., "pleasant" voices being on one side and "unpleasant" voices on the other side). Moreover, these localizations may even change over time. Voices that were initially heard as coming from outside via the ears may eventually be perceived as being located within the hearer's own head or body (Romme, Honig, Noorthoorn, & Escher, 1992). Such changes can also occur according to the hearer's mental and emotional state. For example, when people are stressed or upset, they may experience the voices they hear as being loud and as coming from outside. Finally, there is no evidence that perceived location of hallucinations (i.e., internal, external, or both) has any clear meaningful relationship with demographic, clinical, structural, or other factors (Copolov, Trauer, & Mackinnon, 2004).

Chadwick, Birchwood, and collaborators (Birchwood & Chadwick, 1997; Chadwick & Birchwood, 1994, 1995) have shown that those who experience verbal hallucinations often describe them in terms of the voices' supposed power and authority, in particular, in terms of their degree of omnipotence (e.g., "My voice is very powerful"), malevolence (e.g., "My voice is punishing me for something I have done"), and benevolence (e.g., "My voice wants to protect me"). For instance, Birchwood and Chadwick (1997) found that 45% of patients with schizophrenia or schizoaffective disorder regarded their voices as malevolent, 27% as benevolent, and 27% as benign.

Auditory hallucinations described by patients have often a negative, maladaptive quality (Close & Garety, 1998; Davies, Griffin, & Vice, 2001; Delespaul et al., 2002; Johns, Hemsley, & Kuipers, 2002). Voices may insult and criticize the patient, tell the patient to do something unacceptable (e.g., to commit suicide or to harm someone), or threaten the patient. Chadwick and Birchwood (1994) observed that 46% of their schizoaffective and schizophrenic patients with hallucinations believed their voices to be malevolent. Close and Garety (1998) found that 53% of participants with hallucinating schizophrenia heard voices that were negative in content. In a study including patients with psychosis suffering from hallucinations and delusions, Boschi et al. (2000) found that a majority of patients (57%) indicated that their symptoms were highly stressful. Johns, Hemsley, and Kuipers (2002) observed that the majority of their schizophrenic patients with a history of auditory hallucinations reported negative emotional responses to their hallucinations.

It is not always the case that auditory hallucinations are perceived as negative by patients, and some of them may even state that their voices serve an adaptive function. A number of early studies described hallucinations that made patients feel privileged or protected (Esquirol, 1845/1965), praised them (Kraepelin, 1919/1971), relieved boredom (Esquirol, 1845/1965; Jaspers, 1923/1962), or provided an outlet for hostility (Bleuler, 1908/1950). More recently, Romme and Escher (1989) noted in their questionnaire study of people who heard voices that some of them experienced the voices as positive. For example, those people who began to hear voices after a trauma stated that the voices were helpful and were the beginning of an integrative coping process. Furthermore, for some of them, their voices were perceived as giving them strength or raising their self-esteem.

Positive attitudes toward hallucinations were also reported in a study by Miller et al. (1993) in which a group of 50 chronically hallucinating patients were interviewed about their attitudes toward their hallucinations. The diagnostic categories of patients included schizophrenia and schizophreniform disorder (46%), mood disorders (bipolar and unipolar; 26%), schizoaffective disorder (14%), and other psychotic disorders (14%). Miller et al. found that the majority of patients (52%) reported that their hallucinations served an adaptive purpose. Furthermore, a sizable minority of subjects (20%) did not want the voices to disappear as a consequence of treatment. For instance, patients reported that hallucinations had a relaxing or soothing function (in 58% of subjects), provided them with companionship (42%) and protection (36%), and ameliorated their self-concept (34%). There was no significant relation between positive attitudes toward hallucinations and the subjects' age, sex, occupational status, marital status, or level of education. Similarly, no association was found between positive attitudes and diagnostic category, duration of illness, length of hospital stay, or whether the subject was taking an antipsychotic medication.

Using an alternative to traditional psychometric assessment of hallucinations (Q-sorts), S. Jones, Guy, and Ormrod (2003) found evidence of positive attitudes toward verbal–auditory hallucinations in a group of 20 voice hearers. The subjects were recruited from a variety of sources (e.g., a hearing voices group, spiritualist churches, local community); 11 were current users of mental health services, 4 had never sought such help, and the remaining 5 had briefly used mental health services in the past although not necessarily regarding voice hearing. They were given a set of 45 statements representing a diversity of beliefs and attitudes concerning voice hearing that could be placed along one of three perspectives: biomedical (e.g., "Hearing voices is a symptom of mental illness"), psychological (e.g., "Voices can begin after a major life event"), or spiritual (e.g., "People who hear voices are making contact with a different spiritual plane of reality"). Subjects were then asked to rank these statements along a continuum of significance ranging from *most agree* (5) to *most disagree* (–5), according to how accurately the statement represented their view. The 20 completed Q-sorts (statements rankings) were analyzed using factor analysis, which resulted in six factors.[5] Among these six factors, the principal component (which accounted for 26.8% of the total variance) was interpreted as representing "a positive spiritual perspective" and included very high rankings for statements such as, "People who hear voices are making contact with a different spiritual plane," "People who hear voices are psychic or have a sixth sense," "Voices are a gift and allow people to develop special abilities," and "Voice hearers rise above most people's awareness and beyond 'normal experiences.'" Furthermore, the largest number of subjects (*n* = 8) loaded significantly on this factor compared with the other five factors.

---

[5]These factors included positive spiritual perspective, personal relevance perspective, resigned pessimist perspective, pragmatic response perspective, passivity to forces perspective, and generic mental illness perspective.

Other more recent studies have confirmed that some patients with schizophrenia react positively to (auditory) hallucinations (Birchwood & Chadwick, 1997; Chadwick & Birchwood, 1994; Close & Garety, 1998; Copolov, Mackinnon, & Trauer, 2004; Davies et al., 2001; Johns, Hemsley, & Kuipers, 2002; Sanjuán, Gonzalez, Aguilar, Leal, & van Os, 2004). Johns, Hemsley, and Kuipers (2002) found that 36% of schizophrenic patients with hallucinations reported positive emotional reactions (e.g., "felt comforted by their voices"). Similarly, Chadwick and Birchwood (1994) revealed that 23% of their schizoaffective and schizophrenic patients with hallucinations described the voices as being benevolent, eliciting such positive emotions as amusement, reassurance, calm, happiness, elation, strength, and confidence. In addition, Davies et al. (2001) showed that the mean ratings of the experience of hearing voices and the perception of voices were on the positive side of the rating scale midpoints (4.5) for both psychotic (remitted schizophrenics) and nonclinical groups. Finally, Sanjuán, Gonzalez, et al. (2004) found in their group of patients with schizophrenia and patients with other psychoses that 26% of them reported their auditory hallucinations as being a pleasurable experience. Furthermore, in 10 of these patients, the experience of pleasure was the norm. The identification of positive, agreeable, or pleasurable voices may have important treatment implications. For instance, such hallucinations may have an essential function in empowerment and ego strength (e.g., Jenner, van de Willige, & Wiersma, 1998). Also, patients with (predominantly) pleasurable hallucinations may have less motivation for change and/or be less treatment compliant. (These issues are presented and discussed in more detail in chap 8, this volume.)

In one study, Stephane et al. (2003) interviewed a group of 100 psychiatric patients (with schizophrenia, schizoaffective disorder, and psychotic depression) regarding the phenomenological characteristics of their auditory–verbal hallucinations. A total of 20 phenomenological auditory–verbal hallucination variables were identified on the basis of the literature and the clinical experience of the authors. Multidimensional scaling was then performed to investigate the dimensional structure underlying 11 of these variables. Results revealed three dimensions: linguistic complexity, self–other attribution, and inner–outer space location. The linguistic dimension ranged from low linguistic complexity (i.e., hearing words) at one end of this dimension, to medium complexity (i.e., hearing sentences), to high complexity (i.e., hearing conversations) located at the other end of the dimension. On the second dimension, attribution of the auditory–verbal hallucinations to self ("I hear my own voice") was situated at one end, and attribution to others ("I hear someone else talking to me") was located at the other end. On the third dimension, inner space and outer space location had maximal separation.

Although the findings from Stephane et al. (2003) are generally in line with the literature (Nayani & David, 1996; Watkins, 1998), their study did contain certain limitations. They submitted a restricted range of variables to the multidimensional scaling analysis. For example, only verbal hallucinations were examined. However, studies examining both verbal and nonverbal stimuli have reported that auditory hallucinations may involve a number of different types of sounds (i.e., varying in complexity), including blowing, rustling, humming, rattling, shooting, thundering, crying, laughing, whispering, and talking (Nayani & David, 1996; Watkins, 1998). Studies looking at nonauditory hallucinations have also found evidence of variations in complexity. Gauntlett-Gilbert and Kuipers (2003) examined various phenomenological characteristics of visual hallucinations in a group of psychiatric patients and found, for example, that visual hallucinations with humanoid content could involve restricted features (e.g., faces, skulls), whole figures, or even groups of figures.

In addition, phenomenological characteristics of auditory hallucinations such as affect (e.g., emotional response to hallucinations and/or affective content of hallucinations) were not adequately examined in Stephane et al. (2003). Although little regard has been paid to the complexity of emotional response elicited by hallucinations in the past, more recent studies have taken this aspect seriously (Copolov, Mackinnon, & Trauer, 2004; Haddock, McCarron, Tarrier, & Faragher, 1999; Hayashi, Igarashi, Suda, & Nakagawa, 2004). Copolov et al. (2004) used a comprehensive structured interview schedule to examine various characteristics of auditory hallucinations, in particular their affective impact, in a group of 199 patients. Patients' responses to auditory hallucinations were combined into two (uncorrelated) indexes: one assessing total affective impact (i.e., the strength of affective response) and the other assessing the affective direction (i.e., the degree of positivity or negativity). The authors argued that this suggests that (at least) two dimensions are required to characterize subjects' positive and negative experiences of and responses to auditory hallucinations. That is, even subjects who assess the tone, content, and feeling of their auditory hallucinations as extremely negative may also rate part of their experience in positive terms. Also, in this study, various differential associations (too many to detail here) were found based on this more sophisticated dimensional assessment of affective impact. For instance, it was found that frequent, long, and loud auditory hallucinations were more often perceived as negative. The auditory hallucinations of patients with grandiose delusions were found to be more pleasant than those of patients without such delusions. Also, auditory hallucinations addressing the patient in the second person were found to be significantly more unpleasant than those that did not address the patient in the second person.

Command Hallucinations

Command hallucinations may be considered as a particular subtype of auditory hallucinations in that the voice is experienced as commanding rather than commenting. It is important to specifically examine command halluci-nations as they are often drug resistant and may present a serious social threat to the individuals themselves or to others (Braham, Trower, & Birchwood, 2004). Studies have reported that they are relatively common in voice hear-ers, with between 33% and 74% reporting such activity (Birchwood & Chadwick, 1997; Hellerstein, Frosch, & Koenigsberg, 1987; Mackinnon, Copolov, & Trauer, 2004; Rudnick, 1999; Thompson, Stuart, & Holden, 1992). Shawyer, Mackinnon, Farhall, Trauer, and Copolov (2003) found eight studies reporting the prevalence of command hallucinations in samples of adult psychiatric patients with auditory hallucinations, and they found that the median prevalence rate for these studies was 53% but that there was a wide range (18% to 89%). In the same study, compliance to the command hallucination was found to be 31% in community samples, again with a wide range (0% to 92%), suggesting that patients do not always comply with their commanding voices. The perceived commands range from making a rela-tively harmless gesture (e.g., wash dishes, masturbate, take a bath) to com-mitting minor social transgressions (e.g., break windows, shout out loud, swear in public) to performing potentially injurious or lethal actions to others (e.g., cut her throat, kill someone, beat that person, rape your neighbor) or self (e.g., burn yourself, go into the road, hang yourself, stab yourself, slash your wrists; Byrne, Birchwood, Trower, & Meaden, 2006).

Visual Hallucinations

Although visual hallucinations can occur in a number of populations, they are frequently observed in people with brain disorders (Berrios, 1985) and are a prominent feature of late onset schizophrenia (Howard & Levy, 1994) and major neurodegenerative disorders (Brasić, 1998). Surveys of the general population (Tien, 1991) also find visual hallucinations to be the most common type of hallucination. Tien (1991) compared age-group inci-dence rates for visual, auditory, somatic, and olfactory hallucinations in a randomly selected general population sample ($N = 18,572$). Results revealed that the incidence of visual hallucinations was the highest for six of the eight age groups.[6] The exceptions were that auditory hallucinations (followed by visual hallucinations) represented the highest incidence rates for 18- to 19-year-olds and that 20- to 29-year-olds reported the highest incidence rates for somatic hallucinations (followed by visual hallucinations).

In addition, although visual hallucinations are less prominent in schizo-phrenia (compared with auditory hallucinations), reports of these symptoms actually do exist in the literature (Bracha et al., 1989; D. W. Goodwin et al., 1971; Mueser et al., 1990; Phillipson & Harris, 1985). Some studies have

---

[6]The eight age groups in this study were 18–19, 20–29, 30–39, 40–49, 50–59, 60–69, 70–79, and 80+ years.

reported that up to 40% of schizophrenic patients have visual hallucinations (Mueser et al., 1990; Phillipson & Harris, 1985), and one study even estimated the prevalence of visual hallucination in chronic schizophrenia to be as high as 72% (Goodwin et al., 1971). Bracha et al. (1989) carried out a detailed investigation of the prevalence of visual hallucinations in schizophrenia. When organic causes were carefully excluded by endocrine and metabolic workup, toxicology screen, electroencephalogram, computed tomography, or magnetic resonance imaging, and when strict phenomenological criteria were applied by two raters, 54% of patients were found to have visual hallucinations. This is a much higher rate than what is usually detected in psychiatric settings. Furthermore, in 43% of patients, visual hallucinations were first documented by the researchers (i.e., they were not detected by the referring psychiatrists), suggesting that in a substantial number of cases, visual hallucinations go undetected when assessed by traditional clinical means. Finally, Delespaul et al. (2002) carried out an experience-sampling study that showed that during a week's duration, patients with schizophrenia experienced more visual hallucinations (62.5%) than auditory hallucinations (49.1%). These relatively high prevalence rates suggest that visual hallucinations are probably more common in schizophrenia than traditionally thought. One study has found that visual hallucinations in schizophrenic patients are more frequently perceived in the visual hemifield processed by the dominant cerebral hemisphere (e.g., left-cerebral-dominant patients tended to perceive them in the right hemifield; Bracha, Cabrera, Karson, & Bigelow, 1985).

Gauntlett-Gilbert and Kuipers (2003) examined various phenomenological characteristics of visual hallucinations in a group of psychiatric patients ($N = 20$). In this study, the psychiatric patients were selected on the basis of the fact that they were currently or recently (i.e., in the past 12 months) experiencing visual hallucinations. The participants had the following diagnoses (note that some had multiple diagnoses): schizophrenia or schizoaffective disorder (60%), bipolar affective disorder (15%), depression or psychotic depression (25%), and borderline personality (15%). Results revealed that visual hallucinations were usually humanoid in content, with a minority consisting of animals or objects. In addition, they rarely consisted of something the person had seen before. A majority of patients reported that the initial onset of visual hallucinations was associated with stress (85%), tiredness (60%), loneliness (55%), and relationship problems (50%). They were also asked about the conditions that were currently associated with the onset of a visual hallucination. In 45% of the cases, patients claimed that a psychological factor triggered the hallucinations, and for all patients the trigger was affect. Visual hallucinations were associated with conditions of low sensory and social stimulation. In particular, 75% of visual hallucinations occurred when participants were alone, 65% when they were in a quiet place, and 55% in dim lighting conditions. In terms of affective responses, a large majority of patients (80%) reported fear (i.e., feeling anxious, frightened, or helpless), whereas a relatively smaller number (60%) reported misery (i.e., feeling depressed, sad, or hopeless), and 45% reported more positive emotional reactions (i.e., feeling reassured, happy, or inspired). In addition, a majority (55%) perceived the visual hallucination as a supernatural event rather than as a concrete physical presence. Although the results revealed that few of the visual hallucinations were chronic and persistent (with nearly half occurring in less than 2 weeks), they nonetheless had an impact on patients long after their offset. For example, more than half of the participants reported that visual hallucination affected their beliefs and, in 55% of cases, the visual hallucination helped underpin a delusion (e.g., "It is Jesus telling me I must kill a man").

Musical Hallucinations

Musical hallucinations (hearing tunes, melodies, harmonies, rhythms, and timbres in the absence of an acoustic stimulus) may be experienced under a variety of conditions, including diseases of the ear (Fénelon, Marie, Ferroir, & Guillard, 1993; Tanriverdi, Sayilgan, & Özçürümez, 2001; Terao & Matsunaga, 1999), neurological disorders (Terao & Tani, 1998), psychiatric disorders (Hermesh et al., 2004), and toxic states and as a side effect of antidepressant treatment (Terao, 1995). As the reader will see in chapter 3, this volume, musical hallucinations often occur in older persons with partial or total hearing loss. They seem to be more common in females. Studies also show that age tends to play an important role in that musical hallucinations are more prevalent in older adults (Berrios, 1990) and are rarely observed before middle age (Schielke, Reuter, Hoffmann, & Weber, 2000; Tanriverdi et al., 2001; Terao, 2001).

Musical hallucinations usually consist of songs (usually popular songs, accompanied either by instruments or a cappella), hymns (religious or patriotic), or pieces of classical or instrumental music (including tonal or atonal Western, African, or Eastern music). Subjects are commonly very familiar with the pieces of music they hear (e.g., music from their childhood or pieces of music they play themselves). There have been few reports of musical hallucinations in schizophrenia (Baba & Hamada, 1999; Saba & Keshavan, 1997), although this may be because few patients with schizophrenia spontaneously complain about them and mental health professionals have little interest in them (Baba & Hamada, 1999). Nevertheless, Hermesh et al. (2004) assessed the presence of musical hallucinations in a large group of patients with varying psychiatric diagnoses and found the following lifetime rates of musical hallucinations (in descending order): obsessive–compulsive disorder (41%), schizoaffective disorder (40%), social phobia (35%), major depressive disorder (29%), schizophrenia (26%), panic disorder (23%), and bipolar disorder (20%).

A few studies have reportedly observed the coexistence of musical and verbal–auditory hallucinations in the same patient (Berrios, 1990; Fischer, Marchie, & Norris, 2004; Griffiths, 2000). Although hearing loss, social isolation, advanced age, female sex, and organic brain damage seem to play a major role in the etiology of musical hallucinations (Evers & Ellger, 2004), the relative importance of each factor remains unclear, and research has yet to directly examine other possible contributing factors. Fischer et al. (2004) presented 2 older, female patients (with mild to moderate cognitive impairment, senorineural hearing loss, and who were socially isolated) who initially presented with musical hallucinations and later both went on to develop auditory hallucinations (command hallucinations were also developed in 1 patient). The authors observed that the degree of insight and treatment response declined as the hallucinations changed to voices, suggesting a possible link between musical and auditory hallucinations in older patients in which musical hallucinations may evolve into more serious voice hallucinations over time.

Hypnagogic and Hypnopompic Hallucinations

Hypnagogic hallucinations are vivid perceptual experiences occurring at sleep onset, whereas *hypnopompic* hallucinations are similar experiences that occur on awakening. Here, the use of the term *hallucination* is appropriate because the experiences occur while one is awake and aware of the immediate surroundings. The term *hallucination* was first used in the English language in 1572 to refer to "ghostes and spirites walking by nyght" (Sarbin & Juhasz, 1975; see chap. 1, this volume). Hypnagogic and hypnopompic hallucinations may include experiences in many modalities, including a sensed presence, visual and auditory hallucinations, being touched, falling, flying and floating sensations, and out-of-body experiences (Cheyne, Newby-Clark, & Rueffer, 1999; Cheyne, Rueffer, & Newby-Clark, 1999). They are observed primarily in sleep-related disorders such as narcolepsy, cataplexy, sleep paralysis, and excessive daytime sleepiness (Ohayon, Priest, Caulet, & Guilleminault, 1996).[7] For instance, these experiences may occur in 25% to 30% of narcoleptics (Broughton, 1982). These hallucinations are included in the so-called "narcoleptic tetrad" on which clinical diagnostic criteria for narcolepsy are based (Yoss & Daly, 1960).

However, studies have also demonstrated high prevalence rates of hypnagogic and hypnopompic hallucinations in the general population. For example, Ohayon et al. (1996) observed that 37% of normal subjects reported

---

[7]*Narcolepsy* is a sleep disorder consisting of recurring episodes of sleep during the day, and often disrupted nocturnal sleep. *Cataplexy* is a transient attack of extreme generalized muscular weakness, often precipitated by an emotional state such as laughing, surprise, fear, or anger. *Sleep paralysis* is a brief episodic loss of voluntary movement that occurs when falling asleep or when awakening. All definitions are from *Stedman's Medical Dictionary* (1995).

experiencing hypnagogic hallucinations and 12% reported hypnopompic hallucinations. Although both types of hallucinations were more common among subjects with sleep-related disorders (insomnia, excessive daytime sleepiness) in this study, the prevalence of these hallucinations far exceeded that which can be merely explained by the association with these disturbances. Similar rates were reported in a study investigating the prevalence of hallucinations in the general population in three countries (the United Kingdom, Germany, and Italy), with 24.8% of subjects reporting hypnagogic hallucinations and 13.8% reporting hypnopompic hallucinations (Ohayon, 2000).

Finally, studies reveal that subjects perceive hypnagogic and hypnopompic experiences as predominantly negative (Cheyne, Newby-Clark, & Rueffer, 1999; Ohayon, 2000). For example, Cheyne et al. found that hypnagogic and hypnopompic hallucinations were consistently associated with a strong affective response, with fear being the most frequently described emotion in their nonclinical participants. Similarly, Ohayon observed that half of the participants were frightened by their hypnagogic and/or hypnopompic hallucinations. Finally, Larøi and Van der Linden (2005b) reported that nonclinical participants perceived hypnagogic and hypnopompic hallucinatory experiences as predominantly negative experiences. In particular, 47% and 45% of nonclinical participants responded that these experiences elicited a negative response for items concerning hypnagogic and hypnopompic hallucinations ("Sometimes, immediately prior to falling asleep or upon awakening, I have had a sensation of floating or falling or that I left my body temporarily," and "Sometimes, immediately prior to falling asleep or upon awakening, I have had the experience of having seen or felt or heard something or someone that wasn't there or the feeling of being touched even though no one was there," respectively).

Multimodal Hallucinations

The term *multimodal hallucinations* refers to hallucinations occurring simultaneously in more than one modality. Other descriptive labels have been applied to these (or similar) experiences, such as *complex hallucinations; dissociative hallucinations; visions; fantastic* or *scenic hallucinations;* or *multiple, mixed, polymodal,* and *polysensory hallucinations.* Many psychiatric patients experience multimodal hallucinations in the same phase of a psychotic illness. For example, D. W. Goodwin et al. (1971) found that 75% of 117 consecutively admitted hallucinating patients (with diagnoses of schizophrenia, affective disorder, organic brain syndromes, and hysteria) hallucinated in more than one sensory modality. The multiple hallucinations did not usually occur simultaneously, but when they did, they tended to involve simultaneous auditory and visual hallucinations. Silbersweig et al. (1995) described a patient with schizophrenia experiencing simultaneous auditory and visual hallucinations. In particular, these hallucinations consisted of seeing moving, colored scenes with rolling, disembodied heads speaking to the patient and giving him instructions. Hoffman and Varanko (2006) reported on 2 patients who described visual hallucinations of speechlike lip and mouth movements fused with simultaneous auditory–verbal hallucinations superimposed on perceptions of faces of actual persons in their immediate environment.

EMOTION AND HALLUCINATIONS

Emotional factors may play a significant role in the experience of hallucinations (Kuipers et al., 2006). This is particularly the case for psychiatric hallucinations, and much less so for neurological and pharmacological hallucinations. The emotional connotation is an integral part of the hallucinatory experience and has been described above for a number of hallucinations. With regard to emotion and hallucinations, three aspects can be distinguished: emotional antecedents, emotional content, and emotional consequences. A different question concerns whether hallucinations are associated with affective processing deficits. We address these aspects in turn. A final issue concerns the effect of emotional salience on cognitive processing distortions that may be involved in hallucinations. This is discussed in chapter 5, this volume, which examines metacognitive processes.

Emotional Antecedents

Notably, certain affective states have been associated with the onset of psychotic symptoms. A stage of heightened awareness and emotionality combined with a sense of anxiety and impasse has consistently been described as preceding psychosis (for a review, see Freeman & Garety, 2003). A study among 327 people from a nonclinical sample found higher levels of anxiety to be associated with hallucinatory predisposition (Allen et al., 2005). van't Wout, Aleman, Kessels, Larøi, and Kahn (2004) observed higher self-report ratings of emotionalizing in hallucination-prone subjects. *Emotionalizing* refers to a subscale of an alexithymia questionnaire and concerns ratings of subjective arousal in response to emotion-inducing events. The role of stress and arousal in the elicitation of hallucinations was hypothesized by Slade (1976). Recent models of hallucination (Behrendt & Young, 2004) and emotion (Aleman & Kahn, 2005) in schizophrenia also take this into account.

As for the autonomic arousal, increased skin conductance levels and fluctuations have been reported in hallucinating patients compared with control patients (Toone, Cooke, & Lader, 1981). Moreover, evidence has been reported of an increase in anxiety preceding the onset of hallucinations. Delespaul et al. (2002) studied 94 psychiatric patients with and without hallucinations using the experience sampling method over a period of 1 week. This method requires participants to fill in questionnaires, contingent on a randomly signaling beep, several times a day. The authors found that anxiety was the most prominent emotion during hallucinations. Notably, reports of anxiety intensity exceeded baseline levels before the first report of auditory hallucinations. In a prospective study of 80 twelve-year-old children with hallucinatory experiences, Escher, Romme, Buiks, Delespaul, and van Os (2002b) reported associated anxiety–depression to be an important predictor of the persistence of voices.

Emotional Content

The negative content of hallucinations has already been described above, especially for auditory and command hallucinations. In their phenomenological survey of the experience of hallucinations in 100 psychotic patients, Nayani and David (1996) reported that the hallucinations were distressing for a majority of patients because of their abusive and emotionally threatening content. In a study of 100 psychotic patients, B. Smith et al. (2006) found that individuals with more depression and lower self-esteem had auditory hallucinations of greater severity and more intensely negative content and were more distressed by them. Mosimann et al. (2006) studied complex visual hallucinations in 56 patients with either Parkinson's disease or dementia with Lewy bodies. Most patients experienced complex hallucinations daily, normally lasting minutes. They commonly saw people or animals, and the experiences were usually perceived as unpleasant. Neuropsychiatric symptoms coexisting with hallucinations were apathy, sleep disturbance, and anxiety. In Charles Bonnet syndrome, emotion plays a far less prominent role. After screening 505 visually handicapped patients, Teunisse, Cruysberg, Hoefnagels, Verbeek, and Zitman (1996) found that 60 of them met diagnostic criteria for this syndrome. They observed that in 77% of patients, hallucinations lacked a personal meaning. The hallucinations caused considerable distress in only 28% of patients. Finally, as has also been described above, hallucinations can be experienced as positive. Some people have described them as providing support or guidance.

Emotional Consequences

As mentioned earlier in this chapter, hallucinations have been reported to be distressing in a large number of patients with psychiatric conditions such as schizophrenia and also in neurogenerative conditions. Krabbendam, Myin-Germeys, Hanssen, et al. (2005) reported that individuals who react with negative emotional states (e.g., depression) to their initial psychotic or psychosis-like experiences were more likely to develop clinical psychosis later on.

Hallucinations and Affective Processing Deficits

Rossell and Boundy (2005) hypothesized that auditory–verbal hallucinations would be associated with auditory affective processing deficits. To evaluate this, they used measures of emotional information processing and compared performance of three groups: schizophrenia patients with and without a history of hallucinations and control subjects matched for age, sex, and education. Their hypothesis was derived from the fact that hallucinations are frequently emotional in content and proposals by Woodruff (2004) that emotional aspects of speech might be disturbed in individuals predisposed to auditory–verbal hallucinations and increase a person's liability to experience them. Rossell and Boundy used two different kinds of tasks. One task required the recognition of emotional environmental sounds (happy sighs, grunts, and shrieks) and thus used nonverbal–nonsemantic stimuli. The other tasks used verbal–semantic stimuli, for example, asking subjects to indicate in which emotional tone of voice a certain sentence was spoken by an actor. Patients with hallucinations showed significant impairments on the nonverbal task, particularly for the affective stimuli and not the neutral valence stimuli. For the auditory affect tasks that used verbal–semantic stimuli, both patient groups (with and without hallucinations) were impaired. Rossell and Boundy suggested that semantic deficits in schizophrenia in general may have masked additional auditory affect deficits in the hallucination group in the latter task. They concluded that their findings support the notion of increased liability for auditory affect perception deficits in patients with auditory hallucinations. Other examples of affective processing deficits in hallucinations are described in chapter 5, this volume, where studies including source monitoring tasks are described in detail.

CONCLUSION

Hallucinations are clearly heterogeneous and multifaceted phenomena. On a theoretical level, various cognitive and biological mechanisms may vary, at least in part, according to certain phenomenological characteristics of hallucinations. For instance, neuroimaging studies suggest that hallucinations in a given modality involve areas that normally process sensory information in that modality. Thus, although certain brain areas may be activated during both auditory and somatic hallucinations, the former will also exclusively involve auditory areas, whereas the latter will specifically involve somatosensory cortical areas.

On a clinical level, taking into account the phenomenological diversity of hallucinations may help provide the patient with important information (e.g., provide new insights regarding the experiences, offer new or different coping strategies), improve patient–clinician relations (e.g., revealing to the patient that the clinician is taking his or her experiences seriously), help individualize treatment, open up new therapeutic avenues, and provide information concerning changes in the patient's mental and emotional condition (e.g., characteristics of hallucinations such as volume, localization, and content may reflect important changes in the patient's emotional state). For more detailed information concerning the theoretical and clinical importance of assessing the phenomenological characteristics of hallucinations, see Larøi (2006) and Larøi and Woodward (2007). The clinical implications are also discussed in the Appendix.

Finally, to fully take into account the heterogeneous nature of hallucinations, comprehensive, valid and reliable methods of recording patients' experiences must be developed and used. A varying number of the phenomenological characteristics of hallucinations have been integrated into selected assessment strategies (these instruments are described in the Appendix). These include the Launay–Slade Hallucination Scale (LSHS; Launay & Slade, 1981), the Mental Health Research Institute Unusual Perceptions Schedule (MUPS; Carter et al., 1995), the Psychotic Symptom Rating Scale (Haddock et al., 1999), the Beliefs About Voices Questionnaire (BAVQ; Chadwick & Birchwood, 1995), and the Verbal Hallucinations Questionnaire (Barrett & Etheridge, 1992; Posey & Losch, 1983). It is important to mention that these scales vary in terms of the degree to which they assess the many phenomenological characteristics of hallucinations. For instance, a large majority exclusively assess auditory–verbal hallucinations, with only one scale (i.e., the revised version of the LSHS; Larøi, Marczewski, & Van der Linden, 2004; Larøi & Van der Linden, 2005b) providing assessment of other hallucination modalities (e.g., auditory, visual, olfactory, tactile, hypnagogic, and hypnopompic hallucinations). In addition, certain assessment tools contain relatively more questions concerning (physical) characteristics of hallucinations (e.g., the MUPS), whereas other instruments are more detailed in terms of how people perceive and respond to their verbal auditory hallucinations (BAVQ). Also, some measures (e.g., the LSHS) contain fairly general items (e.g., "I often hear a voice speaking my thoughts aloud"), whereas others (e.g., the Verbal Hallucinations Questionnaire) include questions about relatively specific situations. An example of the latter is the following item: "Sometimes when I am driving in my car, I hear my own voice from the backseat. It sounds like it is little short statements usually soothing like 'It'll be all right' or 'Now, just calm down.' Similar things happen to you?" If, however, for practical reasons it is not possible to assess many of the phenomenological characteristics described in this chapter, an evaluation should as a minimum include frequency of hallucinations and the degree of distress that the hallucinations elicit in individuals, and this for the major hallucination modalities (auditory, visual, tactile, olfactory).

In the next chapter, which describes the different groups of hallucinators, it is important to keep in mind the various phenomenological characteristics of hallucinations that have been described in the current chapter. Studies suggest that although a number of these groups of hallucinators will share certain phenomenological characteristics (e.g., negative content of hallucinations is common in patients with posttraumatic stress disorder and in patients suffering from various psychotic disorders such as schizophrenia, affective disorders, and postpartum psychosis), some groups may differ (e.g., negative content of hallucinations is relatively rare in patients with neurological conditions, such as those suffering from tumors or epilepsy).

CHAPTER HIGHLIGHTS

- Hallucinations may occur in a number of different modalities (auditory, visual, tactile, olfactory, etc.) and, more rarely, in multiple modalities at the same time.
- Phenomenological characteristics often include physical (e.g., frequency, volume, clarity) and personal (e.g., emotional content of the hallucination; whether in first, second, or third person; number of voices; known voice or not) characteristics.
- Emotion plays an important role in hallucinations. For example, as an antecedent to hallucinations, hallucination content is often highly emotional, there are often emotional reactions associated with the presence of hallucinations, and hallucinations are related to affective processing deficits.

3

GROUPS OF HALLUCINATORS

Numerous studies have revealed that hallucinations may occur in a number of populations, including psychiatric patients, nonpsychiatric patients, and even normal subjects. These findings question the diagnostic specificity of hallucinations and also challenge the idea that hallucinations are necessarily a sign of mental illness or pathology (Brasić, 1998; David, 1999; Johns, 2005). Moreover, these findings provide evidence for the so-called *continuum hypothesis of hallucinations*, that is, that both clinical and nonclinical hallucinations lie as points on a continuum and do not differ qualitatively from each other. This hypothesis is presented and discussed at the end of the chapter.

HALLUCINATIONS IN PSYCHIATRIC DISORDERS

Hallucinatory experiences have been reported in a number of psychiatric disorders and are therefore not limited to a single diagnostic category, such as schizophrenia. These categories include affective disorders (e.g., psychotic depression, bipolar disorder), dissociative disorders, borderline personality disorder, delirium, posttraumatic stress disorder (PTSD), obsessive–compulsive disorder, multiple personality disorder, alcoholic hallucinosis, delirium tremens, postpartum psychosis, and conversion disorder (Watkins, 1998). Descriptions of hallucinations in some of these disorders follow. In particular, those psychiatric disorders in which hallucinations are most commonly reported and relatively well documented in the literature (schizophrenia, affective disorders, posttraumatic stress disorder, postpartum psychosis, delirium tremens, alcoholic hallucinosis, and borderline personality disorder) are described below.

Schizophrenia

Hallucinations are common in patients with schizophrenia. A multinational study conducted by the World Health Organization estimated that approximately 70% of patients who met the diagnostic criteria for schizophrenia experienced hallucinations (Sartorius, Shapiro, & Jablensky, 1974). Similarly, in 16 published reports including 2,924 cases, the prevalence of auditory hallucinations was reported as being 60.2% (Slade & Bentall, 1988). Andreasen and Flaum (1991) reported similar base rates for auditory hallucinations in two Iowa samples of patients with schizophrenia (56% and 70%) diagnosed using the *Diagnostic and Statistical Manual of Mental Disorders* (3rd ed., rev.; American Psychiatric Association, 1987) criteria. The most common hallucinations in schizophrenic patients are auditory followed by visual hallucinations. Tactile, olfactory, and gustatory hallucinations also have been reported, although these types are less frequent in schizophrenic patients.

Relatively little research has examined the characteristics of hallucinations in deaf people with a schizophrenia diagnosis (Atkinson, 2006). In a review of the literature, Atkinson (2006) pointed out that the prevalence of schizophrenia within the deaf community is roughly equivalent to the general population and that around half of all deaf people diagnosed with schizophrenia report auditory verbal hallucinations, which also parallels prevalence rates of auditory verbal hallucinations in hearing people with schizophrenia. Although there does not seem to be evidence for increased frequency of psychotic hallucinations in congenitally deaf people, studies have shown that there is a greater proportion of visual (around 50%) and tactile or somatic hallucinations (also around 50%) in these patients. Furthermore, both types of hallucinations usually co-occur with reports of voices.

du Feu and McKenna (1999) recorded the accounts of 17 patients with schizophrenia or schizoaffective psychosis, all of whom had profound deafness. The age of onset of deafness ranged from birth to some time before 2 years of age. Of the 17 patients, 10 (59%) gave accounts of current verbal auditory hallucinations with description of content. Furthermore, the patients' auditory hallucinations showed the same breadth of phenomenological attributes as those in nondeaf patients. In particular, their voices were in both the second and third person, were single and multiple, were located outside and inside the head (or both), and were verbal and nonverbal. Two patients even described hearing voices from their hearing aids. The content of patients' voices often was quite pleasant and supportive. Seven patients also experienced nonverbal auditory hallucinations (e.g., rumbling, drumming, and laughing and talking in which words could not be deciphered). Nine (53%) of the patients experienced visual hallucinations (in most cases in patients who also experienced auditory hallucinations), 8 experienced somatic hallucinations, and 3 had olfactory hallucinations. Other psychotic symptoms were also described by patients (e.g., thought insertion), but patients seemed to be able to distinguish these from hallucinations.

More recently, Atkinson et al. (2007) wished to examine hallucination phenomenology in relation to individual differences in experiences with language and residual hearing in a group of 27 deaf participants with schizophrenia. All participants had experienced voice hallucinations within the past 6 months prior to the study and reported being able to remember the experiences clearly. Hearing loss in participants varied from mild to profound, and participants varied in terms of their age of language (e.g., British sign language or sign supported English) acquisition and fluency. A comprehensive sampling of all known perceptual characteristics relevant to deaf people and patients with hallucinations was collected. Ninety-four sort cards with statements were presented, and participants were asked to sort the cards into three piles according to whether they had ever experienced the phenomenon described ("yes," "no," or "don't know/not sure") and according to the frequency of the phenomena ("always," "sometimes," or "rarely"). Participants were assigned the status of variables and were then factor analyzed to obtain clusters of individuals who sorted statements in the most similar way. Principal-components factor analysis resulted in six factors. The results revealed that the perceptual characteristics of voice hallucinations map closely onto an individual's real-life communication preferences and experience of language and sound. For instance, individuals born profoundly deaf converged on Factor A (nonauditory voices), whereas those who had experience of hearing speech (either because they had acquired deafness or had residual hearing) converged on Factors B (consisting of individuals who were uncertain whether they were really hearing sound when the voices were present) and D (auditory voices).

Affective Disorders

Severe depression is sometimes accompanied by hallucinations, usually auditory hallucinations. The voices, which are usually transient and limited to single words or short phrases, are generally heard saying things consistent with the person's depressed mood. A psychotically depressed person may hear voices that are mocking and humiliating and that criticize him or her for various failures, shortcomings, and sins (which may be real or imagined). A depressed person may be accused of various wrongdoings and might be further ordered by the voices to "make up" for these by performing acts of self-mutilation or even suicide (Watkins, 1998). Although psychotic depression is considered to be the most severe form of depression, it is not uncommon: As many as one quarter of all depressed persons may be suffering from psychotic depression (Schatzberg & Rothschild, 1992).

A number of studies have examined the prevalence of hallucinations in patients with unipolar and bipolar affective disorder. For example, Black and Nazrallah (1989) found that 27% of 1,715 patients with unipolar and bipolar affective disorder reported having visual hallucinations. A somewhat lower figure was reported by F. K. Goodwin and Jamison (1990), who reviewed 20 studies conducted between 1922 and 1989 investigating the prevalence of hallucinations in patients with bipolar disorder and calculated a weighted mean average of 18%. Hammersley et al. (2003) reported that 47% of their adult bipolar affective disorder patients had experienced hallucinations during their lifetime. Among these patients, 30 had auditory hallucinations, 25 had visual hallucinations, 11 heard voices commenting on their actions, and 9 experienced other (tactile, somatic, or olfactory) hallucinations. Furthermore, Hammersley et al. examined the relationship between childhood sexual abuse and hallucinations in this population and found that those subjected to child sexual abuse were twice as likely to have auditory hallucinations in general and 6 times more likely to hear voices commenting. There was also evidence of a dose effect. It is interesting that only 1 of the severely abused patients (*severe abuse* defined as occurring before age 6, with multiple incidents or intrafamilial) did not experience auditory hallucinations.

Hallucinations may also occur during the manic phase of bipolar disorder. For example, Taylor and Abrams (1975) found that 47% of manic patients reported auditory hallucinations. The auditory hallucinations in manic episodes usually involve voices that speak directly to the person and whose content is congruent with the person's abnormally elevated mood.

Posttraumatic Stress Disorder

Posttraumatic stress disorder (PTSD) is a syndrome that some people may develop as a consequence of having been exposed to an extremely traumatic stressor sufficient to provoke intense fear, helplessness, or horror. The characteristic symptoms of PTSD involve the avoidance of stimuli associated with the original event, the numbing of emotional responsiveness, increased arousal, and the reliving of the traumatic event (e.g., intrusive dreams, flashbacks; see American Psychiatric Association, 1994). Flashbacks, or intrusive recollections, often appear to take the form of auditory, visual, tactile, and/or olfactory hallucinations (Morrison, Frame, & Larkin, 2003). Research has noted marked similarities between PTSD and (symptoms of) schizophrenia (Hamner et al., 2000; Muenzenmaier et al., 2005).

Evidence suggests a specific association between hallucinations and childhood sexual abuse in patient (Ellason & Ross, 1997; Read & Argyle, 1999; Ross, Anderson, & Clark, 1994) and nonpatient samples (Bryer, Nelson, Miller, & Krol, 1987; Ensink, 1992; Ross & Joshi, 1992; Startup, 1999). Studies have reported that combat veterans with PTSD have more schizophrenic symptoms, particularly hallucinations and paranoia, compared with those without PTSD (Butler, Mueser, Sprock, & Braff, 1996; Mueser & Butler, 1987; Sautter et al., 1999; Wilcox, Briones, & Suess, 1991). In particular, some combat veterans with PTSD have reported hearing persistent voices that are usually of a depressive nature and involve cries for help or conversations concerning battle (Wilcox et al., 1991). In some cases of combat-related PTSD, the auditory hallucinations may be directly related to a specific and particularly distressing occurrence (Mueser & Butler, 1987). In Butler et al. (1996), 20 combat veterans with PTSD were compared with 18 combat veterans without PTSD on symptom rating scales. Both groups consisted of subjects with no prior psychiatric hospitalization. In addition, suspected presence of major affective disorder or schizophrenia was an exclusion criterion. Results revealed that the subjects with PTSD exhibited a significantly greater degree of hallucinations than the comparison group. Furthermore, Butler et al. found that the hallucinations described by the subjects could vary from being highly related (e.g., a dead soldier calling to the subject to kill himself) to relatively unrelated to the combat trauma experienced by the veterans. For a more detailed review of much of this research, in addition to theoretical and clinical discussions, consult Read, van Os, Morrison, and Ross (2005); Morrison et al. (2003); Read, Perry, Moskowitz, and Connolly (2001); and W. Larkin and Morrison (2006).

Postpartum Psychosis

Postpartum disorders involve a range of disturbances that women can develop shortly after giving birth. They include affective and organic-like mental disorders and functional psychoses, with depression being the most common. Disturbances that involve psychotic manifestations such as hallucinations have often been described as rare, only occurring in about 1 or 2 out of every 1,000 deliveries (Kaplan & Sadock, 1981). Nonetheless, in one study of 100 women with a variety of postpartum disorders, 12 appeared to have *conversion hallucinations* (i.e., hallucinations occurring in the context of conversion disorders; Farley, Woodruff, & Guze, 1968). Symptoms of postpartum disorders center on the woman's feelings about the newborn baby and her role as a mother. A mother who hallucinates during a postpartum psychotic disturbance may hear voices telling her to kill her baby, or she may hear voices accusing her of not being a competent mother. In contrast, some women may simply hear their baby crying.

Delirium Tremens

Hallucinations may occur in the context of *delirium tremens*, which is an acute (and sometimes fatal) episode of delirium usually caused by withdrawal or abstinence from alcohol following habitual excessive drinking but that may also occur during an episode of heavy alcohol consumption (Asaad & Shapiro, 1986; Watkins, 1998). Delirium tremens is usually preceded by disturbed sleep, irritability, and malnutrition and generally takes from 1 day to several days to develop after discontinuation of alcohol consumption. Symptoms include body tremors, convulsions, psychomotor agitation, nausea, increased heart rate and body temperature, grand mal seizures, anxiety, disorientation, and (transient) hallucinations. Hallucinations in delirium tremens usually involve visual hallucinations, which typically involve different types of animals (e.g., cats, dogs, insects, snakes, rats) or signs and shapes (e.g., chalk writing on a slate, multicolored patterns, technical drawings; Platz, Oberlaender, & Seidel, 1995). Tactile hallucinations are often associated with the visual hallucinations. Auditory hallucinations may also occur, in addition to musical hallucinations. Delirium tremens usually lasts 3 to 10 days, although hallucinations may develop independently of delirium tremens and may last from days to weeks. The condition is related to the abrupt drop in blood alcohol level after drinking ceases. In the *Diagnostic and Statistical Manual of Mental Disorders* (4th ed.; *DSM–IV*; American Psychiatric Association, 1994), the term *delirium tremens* has been replaced with *alcohol withdrawal delirium* (and *alcohol withdrawal delirium with perceptual disturbances* when hallucinations or illusions are observed).

Alcoholic Hallucinosis

Alcoholic hallucinosis is a rare complication of chronic alcoholism that may occur during intoxication by a substance or during withdrawal from a substance. In a cohort of 643 alcoholic patients, Tsuang, Irwin, Smith, and Schuckit (1994) reported a prevalence rate of 7.4%. Alcoholic hallucinosis should be distinguished from delirium tremens in that the former does not carry a significant mortality, recurrent or persistent hallucinations are the predominant or only symptom, and symptoms of delirium tremens such as clouding of sensorium or disorientation are not present. In the *DSM–IV*, the term *alcohol hallucinosis* has been replaced by *substance-induced psychotic disorder with hallucinatory features*. The syndrome is characterized by hallucinations (typically auditory, but also visual and tactile), delusions, misidentification, psychomotor disturbances, and abnormal affect. A state of alcoholic hallucinosis may be as brief as a few hours or days or may persist for several months. In some cases, it may become chronic, suggesting that there is an increased genetic loading for schizophrenia in such individuals, although this view remains controversial (Watkins, 1998).

Borderline Personality Disorder

A multiple-case study by Yee, Korner, McSwiggan, Meares, and Stevenson (2005) showed that hallucinations may also occur in borderline personality disorder. Yee et al. found that of the total of 171 patients with borderline personality disorder included in the study, as many as 50 (29.2%) reported that they "heard voices" on the Symptom Checklist 90. Ten cases were then examined in more detail and revealed that a large majority of patients expressed that the hallucinations were distressing, occurred with great frequency over prolonged periods, took control of actions or behavior (especially self-harming or self-destructive behaviors), and had a critical quality (although some patients also stated that their voices had an element of protectiveness or made positive comments).[1] Although the majority of hallucinations were auditory, visual and olfactory hallucinations were also reported. All of the patients expressed mistrust about sharing information concerning their hallucinations, most probably because of fears that disclosure would result in the diagnosis of schizophrenia.

HALLUCINATIONS IN NONPSYCHIATRIC CLINICAL GROUPS

Hallucinations may also be present in a number of nonpsychiatric patient populations. These populations may include patients with a major neurological disorder, such as cerebrovascular disorder, brain tumor, brain injury, epilepsy, narcolepsy, or migraine. Hallucinations may also occur in major degenerative disorders such as Lewy body dementia (LBD), Parkinson's disease (PD), and Alzheimer's disease (AD). A number of studies have found an association between sensory deficits and the presence of hallucinations.

Neurological Conditions

Several studies have reported hallucinations in various neurological conditions such as brain tumors, epilepsy, traumatic brain injury, syncopes, migraines, narcolepsy, cerebrovascular disorders, encephalitis, and meningiomas (Brasić, 1998). For example, Feinstein and Ron (1990) assessed the presence of psychotic symptoms in a group of neurological patients ($N = 62$) and found that 79% had hallucinations. Closer inspection of the data (carried out by David, 1994) revealed that the majority of these were *second-person verbal hallucinations* (voices talking directly to the hallucinator; 53%) followed by *third-person verbal hallucinations* (two or more voices speaking

---

[1]As the authors of this study commented, hallucinations observed in borderline personality disorder (diagnosed on the basis of *DSM–IV* criteria) are normally considered to be transient in nature, that is, occurring for brief periods and in situations of stress. The results of this study, however, clearly show that this is not necessarily the case and that persistent hallucinations may also occur in this disorder.

among themselves about the hallucinator; 27%), with 20% of patients reporting nonverbal hallucinations.

Furthermore, different types of hallucinations have been associated with various brain diseases and neurological disorders (for a review, see Brasić, 1998). Auditory hallucinations have been associated with brain tumors (primarily affecting the temporal lobes, the diencephalons, and the midbrain), temporal lobe epilepsy, and temporal lobe lobectomy. Similarly, studies have associated visual hallucinations with various neurological disorders such as brain tumors, vascular embolism or thrombosis, epilepsy, migraine, viral encephalitis, narcolepsy, and cortical lesions in the occipital and temporoparietal regions. Musical hallucinations have also been reported in brain stem hematoma, meningiomas, encephalitis, epilepsy, cerebrovascular diseases, and pontine degeneration. Both olfactory and gustatory hallucinations have been observed in various neurological disorders such as in brain tumors (in particular in the temporal lobe), epilepsy, meningioma, migraine, and temporal lobe lesions.

Even though reports of experiencing a complex auditory hallucination during a seizure (or coinciding with an electroencephalogram record of seizure activity) appear to be extremely rare, hallucinations occurring in the postictal period are, on the contrary, relatively common in epileptic patients. A study of 90 patients with temporal lobe epilepsy showed that 18% experienced auditory illusions and hallucinations at some time (Bingley, 1958). Another survey of 666 patients with temporal lobe epilepsy revealed that 16% of patients had auditory hallucinations (Currie, Heathfield, Henson, & Scott, 1971). A study including 20 highly selected patients with electrophysiologically confirmed temporal lobe dysfunction recorded spells of atypical psychotic phenomena (including auditory hallucinations) in 50% of patients (Tucker, Price, Johnson, & McAllister, 1986). Maugière (1999) reviewed ictal presentations of sensory seizures from a file of 3,531 epilepsy patients and found that 18% of patients reported auditory hallucinations and 23% reported musical hallucinations. Bien et al. (2000) selected patients who experienced ictal visual phenomena and whose epileptogenic focus had been determined with sufficient certainty ($N = 20$) and found that 8 of these patients (40%) described elementary hallucinations whereas 3 of the patients (15%) reported complex hallucinations.

Degenerative Disorders

In 1996, the International Psychogeriatric Association officially termed noncognitive problems in dementia as "behavioral and psychological signs and symptoms of dementia" (Finkel, Costa, Cohen, Miller, & Sartorius, 1996). Problems in the behavioral domain include eating disorders, agitation, aggression, abnormal vocalizations, wandering, overactivity, sexual disinhibition, sleep disturbances, and apathy. Problems in the psychological domain include euphoria, depression, and psychosis. One can further distinguish among three types of psychotic symptoms: *delusions* (false, unshakable ideas or beliefs that are held with unshakable conviction and unshakable certainty), *delusional misidentification syndromes* (misidentifications and/or misperceptions of oneself, other people, places, or objects), and hallucinations.

Since this decision by the International Psychogeriatric Association, an increasing number of researchers have studied psychotic symptoms, including hallucinations, in the degenerative disorders. It is important to note, however, that far too many studies have considered psychotic symptoms as one homogeneous category rather than explicitly examining specific symptoms. This is mostly the case with earlier studies. Fortunately, the majority of more recent studies take on a more nuanced and refined approach to the exploration of psychotic symptoms in the dementias.

Because most assessment strategies of psychotic symptoms in the dementias do not ask the patient directly for information but rather ask an informant (usually the spouse or another family member), one should be cautious as to the exactness of these reports. Aspects such as the reliance on the informant, the relationship of the informant, the functioning level of the informant, and the degree of the informant's familiarity with the problems to be measured must all be taken into account. For instance, the accuracy of information may be limited because the informant may be trying to protect the patient's integrity by not reporting behaviors (such as hallucinations) that are considered highly bizarre and signs of madness.

It is also important to underline that although neurobiological factors inherent in the degenerative disorders (i.e., cerebral degeneration, pharmacological effects) play an undeniably important role in the development of hallucinations in patients with these disorders, their presence is not sufficient. For instance, pharmacologic treatment of PD using levodopa often results in hallucinations as a side effect, suggesting a causal relation between pharmacological factors and hallucinations. However, a number of studies failed to report evidence pointing to a causal link between hallucinations and levodopa (Aarsland, Larsen, Cummings, & Lake, 1999; Fénelon, Mahieux, Huon, & Ziégler, 2000; Goetz et al., 1998; Graham, Grunewald, & Sagar, 1997; Klein, Koempf, Pulkowski, Moser, & Vieregge, 1997; Rabins, 1982; Sanchez-Ramos, Ortoll, & Paulson, 1996).

Studies including AD patients also suggest that neurobiological factors do not entirely explain the presence of hallucinations. For example, Sweet et al. (2000) compared a group of AD patients with psychotic symptoms (including hallucinations) with a group of AD patients without psychotic symptoms. The results revealed no significant differences between the two groups in terms of their neuropathological features. In addition, not all patients with dementia have hallucinations, suggesting that neurodegenerative factors cannot explain the development of these symptoms. Finally, studies have identified a number of other, nonneurobiological factors as playing an important role in the genesis of hallucinations in patients with dementia. These factors include sensory deficits, life events, personality factors, and cognitive deficits.

Lewy Body Dementia

LBD is acknowledged as the second most common form of degenerative disorder in old age after Alzheimer's disease. According to the First International Consortium on LBD (McKeith et al., 1996), criteria for this diagnosis are cognitive impairment (alertness and attention), spontaneous (nondrug induced) motor features of Parkinsonism, and recurrent visual hallucinations. Because the presence of visual hallucinations is one of the three major inclusion criteria, it is not surprising that studies report high prevalence rates of hallucinations in LBD. For instance, McKeith (1998) found that hallucinations were reported in over 46% of LBD patients during the course of the illness. Similar rates are reported in other studies: 56% by Rockwell, Choure, Galasko, Olichney, and Jeste (2000) and 65% by Ballard et al. (1999).

Although visual hallucinations are the most frequently reported type of hallucination in LBD, auditory or complex hallucinations and even—albeit rarer—olfactory or tactile hallucinations have also been observed. In addition to visual hallucinations, vision-related behavioral symptoms, including visual agnosia and delusional misidentifications, are common in LBD (Ballard, Harrison, Lowery, & McKeith, 1996; Hirono et al., 1999; McKeith et al., 1996). Hallucinations in LBD are often rich, detailed, and personal; they often involve family members and personal experiences. They can evoke highly varying emotional responses that may range from fear to amusement to indifference. In general, hallucinations in LBD appear in the early stages of the disease. Finally, compared with hallucinations in other degenerative disorders, hallucinations in LBD are relatively stable, and patients often have a certain degree of insight into their symptoms.

Parkinson's Disease

Hallucinations are also relatively common in PD. Aarsland et al. (1999) found that 27% of PD patients drawn from a community-based sample had hallucinations. Similar figures are reported in other studies (Graham et al., 1997: 24.8%; Sanchez-Ramos et al., 1996: 25.7%). A somewhat higher rate was reported in Fénelon et al. (2000): 39.8% of their patients with PD experienced hallucinations during the previous 3 months. In addition, three forms of hallucination were distinguished in this study: minor forms, consisting of the sensation of a presence (e.g., a person), present in 25.5% of the patients; formed visual hallucinations, present in 22.2% of patients; and auditory hallucinations, present in 9.7% of patients. The relatively higher rate of hallucinations in the study by Fénelon et al. compared with other studies is likely due to the fact that minor forms of hallucinations were taken into account.

In terms of phenomenological characteristics, hallucinations in PD are commonly visual but can occur in other modalities, including auditory, olfactory, and tactile modalities (Asaad & Shapiro, 1986; Fénelon, Thobois, Bonnet, Broussolle, & Tison, 2002). However, when nonvisual hallucinations occur (especially auditory hallucinations), they are rarely isolated but are instead often associated with the presence of visual hallucinations. For instance, Inzelberg, Kipervasser, and Korczyn (1998) examined the occurrence (past and present) of auditory hallucinations in a group of PD patients and found that hallucinations were reported in 37% of patients. Furthermore, 29% had only visual hallucinations, 8% had both visual and auditory hallucinations, and no patient reported auditory hallucinations unaccompanied by visual hallucinations. Hallucinations in PD are commonly neutral and nonthreatening for patients, and some patients even report being amused by their hallucinations (Henderson & Mellers, 2000). In addition, (visual) hallucinations are typically rich and complex (Barnes & David, 2001). A unique aspect of hallucinations in PD (compared with other degenerative disorders and other neurological and psychiatric conditions) is that hallucinatory experiences may include sensations of the presence of people or animals or feelings of floating. Also, patients reveal adequate levels of insight. For example, Graham et al. (1997) found that 70% of PD patients with hallucinations had retained insight. Finally, hallucinations in PD usually occur in the late phases of the illness.

Alzheimer's Disease

Hallucinations are also observed in AD, with studies reporting prevalence rates ranging from 12% to 53% (Holroyd, 1998). For example, Burns, Jacoby, and Levy (1990) found that 17% of their patients with AD experienced hallucinations. The same figure is reported in Jeste, Wragg, Salmon, Harris, and Thal (1992), with subsequent studies observing similar rates (Della Sala, Francescani, Muggia, & Spinnler, 1998: 24%; Hirono et al., 1998: 11%). Hallucinations in AD most often include those in the visual modality, although auditory, tactile, and olfactory hallucinations have also been observed. For example, Jeste et al. (1992) reported that among the 17% of their patients with AD who experienced hallucinations, 13% of them were visual hallucinations, 7% were auditory, 2% were olfactory, and 1% were tactile. Although the majority of hallucinations in AD are simple and/or isolated, complex or multimodal hallucinations may also occur.

The prevalence of hallucinations in AD seems to vary with the stage of disease. In particular, studies have shown that hallucinations are most prevalent in the moderate to severe stages of the illness and do not seem to occur at the end stage of the disorder (Drevets & Rubin, 1989; Reisberg, Franssen, Sclan, Kluger, & Ferris, 1989). These findings suggest that although some degree of cognitive impairment is needed to develop hallucinations, a severely impaired brain can no longer generate such symptoms. In addition, a number of studies suggest that hallucinations in AD are related to the presence of sensory deficits. For instance, the presence of visual impairments and poor visual acuity in AD patients has been associated with visual hallucinations (Ballard, Bannister, Graham, Oyebode, & Wilcock, 1995; Chapman, Dickinson, McKeith, & Ballard, 1999). In a single-case study, Dary, Eustache, Viader, and Lechevalier (1994) suggested that the auditory hallucinations observed in their AD patient were the result of cumulated factors that included peripheral hearing loss. One study described 3 patients with AD whose visual hallucinations improved when they were given optical aids (Pankow, Pliskin, & Luchins, 1996). It is not clear, however, if the link between sensory deficits and hallucinations is specific to AD because few studies have addressed this question in other degenerative disorders.

HALLUCINATIONS IN NONPSYCHIATRIC CONDITIONS ASSOCIATED WITH SENSORY DEFICIT

A number of studies suggest an association between sensory deficit and the presence of hallucinations. More specifically, they show a relation between visual sensory impairment and the presence of auditory hallucinations. For instance, hallucinations within a scotoma have long been recognized (J. W. Brown, 1985); destructive lesions of the optic nerve, chiasm, and radiation may all result in hallucinations (Kölmel, 1985); 10% to 30% of people who are blind experience hallucinations (Lepore, 1990); and people with poor vision have been found to have more hallucinations. There is also an association between deafness and auditory hallucinations in older adults as well as between deafness and musical hallucinations (David, 1999).

A good example of the association between sensory impairment and hallucinations is Charles Bonnet syndrome (CBS). This syndrome, most common in old age, involves severe visual loss (mostly because of visual diseases such as cataract or senile macular degeneration) but with preserved cognitive status and no sign of psychiatric disorder. One of the most characteristic symptoms of CBS is the presence of (isolated) visual hallucinations, although some reports of auditory hallucinations also exist (e.g., Chédru, Feldman, Améri, Salès, & Roth, 1996; Hori, Terao, & Nakamura, 2001). These visual hallucinations can vary from simple flashes to repetitive patterns to the appearance of people, animals, or scenes. Patients may react positively or negatively to their hallucinations (Schultz & Melzack, 1991), and there is often full or partial retention of insight into the unreal nature of the hallucinations (Eperjesi & Akbarali, 2004). Negative reactions to the hallucinations often happen in association with bizarre or frightening hallucinations, such as grotesque, disembodied, or distorted faces with prominent eyes and teeth (Santhouse, Howard, & ffytche, 2000). One possible distinguishing charac-

TABLE 3.1
Hallucinations and Clinical Disorders: Dominating Modality,
Emotional Content of Hallucinations, and Emotional Reaction

Disorder	Dominant modality/modalities	Emotional content	Emotional reaction
Schizophrenia	Auditory, visual	Yes	Yes
Affective disorders	Auditory, visual	Yes	Yes
Posttraumatic stress disorder	Auditory, visual, tactile, olfactory	Yes	Yes
Postpartum psychosis	Auditory	Yes	Yes
Delirium tremens	Visual, tactile		
Alcoholic hallucinosis	Auditory		
Borderline personality disorder	Auditory	Yes	Yes
Neurological disorders	Auditory, visual		
Lewy body dementia	Visual	No	Possible
Parkinson's disease	Visual	No	No
Alzheimer's disease	Visual	No	No
Charles Bonnet syndrome	Visual	No	Possible

Note. Empty cells indicate that not enough research has been carried out to answer the question.

teristic of hallucinations in CBS is that they disappear when patients close their eyes (Teunisse, Zitman, & Raes, 1994). Table 3.1 summarizes these various clinical disorders in terms of the dominating modality or modalities, whether the content of hallucinations is emotionally negative, and whether their presence elicits negative emotional reactions.

A number of studies have observed hallucinations in persons with partial or total hearing loss. In particular, musical hallucinations have been reported in (often older) persons with moderate or severe acquired deafness but without either neurological or psychiatric disorders and without dementia (Ali, 2002; Fénelon, Marie, Ferroir, & Guillard, 1993; Fenton & McRae, 1989; Griffiths, 2000; Hammeke, McQuillen, & Cohen, 1983; Naccache, Habert, Malek, Cohen, & Willer, 2005) and may thus have been seen as representing an auditory form of Charles Bonnet syndrome.

Important differences between clinical groups of subjects experiencing hallucinations can be suggested. For example, differences exist in terms of characteristics of hallucinations between patients with so-called "late onset" or "very late onset" schizophrenia-like psychosis and patients with AD. Whereas hallucinations in AD patients are more frequently visual than auditory, the reverse is true in older patients with schizophrenia (e.g., with late onset schizophrenia-like psychosis), which fall in approximately the same age group. In addition, Schneiderian first-rank symptoms involving hallucinatory experiences (e.g., hearing a voice speaking one's thoughts aloud, two or more voices conversing with one another, voices that keep a running commentary on the person's thoughts or behavior) are rare in AD patients compared with patients with late onset schizophrenia-like psychosis (Bentall, 2003).[2]

The content of hallucinations may also vary from group to group. For example, although hallucinations often reflect the concerns of schizophrenic patients and are highly personally salient and emotionally charged, hallucinations in nonpsychiatric patients (e.g., those suffering from tumors, epilepsy, or drug or alcohol withdrawal) usually give rise to contentless or arbitrary perceptual phenomena such as noises or flashes of light or color (Healy, 1990). In addition, many of the (auditory) hallucinations described by patients with schizophrenia are negative in content (e.g., persecutory comments, criticisms of the self, instructions to commit violent acts against the self or others; Bentall, 2000), yet this is rarely the case in other subjects with hallucinations (e.g., neurological patients, patients with dementia, nonclinical subjects). Finally, the degree of insight into hallucinations also differs between clinical groups. For instance, most patients with PD have insight into their hallucinations (Graham et al., 1997). This is not the case, however, in patients with schizophrenia, in which studies report a great deal of interindividual disparity in terms of degree of insight into their symptoms (Amador & David, 2004).

Auditory hallucinations observed in severe depression or psychotic depression generally are consistent with the person's depressed mood (e.g., the person hears voices that are mocking and humiliating and that criticize the patient for various failures, shortcomings, and sins). Similarly, the auditory hallucinations in manic episodes usually involve voices that speak directly to the person and whose content is congruent with their abnormally elevated mood. Lowe (1973) observed that paranoid hallucinations were predominantly auditory, whereas manic–depressive hallucinations were predominantly visual. As mentioned earlier, some people with PTSD (e.g., combat veterans) may hear persistent voices that are often directly related to their past experiences (e.g., hear voices that involve cries for help) and hallucinations in a woman with postpartum disorders may be a reflection of her mood and preoccupations (e.g., hearing voices accusing her of being an incompetent mother). In the case of the dementias, in LBD and PD, hallucinations are often rich and detailed, whereas in AD they are commonly simple or isolated. Hallucinations in CBS are often unique, bizarre, or frightening (Santhouse et al., 2000).

---

[2]Kurt Schneider (1887–1967) was a German psychiatrist who was interested in identifying characteristics that were peculiar to schizophrenia. This resulted in the so-called "first-rank" symptoms of the disorder that were all forms of hallucinations (e.g., audible thoughts), delusions, or passivity experience (e.g., the feeling that one's will is being controlled by some external force or agency). As Bentall (2003) pointed out, Schneider was careful to deny that these symptoms were crucially important features of schizophrenia but, rather, to state that they were chosen purely for convenience because they were easy for clinicians to recognize. However, the importance that many diagnostic systems (e.g., various editions of the *DSM*) attribute to these symptoms suggests that this fact has not been taken into consideration.

On the basis of much of what has been presented in terms of hallucinations in various clinical groups, it might be suggested that at least three groups of hallucinations may be distinguished: those observed in psychotic disorders, those seen in neurological disorders, and those seen in the context of substance use. Although these three types of (clinical) hallucinations may share common mechanisms, their distinguishing characteristics seem nonetheless to dominate, not only in terms of their phenomenological characteristics (described in the preceding paragraphs) but also in terms of potential psychological and biological mechanisms involved in the genesis of hallucinations. This issue is described in more detail in chapter 7, this volume.

HALLUCINATIONS IN NONCLINICAL GROUPS

Not only are hallucinations observed in the various clinical populations described above, numerous studies have also found that normal, healthy individuals (i.e., who do not suffer from any neurological or psychiatric disorders or who have not suffered from any neurological or psychiatric disorders) may experience hallucinations. Furthermore, these may occur in adults, in children and adolescents, and in older individuals. A description of the studies that have examined the presence of hallucinatory experiences in individuals from these age-groups follows.

Hallucinations in Nonclinical Adult Groups

Several studies reveal that a substantial number of nonclinical participants (i.e., people who have not been clinically referred or have never received a psychiatric or neurological diagnosis) report having typical hallucinatory experiences (Aleman, Böcker, & de Haan, 2001; Allen et al., 2005; Barrett & Etheridge, 1992; Bentall & Slade, 1985b; Eaton, Romanoski, Anthony, & Nestadt, 1991; Johns et al., 2004; Johns, Nazroo, Bebbington, & Kuipers, 2002; Larøi, DeFruyt, van Os, Aleman, & Van der Linden, 2005; Larøi, Marczewski, & Van der Linden, 2004; Larøi & Van der Linden, 2005b; McKellar, 1968; Milham & Easton, 1998; Morrison, Wells, & Nothard, 2000; Ohayon, 2000; Ohayon, Priest, Caulet, & Guilleminault, 1996; Olfson et al., 2002; Romme & Escher, 1989; Serper, Dill, Chang, Kot, & Elliot, 2005; Sidgewick, 1894; Tien, 1991; van Os, Hanssen, Bijl, & Ravelli, 2000; Waters, Badcock, & Maybery, 2003; D. J. West, 1948; Young, Bentall, Slade, & Dewey, 1987).

The first systematic attempt to determine whether hallucinations might occur in people without physical or mental illness was conducted at the end of the 19th century (Sidgewick, 1894). In total, 7,717 men and 7,599 women were interviewed. Of the total sample, 7.8% of the men and 12.0% of the women reported at least one vivid hallucinatory experience, the most common type being a visual hallucination of a living person who was not present at the time of the experience. Hallucinations with a religious or supernatural content were also reported, and auditory hallucinations were found to be less common than visual hallucinations. Finally, hallucinations appeared to occur most commonly in people between 20 and 29 years of age. In a follow-up study, D. J. West (1948) distributed a questionnaire covering the same area surveyed in Sidgewick's study. Out of the 1,519 subjects who responded, 217 (14.3%) reported having experienced hallucinations. Here, too, visual hallucinations were more commonly reported than auditory hallucinations, and women respondents were more likely to have experienced hallucinations than men.

McKellar (1968) found that 125 out of 500 normal people (25%) reported having had at least one hallucinatory experience. In a later study, Posey and Losch (1983) questioned 375 college students and found that 39% reported experiencing the Schneiderian first-rank symptom of hearing a voice out loud, and 5% reported holding conversations with their hallucinations.

Tien (1991) conducted one of the first and most comprehensive surveys of hallucinations in the general population. The data were collected from the Epidemiological Catchment Area (ECA) study, a large interview survey of psychiatric symptoms in a randomly selected general population sample. A total of 18,572 people were assessed, and 15,258 of them agreed to be reassessed 1 year later. Results revealed that hallucinations occurred in at least 10% to 15% (prevalence) and in 4% to 5% (annual incidence) of the sample. Tien also compared the ECA data with Sidgewick's (1894) data (described above), which he submitted to a reanalysis. The data from the two studies proved to be remarkably similar. Estimates of the lifetime prevalence of hallucinations in the ECA study were 13.0% at the first assessment and 11.1% at the second, figures that did not differ significantly from Sidgewick's findings. There were two main differences between the two studies. The first concerned the age prevalence of hallucinations, in which the ECA data revealed that hallucinations occurred across the age spectrum but most often in older adults, whereas Sidgewick's data showed a higher prevalence of hallucinations in subjects between ages 20 and 29. The second difference centered on the prevalence of visual hallucinations, which were reported more often by Sidgewick's respondents compared with the ECA data.

Another comprehensive investigation of the occurrence of hallucinations in the general population was conducted by Ohayon (2000). In this study, representative samples of the noninstitutionalized general population with ages between 15 and 100 (N = 13,057) in three countries (the United Kingdom, Germany, and Italy) were surveyed by telephone. Various types of hallucination (visual, auditory, olfactory, haptic, gustatory, hypnagogic, and hypnopompic) were investigated. Results revealed that 38.7% of the sample reported hallucinatory experiences (19.6% less than once a month, 6.4% monthly, 2.7% once a week, and 2.4% more than once a week). Furthermore, these proportions were comparable across the three countries.

TABLE 3.2
Mean Rates of Hallucinations in General Population
or Epidemiological Studies

Study	N	Assessment strategy	Hallucinations (%)
Tien (1991)	18,572	NIMH Diagnostic Interview Schedule	10.0–15.0[a]
Ohayon (2000)	13,057	Sleep-EVAL	38.7
van Os, Hanssen, Bijl, and Ravelli (2000)	7,076	Composite International Diagnostic Interview	1.7–6.2[b]
Olfson et al. (2002)	1,005	Mini International Neuropsychiatric Interview	13.0
Johns et al. (2004)	8,520	Psychosis Screening Questionnaire	4.2

Note. NIMH = National Institute of Mental Health.
[a]Indicates men and women, respectively. [b]Indicates those with true hallucinations and those whose hallucinations were not associated with distress, respectively.

van Os et al. (2000) conducted psychiatric interviews of 7,076 people randomly selected from the Dutch general population. When abnormal experiences secondary to drug taking or physical illness were excluded, 1.7% of participants were found to have experienced "true" hallucinations, but another 6.2% had experienced hallucinations that were judged not clinically relevant because they were not associated with distress.

Olfson et al. (2002) asked a group of adult primary care patients (*N* = 1,005) from an urban general medicine practice to complete the Mini International Neuropsychiatric Interview (Sheehan et al., 1998). They found that around 21% reported one or more current psychotic symptoms, including 13% of participants who reported one or more current auditory hallucinations and 10% who reported one or more current visual hallucinations.

Johns et al. (2004) used data from another large cross-sectional survey of the British population to examine the distribution and correlates of self-reported hallucinatory experiences. After excluding people with probable psychosis, data were available for 8,520 individuals. Of this sample, 5.5% reported one or more psychotic symptoms as measured by the Psychosis Screening Questionnaire (Bebbington & Nayani, 1995). For hallucinations, 4.2% of the sample said there had been times when they heard or saw things that other people could not, but only 0.7% reported hearing voices saying words or sentences when there was no one around who might account for it. Table 3.2 lists the mean rates of hallucinations in the general nonclinical adult population and in epidemiological studies.

In a study involving a university sample, Larøi and Van der Linden (2005b) found that 34% of the 236 participants responded affirmatively (i.e., *possibly applies* or *certainly applies*) that they had heard a person's voice even

TABLE 3.3
Mean Rates of Hallucinations in Young Adult (University) Samples

Study	N	Assessment strategy[a]	Hallucinations (%)
Aleman, Böcker, and de Haan (2001)	243	LSHS	11[b]
Waters, Badcock, and Maybery (2003)	562	LSHS	30[b]
Larøi, Marczewski, and Van der Linden (2004)	265	Revised LSHS	13[b]
Larøi and Van der Linden (2005b)	236	Revised LSHS	19[b]
Larøi, DeFruyt, et al. (2005)	230	Revised LSHS	17[b]
Barrett and Etheridge (1992)	586	Verbal Hallucinations Questionnaire	37[c]

Note. LSHS = Launay–Slade Hallucinations Scale.
[a]These instruments are described in the Appendix.
[b]Percentage of participants who responded affirmatively (i.e., *possibly applies* or *certainly applies*) to the item, "I often hear a voice speaking my thoughts aloud."
[c]Percentage of participants who responded affirmatively to the item, "I sometimes hear my thoughts aloud. I actually hear them spoken outside my head when no one really said anything."

though no one was there, and 19% responded affirmatively to an item related to the first-rank symptom of hearing a voice speaking their thoughts aloud (see Table 3.3). Other studies using student populations have reported similar figures (Aleman, Böcker, & de Hann, 2001; Barrett & Etheridge, 1992; Bentall & Slade, 1985b; Larøi, DeFruyt, et al., 2005; Larøi, Marczewski, & Van der Linden, 2004; van't Wout, Aleman, Kessels, Larøi, & Kahn, 2004; Young et al., 1987). Furthermore, studies have found that reports of hallucinations in student populations are not related to measures of social conformity (Barrett & Etheridge, 1992; Larøi & Van der Linden, 2005b), overt symptoms of psychopathology (Barrett & Etheridge, 1992), or alcohol and/or drugs (Larøi & Van der Linden, 2005b).

Hallucinations in the general population are associated with certain risk factors. It is important to note that these risk factors often mirror those observed in clinical populations. In a large, general population study, Johns et al. (2004) found that neurotic disorder, victimization experiences, average and below average IQ, alcohol dependence, and female gender were independently associated with self-reported hallucinatory experiences. There was also a trend for an association between hallucinations and Black ethnic group, replicating the finding of Johns, Nazroo, et al. (2002).

A large body of evidence indicates an association between exposure to trauma and the development of hallucinations in nonclinical participants (Read et al., 2005). For example, one study found that 27% of a group of survivors of childhood incest heard voices later in life (Ensink, 1992). In a community survey, Ross and Joshi (1992) reported that 46% of those who reported three or more Schneiderian symptoms had experienced childhood physical or sexual abuse compared with 8% with no such symptoms. Surveys of schizotypal traits in the normal population have also found that reports of unusual experiences correlate with a reported history of childhood sexual abuse (Bryer et al., 1987; Startup, 1999). Finally, in a sample of 200 community patients, Read, Agar, Argyle, and Aderhold (2003) found that hallucinations were significantly related to sexual abuse and childhood physical abuse and that this was particularly the case for commenting voices and command hallucinations.

In an extensive epidemiological study, Janssen et al. (2004) reported that childhood abuse is a risk factor for positive psychotic experiences in the general population. Childhood abuse was assessed at baseline, and first-onset incident of positive psychotic symptoms was assessed using the Composite International Diagnostic Interview (CIDI) and the Brief Psychiatric Rating Scale (BPRS) 2 years later. The result revealed that childhood abuse reported at baseline predicted the development of positive psychotic symptoms (unusual thought content and hallucinations). Three levels of psychosis outcome were analyzed: subclinical symptoms, pathologic symptoms, and symptoms associated with need for care. Furthermore, there was a dose–response relationship between the frequency of reported abuse and these psychosis outcomes. In particular, those who had experienced child abuse of mild severity were 2.0 times more likely than nonabused individuals to have a pathological psychosis, compared with 10.6 and 48.4 times more likely than those who had suffered moderate and high severity of abuse, respectively. (The same dose effect was also found for the two other psychosis measures.) The fact that adverse life events predict psychosis has also been reported in another large general population study (Bebbington et al., 2004).

A number of studies indicate that emotional disorders (especially depression and anxiety) are associated with hallucinatory experiences in nonclinical participants (Allen et al., 2005; Lewandowski et al., 2006; Paulik, Badcock, & Maybery, 2006; Verdoux et al., 1998). For instance, Allen et al. (2005) reported that higher levels of anxiety, self-focus, and extreme responding were associated with hallucinatory predisposition in their group of nonclinical participants. In a series of (general population) studies, Krabbendam and collaborators have found that in nonclinical individuals with self-reported hallucinatory experiences the risk for onset of psychotic disorder is mediated by the presence of delusional ideation and the development of depressed mood (Krabbendam et al., 2004; Krabbendam, Myin-Germeys, Bak, & van Os, 2005; Krabbendam, Myin-Germeys, Hanssen, et al., 2005; Krabbendam & van Os, 2005). According to the authors, the relations between hallucinations and depression and anxiety may be mediated by people's interpretations of the voices. For instance, in those who perceive the voice as omnipresent and omnipotent (resulting in feeling overwhelmed or powerless), this may lead to depressed mood. On the other hand, in those who might feel threatened or humiliated by the voice, the development of delusional ideation may be an outcome. Finally, as pointed out by Johns (2005), these findings from studies including nonclinical populations revealing clinical outcome predictors (e.g., beliefs, appraisals, mood) suggest targets for intervention in those individuals who have hallucinatory experiences and who seek help.

A multitude of circumstances or contexts can trigger hallucinations in nonclinical participants (Brasić, 1998; Watkins, 1998). Again, it is important to note that these triggers will apply equally to clinical subjects with hallucinations. These may include deprivation (e.g., food, sensory, sleep), fatigue, sleep and related states, life-threatening stress, bereavement and grief reactions, prolonged perceptual isolation, sexual abuse, and religious and ritual activities both in the major religions (e.g., in Muslim, Christian, and Jewish traditions) and in nondenominational spiritual experiences (e.g., trance channeling, shamanism).

One major external factor, external stimulation, is known to influence hallucinations although its influence may differ depending on the case. For example, subjects may report hallucinations in conditions of increased external stimulation (e.g., when in a crowd), of decreased external stimulation (e.g., when alone at night), or in conditions when there is a particular, usually repetitive, background noise (e.g., being close to electrical machinery such as fans and washing machines). Also, a number of studies suggest an association between sensory deficit and the presence of hallucinations, in particular, a relation between visual sensory impairment and the presence of auditory hallucinations. Studies also reveal an association between deafness and auditory hallucinations in older adults, and between deafness and musical hallucinations (David, 1999). A number of general population studies have reported that hearing impairment acts as a risk factor for psychotic experiences (Stefanis, Thewissen, Bakoula, van Os, & Myin-Germeys, 2006; Thewissen et al., 2005; van der Werf et al., 2007). For a review of studies examining relations between sensory impairment and hallucinations, the reader may consult Behrendt and Young (2004). A lack of external stimulation due to sensory deficits in subjects with hallucinations can be related to the fact that the brain may generate sensory experiences to compensate for sensory loss or loss of external stimulation. Furthermore, this suggests that a person's ability to distinguish between external and internal experiences depends on adequate external stimulation. That is, decreased external stimulation due to sensory loss or diminished social engagement may leave the subject overly influenced by internal stimuli and beliefs.

A recurring theme of many of the above-mentioned contextual factors is the presence of stress. For instance, Johns, Hemsley, and Kuipers (2002) found that a majority of nonpsychiatric participants (tinnitus patients suffering from musical hallucinations) had experienced stress when their hallucinations first started and that stress was the most important factor in triggering hallucinations. Further evidence that stress may play a specific role in hallucinations in nonclinical subjects has emerged from case studies of individuals exposed to extraordinary or life-threatening circumstances, such as mining accidents (Comer, Madow, & Dixon, 1967), sustained military operations (Belenky, 1979), and terrorist attacks (Siegel, 1984). Finally, Larøi and Van der Linden (2005b) found that almost one fourth of nonclinical participants indicated that their hallucinatory experiences occurred in the context of a particularly difficult or stressful life event.

Grief and mourning are part of the normal process of bereavement that follows the loss of a loved one. Research has revealed that it is common for people to see, hear, or feel the presence of the deceased person during bereavement. In a detailed study about the hallucinations and illusions of a group of 293 widows and widowers (young, middle-aged, and older subjects), Reese (1971) found that nearly half had experiences of this kind. In total, the sense of the deceased's presence was most common (39%), followed by visual and auditory hallucinations (14% and 13%, respectively). Twelve percent of the subjects said they had talked with, and 3% said they had been touched by, the deceased. Furthermore, 53% still reported having hallucinations 10 years after their spouse died, and 43% said they still had them after 20 years. Finally, 40 years afterward, 32% still had some kind of sensory experience involving their loved ones. These results reveal that the closer the subjects were to bereavement in time, the more common such experiences were. Findings also showed that younger people hallucinated to a lesser extent than older adults. The type of hallucination also varied with age: The older adults (more than 60 years of age) had more visual hallucinations and more frequently talked with the deceased. Reese also found that a long, happy marriage increased the probability of experiencing hallucinations, as did the existence of children. A large majority of the subjects had a positive attitude to their experiences and felt helped by them, with only 6% of subjects finding them unpleasant. Finally, none of the subjects had told a doctor about their experiences previously, and only 1 had confided in a priest. One quarter had, however, told some close friend or relative about the experiences. The most common reason for keeping their experiences to themselves was the fear of being made fun of.

Likewise, Olson, Suddeth, Peterson, and Egelhoff (1985) showed that nearly two thirds of 46 widows (average age 80 years) residing in nursing homes had experienced hallucinations or illusions. As many as 79% had visual and 50% had auditory experiences of the deceased, whereas 21% had had a tactile experience, 32% had a feeling of presence, and 18% had spoken with the deceased. They also reported that these phenomena were usually experienced at night (61%) and were less common during the day (7%). However, 32% had both nighttime and daytime experiences. In addition, a study of 50 bereaved people in their early 70s revealed that 82% of respondents reported having felt the presence of the deceased person (Grimby, 1993,

1998). Many of them also said they spoke to, heard, and saw the deceased person during the first month of bereavement. Thirty-six percent had experienced one type of hallucination, whereas 30% had experienced two, 12% three, and 2% four or five different types. After 1 month postbereavement, the most common experience was the feeling that the deceased person was present (52%), followed by reports of having heard the voice of the deceased person (30%), having spoken to the deceased person (30%), having seen the deceased person (26%), and having the sense of being touched by the deceased person (6%). When interviewed again after 3 months, 71% of the subjects reported hallucinations and/or illusions, and after 12 months had elapsed, 52% of the subjects were still having these experiences. Significantly more women than men had illusions and/or hallucinations at each of the successive interviews.

Also, consistent with previous studies (Reese, 1971), these bereavement hallucinations seemed to be especially common among people who had long and happy marriages (Grimby, 1993, 1998), and these hallucinations were not associated with depression or any kind of psychological or physical abnormality. The majority of widows and widowers actually found the experience of hearing the voice of a deceased spouse pleasant and helpful. Despite the fact that these kinds of experiences are a normal and often helpful aspect of bereavement, most people who have them do not disclose them to anyone—not even to relatives, close friends, clergy, or medical personnel—for fear of possible negative reactions such as being judged as mentally abnormal. In contrast, in cultures such as Japan where no stigma is associated with such experiences, bereaved persons who have them do not needlessly become fearful about their sanity (Yamamoto, Okonogi, Iwasaki, & Yosimura, 1969). In Yamamoto et al.'s study (1969), nearly all (90%) in a group of Japanese widows had experiences involving their dead husbands in some way. As a matter of fact, because these experiences may be expected to occur in the newly bereaved, both the bereaved person and others concerned should be counseled to accept them as a normal phenomenon to alleviate fear and prevent unnecessary worry and other negative reactions.

A number of chemical substances (both naturally occurring and synthetic) can elicit hallucinations in nonclinical individuals. These substances include LSD, cannabis, opiates, PCP, amphetamine, mescaline, and cocaine (Watkins, 1998). Some of these drugs are in fact known primarily for being hallucinogenic and are commonly labeled as such. Chronic cocaine abuse can result in the development of *cocaine psychosis*, a subacute delirious state characterized by auditory hallucinations with persecutory content. Ingestion of large quantities of cannabis over a long period of time can also precipitate an acute psychotic state in which persecutory voices may be a prominent feature. Following the use of a hallucinogenic drug such as LSD, some people may later reexperience one or more of the perceptual experiences that occurred while they were under the influence of the drug. These experiences (sometimes known as *flashbacks*) may include auditory hallucinations of sounds or voices, although they typically only last a few seconds. Tactile hallucinations (in the form of the sensation of insects crawling up the skin) are rare, but when they occur, it is usually in the context of cocaine and amphetamine intoxication. Subjects under the influence of psychedelic drugs may experience synesthetic hallucinations, whereby they perceive a colorful visual hallucination after hearing a loud noise or may have auditory hallucinations in response to a bright light.

Important to note is that the same drug may not produce the same hallucinatory effect every time. These effects may vary according to the person, dose, mood, and social setting (Asaad & Shapiro, 1986). It is necessary to emphasize, however, that the typical phenomenology of drug-induced hallucinations—which often consists of visual experiences incorporating intense colors as well as explosive, concentric, rotational, or pulsating movements—is quite different from that of hallucinations that occur in the absence of intoxication (Bentall, 2003). In addition, visual hallucinations induced by drugs tend to change if the eyes are closed or open. That is, these experiences are more readily seen with the eyes closed or in darkened surroundings. Moreover, if auditory hallucinations do occur in the context of chemical substances, they tend to be elemental or unformed (e.g., indistinct noises), although more complex experiences, including voices, do sometimes occur. An increase in the likelihood of hallucinations occurring in otherwise normal subjects is observed only when chemical substances are taken frequently, in large amounts, and over long periods of time. Also, as described earlier in this chapter, withdrawal from certain chemical and alcoholic substances may also provoke hallucinations (Asaad & Shapiro, 1986; Watkins, 1998).

Hallucinations in Nonclinical Children and Adolescents

Studies examining rates of hallucinatory experiences in general, nonclinical populations have reported that a substantial percentage of individuals have had such experiences. A summary of prevalence rates reported in studies are presented in Table 3.4. Prevalence of hallucinations varies from 6% to 33%; for having hallucinations and delusions, 11%; and for having either a hallucination or delusion, 13%. Variations between studies most probably reflect differences in sample characteristics and the assessment strategies used.

Information concerning the types and modalities of hallucinations is provided in some of these studies. In general, auditory and visual hallucinations are the most frequently reported types of hallucinations (Dhossche, Ferdinand, Van der Ende, Hofstra, & Verhulst, 2002; McGee, Williams, & Poulton, 2000). In the most complete study to date, Yoshizumi, Murase, Honjo, Kaneko, and Murakami (2004) found that in a group of 761 children

TABLE 3.4

Mean Rates of Hallucinations (Hall.) and Delusions (Del.) in Children and Adolescents in the Nonclinical Population

Study	N	Mean age (in years) of participants (range)	Assessment strategy[a]	Hall.	Hall. or del.	Hall. and del.
Dhossche, Ferdinand, Van der Ende, Hofstra, and Verhulst (2002)	913	14 (11–18)	Youth Self Report	6%	—	—
McGee, Williams, and Poulton (2000)	788	11	DISC	8%	—	—
Yoshizumi, Murase, Honjo, Kaneko, and Murakami (2004)	761	11–12	Designed by authors	21%	—	—
Altman, Collins, and Mundy (1997)	38	16 (13–21)	DIS[b]	33%	—	11%
Poulton et al. (2000)	789	11	DISC	—	13%	—

Note. Dashes in cells indicate that the studies did not examine the aspect indicated. DISC = Diagnostic Interview Schedule for Children; DIS = Psychotic Symptom Module from the Diagnostic Inventory Schedule; From "Hallucinations and Delusions in Children and Adolescents," by F. Larøi, M. Van der Linden, and J.-L. Goëb, 2006, *Current Psychiatry Reviews, 2,* p. 474. Copyright 2006 by Bentham Science Publishers Ltd. Adapted with permission. [a]Many of these instruments are described in the Appendix. [b]Psychotic Symptom Module from this instrument.

(ranging from 11 to 12 years of age), 9% had isolated auditory hallucinations, 6% had isolated visual hallucinations, and 7% had combined auditory and visual hallucinations. Of those who had auditory hallucinations, 58% heard their names called or were addressed by a single word (e.g., "Hey" or "Hello"), and in 13%, the voices attempted to interfere with the subject's actions or situation using longer sentences (e.g., "You are not concentrating now" or "Please come here"). In addition, singing voices (5%), laughing voices (5%), aspersions (3%), thought hearing (2%), screaming voices (2%), and groaning voices (2%) were recorded. Of those who had visual hallucinations, 61% reported seeing a human figure such as a friend; a deceased person; an unknown person; or a human hand, head, or foot. In 20%, lights, lines, or colored objects were seen. Visions of ghosts (4%), plants (4%), shadows (2%), animals (2%), fog (2%), geometric objects (2%), and dots (2%) were also reported.

There is much evidence that other psychopathological symptoms coexist with the presence of hallucinatory experiences in nonclinical children and adolescents (Altman, Collins, & Mundy, 1997; Dhossche et al., 2002; McGee et al., 2000; Yoshizumi et al., 2004). For instance, Altman et al. (1997) reported significant correlations of hallucinations with self-reports of dissociative experiences, depressive symptoms, and odd (schizotypal) thought processes. Furthermore, a relation between type of hallucination and extent of comorbidity risk was observed in Yoshizumi et al. (2004). Results revealed that children who had experienced hallucinations (in particular, combined auditory and visual hallucinations) also had significantly higher psychopathology scores (i.e., higher scores on the anxiety and dissociative experiences measures) compared with children with a single modality of hallucination (and especially compared with those with isolated auditory hallucinations) and those without hallucinations. Furthermore, with regard to the content of the visual hallucinations, children with concrete content of visual hallucinations had significantly higher levels of depression, anxiety, and dissociation than those with no concrete or abstract content of visual hallucinations.

HALLUCINATIONS IN CHILD AND ADOLESCENT CLINICAL POPULATIONS

Hallucinations may also present themselves in children and adolescents in a number of different psychiatric disorders (both psychotic and nonpsychotic) and nonpsychiatric disorders. In terms of nonpsychiatric disorders, hallucinations have been observed in disorders such as thyroid and parathyroid disease, adrenal disease, Wilson's disease, beriberi, electrolyte imbalance, porphyria, meningitis, encephalitis or febrile illness, migraine, Tourette's syndrome, and velo–cardio–facial syndrome. Concerning psychiatric disorders, studies have examined their presence in individuals with schizophrenia, mood, and anxiety disorders and in children and adolescents with emotional or conduct disorders. For a detailed review of these studies, see Larøi, Van der Linden, and Goëb (2006).

Predictive Value of Hallucinations in Children and Adolescents

Dhossche et al. (2002) provided follow-up data in their group of nonclinical individuals. They reevaluated 86% of their original sample of children and adolescents after 8 years (mean age of subjects at follow-up was 23 years). Results revealed that no subjects were diagnosed with schizophreniform disorders or schizophrenia, but about half of those with self-reported hallucinations were diagnosed with nonpsychotic psychiatric disorders (i.e., depressive disorders, substance use disorders, PTSD, and social phobia). The risk for being diagnosed with a *DSM–IV* Axis I (i.e., nonpsychotic) disorder was almost 4 times higher in adolescents with self-reported hallucinations than in controls.

In Poulton et al. (2000), prospective data from a birth cohort were collected in which nonclinical children were asked about delusional beliefs and hallucinatory experiences at age 11 years ($N = 789$) and then at 26 years of age ($N = 761$, or 97% of the original sample). Results showed that self-reported psychotic symptoms at age 11 years increased the odds for psychotic illness at age 26 years by 16.4 times, but the actual number of children who developed a psychotic disorder was very small. Furthermore, childhood psychotic experiences had predictive value independent of childhood psychiatric diagnosis.

In a retrospective design, Garralda (1984) collected demographic and clinical data of 4,767 children. Among these, 20 children who had experienced hallucinations and who had diagnoses of emotional or conduct disorder were selected along with a control group of 20 matched individuals. Auditory hallucinations were present in 85% of the children. In 20% of children with hallucinations, bereavement was a precipitant, and in 15% of cases, there was evidence of inadequate social stimulation and/or social deprivation. The two groups did not differ in terms of vivid imagination, daydreaming, insomnia, and deafness. When the two groups were compared in terms of clinical factors, there were significantly higher levels of depressive symptoms and family history of mood changes in the children with hallucinations. Anxiety symptoms were more common in the children with hallucinations, although the difference was not statistically significant. These two groups were also followed up (mean follow-up was 17 years, and the mean age at follow-up was 30 years; Garralda, 1984). Sufficient information to make an assessment of psychiatric functioning was available for 87.5% of the original sample. Results did not show an increased risk for psychotic disorders, depressive illness, or organic brain damage in adulthood for those individuals who had experienced hallucinations in childhood. Furthermore, there were no significant differences between the two groups in terms of social adjustment.

Escher, Romme, Buiks, Delespaul, and van Os (2002b) studied a group of 80 children who were hearing voices (around 50% of these children were not receiving mental health care) and collected information such as voice characteristics, voice attributions, psychopathology, stressful life events, coping mechanisms, and receipt of professional care. These participants were also followed up three times over a period of 3 years. It was found that the rate of voice discontinuation over the 3-year period was 60%. Predictors of persistence of voices were severity and frequency of the voices, associated anxiety and depression, and lack of clear triggers in time and place. Need for care in the context of the experience of voices was associated with the appraisal of the voices in terms of intrusiveness and omnipotence rather than the perception itself or the presence of a diagnosis.

In another study including the same group of 80 children, Escher et al. (2002a) also looked at possible factors involved in delusion formation in the presence of hallucinatory experiences. Results revealed that 16% displayed evidence of delusional ideation over at least one of the three follow-up periods. In 9% of the sample, the delusions appeared de novo. Delusion formation over the follow-up period was associated with baseline voice appraisals and attributions such as tone of the voice, perceived location of the voice, and whether the voice resembled that of a parent. Other predictors were baseline BPRS anxiety and depression, baseline BPRS disorganization, and the baseline amount of reported recent stressful life events. In addition, in older children, the perceived influence of the voices on emotions and behavior was strongly associated with delusion formation.

In general, studies have revealed that a substantial number of children and adolescents report hallucinations, both in clinical and nonclinical populations. The presence of hallucinations may increase the likelihood of the presence of various psychopathological conditions (but these do not exclusively include psychotic disorders) in childhood and adolescence and also later in life. However, it is important to note that many of these hallucinations may be of a transient nature and therefore may disappear shortly after their apparition. Also, a substantial number of children and adolescents experiencing hallucinations will not necessarily develop any major psychopathological conditions later in life.

Certain studies have found that hallucinations may predict future psychopathological conditions. In a nonclinical general population study, Poulton et al. (2000) showed that high scores on a composite measure of self-reported psychotic symptoms predicted a diagnosis of schizophreniform disorder at age 26. Dhossche et al. (2002) found that hallucinations had predictive value in a nonclinical sample, albeit for Axis I (i.e., nonpsychotic) disorders. In contrast, Garralda (1984) concluded that hallucinations had no prognostic value for psychosis or any other psychiatric disorder in a sample of child psychiatric outpatients with nonpsychotic disorders (i.e., conduct and emotional disorders). Possible reasons for these differences in findings are described in detail in Larøi, Van der Linden, and Goëb (2006). Furthermore, researchers (Laurens et al., 2007) have argued that to identify children at risk of developing schizophrenia spectrum disorders, one must screen not only for the presence of psychotic-like experiences (e.g., hallucinations) but also for the presence of speech and/or motor development lags or problems and social, behavioral, or emotional problems.

Traumatic Life Events in Children and Adolescents

A large body of evidence reports an association between childhood abuse and hallucinations. In particular, multiple case studies have revealed that traumatic events such as physical or sexual abuse, bereavement, and separation represent important triggers for hallucinations in otherwise normally functioning children and adolescents (Kaufman, Birmaher, Clayton, Retano, & Wongchaowart, 1997; Murase, Honjo, Inoko, & Ohta, 2002; Murase, Ochiai, & Ohta, 2000; Schreier & Libow, 1986; Semper & McClellan, 2003). Important to add is that in the large majority of these cases, the hallucinations are highly transitory, no medication is required, and interventions usually involve supportive therapy and reassuring the family.

In a study that investigated relations between life events and psychotic ideation in detail, Escher et al. (2004; the same cohort was included in this study as in Escher et al., 2002a, 2002b) found that in about 75% of participants who heard voices, traumatic events or circumstances beyond their control had occurred at the onset of hearing voices. These included the death of a close family member or friend, problems in the home situation (e.g., tensions between parents or between siblings), problems at school (e.g., bullying, problems with teachers, learning ability problems), or circumstances beyond the child's control (e.g., sexual abuse, birth trauma, long-term physical illnesses). In many cases, the voices disappeared when these problems were resolved, and the children's development took a positive turn. During the 3-year research program, 60% of the children stopped hearing voices. Furthermore, whether the child was receiving professional mental health care did not itself influence the probability of voice discontinuation. (This latter finding is described in more detail in chap. 8, this volume.)

A number of epidemiological or general population studies also report an association between exposure to victimization during childhood and psychotic experiences. Janssen et al. (2004) reported that childhood abuse predicts psychotic symptoms in adulthood and that this association remained after adjustment for demographic variables, reported risk factors, and presence of any lifetime psychiatric diagnosis at baseline. Lataster et al. (2006) found that both serious traumatic experiences (e.g., being a victim of unwanted sexual experiences) and apparently mild traumatic experiences (e.g., being a victim of bullying) were associated with nonclinical psychotic experiences in early adolescence. Similarly, in a recent study including a large, representative, nonclinical community sample, Shevlin, Dorahy, and Adamson (2007) observed an association between traumatic childhood experiences and auditory, visual, and tactile hallucinations. In particular, four types of childhood abuse (physical abuse, neglect, rape, and molestation) were all associated with an increased likelihood of experiencing visual hallucinations, auditory hallucinations were associated with two of these types of childhood abuse (rape and molestation), and tactile hallucinations were associated with three of these (physical abuse, rape, and molestation).

HALLUCINATIONS IN OLDER NONCLINICAL ADULTS

A number of recent studies have examined hallucinations in the older nonclinical population. These studies are presented in Table 3.5. Turvey et al. (2001) investigated the demographic, medical, and psychiatric correlates of hallucinations (and delusions) reported by proxy informants (reports of hallucinations from caregivers) for 822 older adults (selected from the community) aged 70 and older. Results revealed that 20% of the subjects experienced visual or auditory hallucinations. Marital status, trouble with vision, and cognitive impairment were found to be associated with hallucinations.

Livingston, Kitchen, Manela, Katona, and Copeland (2001) interviewed 720 older subjects (ages 65 and over) from a community sample concerning psychiatric symptoms and diagnosis. In particular, participants were asked about their persecutory symptoms and perceptual distortions. *Perceptual distortions* were defined as "clearly abnormal or puzzling experiences in all sensory modalities" (p. 464). If participants responded affirmatively, they were asked whether the perceptual distortions or persecutory symptoms occurred when they were awake and whether they judged the experience to be real. Results revealed that the 1-month prevalence rate of persecutory and perceptual disturbances was 3.9%. When the presence of dementia was taken into account, persecutory and perceptual disturbances were recorded in 42.9% of those with dementia and in 2.4% of those without dementia. A forward logistic regression analysis for independent predictors of these symptoms found that the significant predictors were dementia, drinking alcohol in the past 6 months, drinking alcohol to help sleep, subjective memory loss, and uncorrected visual impairment.

Cole, Dowson, Dendukuri, and Belzile (2002) examined the presence of auditory hallucinations in a group of older adult subjects with hearing impairment. The sample, comprising 125 subjects (65 years or over), was referred to the auditory department of a university-affiliated primary acute-care hospital. All of the subjects were assessed for the presence of auditory

TABLE 3.5

Mean Rates of Hallucinations in the Older Nonclinical Population

Study	N	Mean age (years)	Assessment strategy[a]	Hallucinations (%)
Turvey et al. (2001)	822	80	Item developed by authors	20
Livingston, Kitchen, Manela, Katona, and Copeland (2001)	720	75	Geriatric Mental State Schedule	3.9[b]
Cole, Dowson, Dendukuri, and Belzile (2002)	125[c]	78	Item developed by authors	32.8[d]
Lyketsos et al. (2000)	329–673[e]	84–81[e]	Neuropsychiatric Inventory	13.7–0.6[e]
Larøi, DeFruyt, et al. (2005)	183	69	Modified version of the Launay–Slade Hallucinations Scale	31[f]

[a]Many of these instruments are described in the Appendix. [b]One-month prevalence rate of persecutory and perceptual disturbance. [c]All subjects had a certain degree of hearing impairment. [d]Rate for auditory hallucinations. [e]Participants with dementia–participants without dementia. [f]Percentage of participants who responded affirmatively (i.e., *possibly applies* or *certainly applies*) to the item, "I often hear a voice speaking my thoughts aloud."

hallucinations during the past month. They were asked if they had heard any sounds, music, or voices when there did not seem to be a source for the sound. Those who reported auditory hallucinations (i.e., those who responded either "possibly" or "probably" to the first item) were asked to describe the sound and to indicate whether it was heard in the left, right, or both ears; whether it originated inside or outside the head; and whether they believed that other people could hear the sound. A hallucination score was computed by summing up the scores of responses to the four questions about hallucinations (i.e., heard sound, location of sound, source of sound, and others can hear sound). Findings revealed that the prevalence of auditory hallucinations (i.e., the percentage of subjects scoring at least 1 point; that is, responding "possibly heard a sound") was 32.8%.

Lyketsos et al. (2000) screened a large community sample of older subjects (65 years and older) for dementia, resulting in a group of participants with dementia (n = 329) and a group of participants without dementia (n = 673). Both groups underwent comprehensive neuropsychiatric examinations, which included being assessed for hallucinations. Results revealed that hallucinations were present in 13.7% of participants with dementia, whereas only 0.6% of participants without dementia reported having hallucinations.

Larøi, DeFruyt, et al. (2005) examined hallucination proneness in a sample consisting of 183 active, noninstitutionalized older adults. To assess hallucination proneness, the researchers asked subjects to complete a modified and elaborated version of the Launay–Slade Hallucination Scale (Larøi, Marczewski, & Van der Linden, 2004; Larøi & Van der Linden, 2005b). The results revealed that a substantial percentage of participants responded affirmatively (i.e., "possibly applies" or "certainly applies") to typical hallucination items. For example, 46% of participants responded affirmatively to the item, "In the past, I have had the experience of hearing a person's voice and then found that no one was there," and 31% responded affirmatively to the item, "I often hear a voice speaking my thoughts aloud."

COMPARISONS BETWEEN AGE GROUPS IN TERMS OF HALLUCINATION EXPRESSION

Tien (1991) compared age groups in terms of hallucination expression. Incidence rates of visual, auditory, somatic, and olfactory hallucinations across the life span (from 18 to 80+ years of age) in a large community population (N = 18,572) suggested general increases in hallucinations with advanced age. In particular, there was an increase in the incidence of visual and auditory hallucinations. In terms of this latter finding, Tien hypothesized that this may be at least partly related to sensory loss with advancing age.

Larøi, DeFruyt, et al. (2005) found differences in prevalence rates between young and older adult subjects in terms of the types of hallucinatory experiences. In particular, young subjects reported more hallucinatory experiences related to vivid daydreams as well as vivid and intrusive thoughts. In contrast, older adult subjects reported more sleep-related hallucinations and auditory and visual hallucinations. The authors also reported differences between the two age groups in terms of the association between hallucination proneness and personality traits as described by the Big Five personality factors. Hallucination proneness was associated with Openness to Experience in both the older and young sample. However, in the young sample, Neuroticism was also significantly associated with hallucination proneness. In contrast, an association between hallucination proneness and Neuroticism was not found in the older sample.

SIMILARITIES BETWEEN CLINICAL AND NONCLINICAL GROUPS OF HALLUCINATORS

Studies comparing hallucinations in a variety of groups of subjects experiencing hallucinations indicate a similarity (at times remarkable) in terms of the phenomenological characteristics of the voices. For example, Honig et al. (1998) compared nonclinical participants without a psychiatric history with schizophrenic patients and patients diagnosed with dissociative disorders, all of whom were hearing voices. Results revealed a number of similarities between all three groups in terms of the characteristics of their hallucinations, namely the different forms the voices took and the fact that the voices spoke in the second or third person. In addition, all three groups perceived their voices as both negative and positive. Finally, all of the groups expressed a certain lack of control in association with their hallucinations. However, the study had some limitations. For example, it only explored auditory hallucinations, and certain important aspects of hallucinations (e.g., frequency, personal salience, and context specificity) were not examined or taken into account.

In a similar comparison of hallucinating schizophrenic patients with nonpsychiatric hallucinators, Leudar, Thomas, McNally, and Glinski (1997) found surprisingly few differences between patients and nonpatients. A group of schizophrenic patients with hallucinations ($n = 14$) and a group of nonclinical participants (students) who heard voices ($n = 13$) were interviewed regarding their experiences of hearing voices. On the basis of these interviews, the pragmatic properties of the verbal hallucinations were ascertained. Results revealed that both groups shared a number of these properties. For instance, in both groups, the majority of the participants reported that their voices attempted to regulate their everyday activities, for example, telling them what to do or not to do and issuing instructions about particular courses of action. Also, the voices were rarely bizarre and were usually aligned to significant individuals in their lives. However, because the study aimed at examining pragmatic–linguistic aspects of hallucinations, the investigation of phenomenological characteristics was limited to auditory hallucinations, leaving other types of hallucinations unexamined.

Johns, Hemsley, and Kuipers (2002) compared auditory hallucinations in a group of psychiatric patients (schizophrenic patients with a history of auditory hallucinations) and in a group of nonpsychiatric participants (tinnitus patients suffering from musical hallucinations). Results revealed that the majority of subjects reported negative emotional responses to their hallucinations, with no significant differences between groups. Subjects in both groups described feelings of anger, irritation, and agitation (especially if their hallucinations occurred frequently) and were distressed by their perceived lack of control over their experiences. Both groups had a common need to find an explanation for the presence of their hallucinations, and 60% of both schizophrenic patients with auditory hallucinations and nonpsychiatric participants experienced stress when their hallucinations first started. Furthermore, stress was the most important factor in triggering hallucinations in both groups. In addition, the physical characteristics of the hallucinations (volume, clarity, and frequency) were similar in both groups. However, it is important to mention that the nonpsychiatric group (tinnitus patients) consisted of patients with a neurological (albeit mild) condition. Thus, findings cannot be generalized to the general, nonclinical population. In addition, each group contained few subjects (16 in the group of tinnitus patients and 14 in the schizophrenia group), and subjects were selected in a nonrandom manner. Finally, the study compared two different types of hallucinations (auditory hallucinations in schizophrenic patients vs. musical hallucinations in tinnitus patients).

Davies, Griffin, and Vice (2001) compared the incidence and subjective experiences of hearing voices in three different groups: schizophrenic outpatients, evangelical Christians, and controls (nonpsychotic, nonevangelical). Evangelical Christians were included (and not simply religious people) because of the importance of spiritual experiences and spiritual rebirth in these religious denominations. Participants were first asked to complete the Launay–Slade Hallucination Scale (Launay & Slade, 1981). Then, those participants who responded affirmatively to the question of whether they had ever experienced hearing a voice outside the head when no one was present completed additional questionnaires, including reported frequency of hearing voices, affective experiences of hearing voices, and perception of voices. Results revealed that the reported occurrence of hallucinations increased significantly from normal controls (27%) to evangelical Christians (57%) to psychotic individuals (100%). Furthermore, the mean ratings of both the experience of hearing voices and the perception of voices were on the positive side of the 8-point rating scale midpoints (4.5) for all three groups, indicating that in general, people's experience of auditory hallucinations was not markedly negative. Group comparisons revealed, however, that the three groups differed significantly from each other: The evangelical group rated the experience of hearing voices as significantly more positive than those of the control group, which in turn were significantly more positive than those of the psychotic group.

Using the Launay–Slade Hallucination Scale, Serper et al. (2005) examined the factorial structure of hallucinatory experiences in three different groups: schizophrenic patients with active hallucinations, schizophrenic patients without hallucinations, and a group of university students. The results revealed a very similar factor-analytic solution for all three groups. In particular, a two-factor solution was extracted, which the authors labeled as representing "subclinical" (which included items referring to vivid intrusive thoughts and daydreams) and "clinical" (which included items representing auditory and visual hallucinations) hallucination factors. Furthermore, the same two salient dimensions of hallucination expression (clinical and subclinical hallucination factors) could be described for all three groups.

THE CONTINUUM HYPOTHESIS

Similarities in both clinical and nonclinical groups suggest that hallucinations may lie on a continuum with normal experiences. This line of reasoning, known as the *continuum hypothesis*, argues that the main difference between pathological and normal groups is quantitative rather than qualitative. Furthermore, researchers supporting this hypothesis have suggested that it may not be the nature of hallucinatory experiences per se that determines whether people become psychiatric patients but the way in which individuals react to their experiences. Thus, findings of similarities between clinical (psychiatric and nonpsychiatric) and nonclinical subjects have led some researchers to doubt the existence of symptoms as discrete entities. The concept of psychiatric symptoms has evolved from being defined dichotomously (qualitative differences between clinical and nonclinical hallucinations) to being situated on a continuum ranging from normal to highly abnormal experiences (quantitative difference between two groups). This continuum may not be restricted to clinical populations because the presence of these symptoms (as described above) is not solely restricted to the abnormal population.

In an influential study of psychiatric patients' responses to a standardized psychiatric interview, J. S. Strauss (1969) argued that it was possible to identify reports that fall between strict hallucinations and normal experiences. In this study, 119 psychiatric patients were interviewed by three psychiatrists with the help of the Present State Examination (Wing, Birley, Cooper, Graham, & Isaacs, 1967). Patients were excluded if they were known to have severe psychotic symptoms, including hallucinations, delusions, or thought disorder continuously for more than 3 years or had 2 years or more of psychiatric hospitalization in the 5 years prior to their current admission. During assessment of delusions and hallucinations, the interviewers were impressed by the frequent number of responses that could not be rated in a dichotomous manner (i.e., present or absent). The authors termed these responses "questionable" in contrast to "definite" responses, which included responses that could be rated in a clear-cut, absent-or-present manner. The results showed that there were half as many questionable delusions as there were definite delusions (i.e., 142 questionable delusions compared with 269 definite delusions for the whole population). For items concerning hallucinations, the results were even more dramatic: Three fourths as many questionable hallucinations as definite hallucinations (i.e., 56 vs. 81 for the total population) were observed. Furthermore, Strauss calculated the number of patients with questionable, compared with definite, hallucinations and delusions. This revealed that 91 patients had definite delusions, and as many as 74 patients had questionable delusions. In terms of hallucinations, once again the findings were striking: A greater number of patients had questionable hallucinations ($n = 41$) than definite hallucinations ($n = 38$). On the basis of these observations, Strauss called for the need for a system describing hallucinations and delusions more accurately than is possible with a present–absent dichotomy. In doing so, he also pleaded for a change in the conceptualization of these symptoms from being considered all-or-nothing phenomena to being considered nondichotomous, dimensional phenomena that lie as points (or series of points) on a continuum with normal functioning.

More specifically, J. S. Strauss (1969) concluded that that the hallucinations could be classified along four dimensions: (a) the strength of the individual's conviction in the objective reality of the experience, (b) the extent to which the experience seems to be independent of stimuli or cultural determinants, (c) the individual's preoccupation with the experience, and (d) the implausibility of the experience. These dimensions were identified after examination of patients' reports of questionable responses. "Full-blown" hallucinations fall at the end of all of these dimensions. Still, there is no doubt that some experiences fall midway along these dimensions. For instance, a person may think but not be certain that he or she has glimpsed someone he or she was hoping to avoid. In addition, it is more probable that one may mistake seeing a car outside one's house than seeing a man from Mars. Similarly, a person without a religious background may doubt the reality of hearing the voice of the Devil yet may be more convinced that his or her mother's voice was heard. In contrast, it is difficult to dichotomize satisfactorily such statements as "The Devil seems to be trying to get me to do bad things" or "I have heard the voice of the Devil" in subjects who come from a fundamentalist religious background.

Data from van Os et al. (2000) confirmed the fact that the findings reported by Strauss (1969) also apply to the general, nonclinical population. In this study, a random sample of 7,076 men and women (ages 18 to 64 years) were interviewed by trained lay interviewers using the CIDI Version 1.1 (Robins et al., 1988; Smeets & Dingemans, 1993; World Health Organization,

1990). Lifetime ratings from the 17 CIDI core psychosis sections on delusions (13 items) and hallucinations (4 items) were used. (In brief, these items concern classic psychotic symptoms involving, for example, persecution, thought interference, auditory hallucinations, and passivity phenomena.) All of these items were rated in six ways: 1 = no symptom; 2 = symptom present, but not clinically relevant (i.e., the subject was not bothered by it and not seeking help for it); 3 = symptom result of ingestion of drugs; 4 = symptom result of somatic disease; 5 = true psychiatric symptom; and 6 = symptom is not really a symptom because there appears to be some plausible explanation for it. Symptom ratings were then further categorized into (a) not clinically relevant symptoms (those rated as Type 2 symptoms), (b) secondary symptoms (rated as Type 3 and Type 4 symptoms), (c) clinical symptoms (Type 5), and (d) plausible symptoms (Type 6).

To be certain of the diagnoses, psychiatrists further interviewed those with evidence of psychosis according to the CIDI (i.e., those individuals who had at least one rating of clinical symptom or plausible symptom). A senior registrar in psychiatry conducted the clinical reinterviews over the telephone using questions from the Structured Clinical Interview for *DSM–III–R* (Spitzer, Williams, Gibbon, & First, 1992). The following demographic variables were included: age (18–24, 25–34, 35–44, 45–54, 55–64 years), sex, urbanicity of place of residence, level of income, years of education, unemployment, and marital status.[3] Analyses included calculating prevalence rates (for the whole population) of the various symptom categories and associating the different types of symptom categories with the various demographic risk factors (using logistic regression). Prevalence rates for the total population for the various categories of hallucinations were as follows: not clinically relevant hallucinations (6.2%), secondary hallucinations (0.3%), clinical symptoms (1.7%), and plausible symptoms (0.5%).

Results also revealed strong associations between symptom categories. This indicates that subclinical phenomena elicited by lay interviewers were continuous with clinical symptoms rated by a psychiatrist. In addition, female sex, younger age, higher level of urbanicity, lower income, lower level of education, unemployment, and single marital status were associated with each type of psychosis rating. These associations did not differ qualitatively as a function of type of rating of the symptom and closely resembled those previously reported for schizophrenia. The fact that participants' (hallucinatory) experiences were continuous in terms of risk factors suggests a developmental mechanism in nonclinical participants that is similar to the one reported in schizophrenia.

It is possible to identify a number of specific and underlying suppositions or components of the continuous hypothesis. The most important of

---

[3]The demographic variables identified by van Os et al. (2000) consisted of variables that have previously been shown to be associated with schizophrenia.

these are the distributional, phenomenological, developmental, and etiological aspects of the continuum hypothesis.

Distributional component: Hallucinations should be present not only in subjects identified as clinical cases but also in a proportion of subjects from the general population who do not fulfill the clinical criteria of a patient. Furthermore, the continuous hallucination phenotype as it exists in nature is expected to be much more prevalent than clinical hallucinations based on narrow medical criteria. Therefore, the clinical definition of hallucinations may be viewed as only a minor segment of the total phenotypic hallucination continuum that exists in nature. For example, it has been proposed that the psychosis phenotype may be 50 times more common than the medical concept (van Os et al., 2000).[4]

Phenomenological component: There should be a sufficient degree of intergroup similarity, in addition to a large degree of within-group variation, in terms of phenomenological characteristics of hallucinations (e.g., prevalence, degree of control, insight, emotional responses, conviction), resulting in some overlapping between clinical and nonclinical groups. In other words, if phenomenological boundaries are opened up and broadened, the hallucination phenotype present in clinical samples is expected to concur with and be continuous with the hallucination phenotype inherent in nonclinical samples.

Developmental component: Developmental aspects associated with the genesis of hallucinations should also be continuous between pathological and nonpathological samples. That is, factors identified as important demographic risk factors in clinical cases of hallucinations (e.g., female sex, younger age, higher level of urbanicity, lower income, lower level of education, unemployment, and single marital status) should also be associated with the presence of hallucinations in nonclinical subjects. This would suggest a developmental mechanism underlying hallucination genesis, which is applicable to both clinical and nonclinical samples.

Etiological component: Clinical and nonclinical populations should share common ground in terms of the cognitive and emotional mechanisms underlying hallucinations. That is, concurrence of prevalence, phenomenology, and risk factors of clinical and nonclinical hallucinations should be expected to share the same underlying etiological mechanisms. These etiological mechanisms may include, for example, biological (e.g., genetic) and/or environmental (e.g., exposure to adverse life events) factors. Important to note is that although a substantial number of studies have examined the influence of various environmental factors in hallucinations (these studies were described in this chapter and also in W. Larkin & Morrison, 2006; Morrison et al., 2003; Read et al., 2001, 2005), the examination of possible biological

---

[4]Although the psychosis phenotype includes such experiences as hallucinations, other experiences (e.g., delusions) are also included in this concept. A discussion of the nature of a specific hallucination's phenotype is included later in this chapter.

(e.g., genetic) etiological factors has received relatively little attention in the literature. In the context of schizophrenia, studies tend to attempt to identify the genetic etiology of this disorder in general, without examining possible specific relations with hallucinations (e.g., by differentiating between those with or without hallucinations; for some exceptions, see Sanjuán, Toirac, et al., 2004; Wei & Hemmings, 1999).

Nevertheless, in this context, the cognitive approach is deemed particularly pertinent and fruitful in the context of hallucinations for at least two reasons. First, it forges links between normal and abnormal functioning (Bentall, 1996). As a result, researchers following this approach are not required to assume a dichotomy between the pathological and nonpathological but rather may view hallucinations as lying on a continuum with normal mental states. Second, the cognitive approach is neutral with regard to biological and environmental factors (Bentall, 1996). This approach's ability to address a number of different levels of explanations is particularly important in light of the broad array of risk factors associated with hallucination genesis and maintenance, ranging from genetic to sociocultural ones. As Garety, Bebbington, Fowler, Freeman, and Kuipers (2007) explained, "Cognitive models are an important link in the chain from phenotype to genotype, providing a psychological description of the phenomena from which hypotheses concerning causal processes implicated in specific symptoms can be derived and tested" (p. 1378).

It is also important to distinguish between two types of continuum: the continuum of experience and the continuum of personality (Bentall, 2003).[5] The continuum of experience suggests that different kinds of experience (e.g., vivid daydreams, hearing voices, intrusive and vivid thoughts) may be related to each other, whereas the continuum of personality indicates that people differ in their propensity to have those experiences. Of course, both types of continuum imply that there is no clear dividing line between normality and abnormality and therefore can be related to the above-mentioned components of the continuum hypothesis. However, given that hallucination proneness and the hallucination phenotype are directly related to the continuum of personality, it is the most pertinent type of continuum. Nevertheless, the continuum of experience is also pertinent, albeit to a lesser extent.

THE TRANSITION FROM A NONCLINICAL HALLUCINATION TO A CLINICAL HALLUCINATION

In the context of hallucinations, it may be argued that the primary goal of the continuum hypothesis is the delineation of the existence of the "hallu-

---

[5]Bentall (2003) argued for a similar distinction but used the term *dimension* rather than *continuum*. For the sake of consistency, we use the term *continuum* throughout, even though we consider the two terms essentially synonymous.

cination phenotype," albeit in a continuous (as opposed to dichotomous) form.[6] Bearers of the hallucination phenotype may be viewed as individuals with an inherent capacity to experience hallucinations, that is, who are hallucination prone. This capacity depends on various internal and dispositional factors, including genetic, neurobiological, and cognitive–emotional. Although the widely used terms *disposition toward hallucinations* and *predisposition toward hallucinations* may be seen as being related to the term *continuous hallucination phenotype* and its expressional counterpart *hallucination proneness*, they are not entirely accurate terms. The problem with the terms *disposition toward hallucinations* and *predisposition toward hallucinations* is that they suggest a latent personality disposition waiting to be expressed or waiting to manifest itself. Furthermore, according to such terms, when the trait finally manifests itself (on the basis of clinical data, this would be expected to occur in late adolescence or early adulthood), there is a sense of permanence; that is, the subject's existence becomes filled with, or dominated by, hallucinatory experiences. However, there are two problems with this statement. First, proneness toward hallucinations is more accurately viewed as a capacity that is present and expressed early in life (i.e., from childhood). There would be, therefore, no manifestation delay. Second, this ability is relatively controllable and usually only expresses itself in the event of specific internal or external triggers.

In contrast, *hallucination proneness* and *hallucination phenotype* are terms that are relatively unambiguous, contain clear assumptions regarding the nature and onset of hallucinations, and consequently will help prompt important discussions within this area of research. To better illustrate the notion of hallucination proneness, let us imagine 2 subjects. One subject, Person A, is a 22-year-old man with a schizophrenia diagnosis and who has hallucinations once in a while. The other, Person B, is a 22-year-old normal subject who experiences hallucinations once in awhile. Both are hallucination-prone subjects and therefore can be viewed as being bearers of the hallucination phenotype. However, these 2 subjects also differ in that the former is a clinical hallucination-prone subject, whereas the latter is a nonclinical hallucination-prone subject. The hallucination phenotype has played its part in the development of these 2 subjects and will continue to do so throughout their lives. However, at one point in time, one subject is considered a clinical hallucination-prone subject whereas the other has become a nonclinical hallucination-prone subject.

---

[6]Note that although research has examined the nature of the psychosis phenotype (see, e.g., van Os et al., 2000), suggesting that this phenotype may be much more common than the medical concept, research has yet to explore the nature of a more specific and limited phenotype, that is, the hallucination phenotype. Ideas expressed in Garety et al. (2007) seem to be in accord with such a view, whereby they argued that issues such as the choice of phenotype and the development of theoretical (cognitive) models should be examined on the level of specific positive symptoms (e.g., persecutory delusions, grandiose delusions, and hallucinations).

Studies have attempted to examine the difference between these 2 subjects, that is, to explore the transition from a nonclinical hallucination to a clinical hallucination (or clinical case in which there may be a need for treatment). Two main psychological mechanisms seem to be involved in this. First, response to abnormal experience seems to be cognitively mediated by beliefs or appraisals (Garety, Kuipers, Fowler, Freeman, & Bebbington, 2001). That is, the mere experience of voices itself might not lead to full-blown psychotic hallucinations, but attributing the voice to an external malevolent source or giving it personal significance does. Another important determinant of the transition to clinical states may be the level of functional coping that the person mobilizes in the face of stressful (psychotic) experiences. Active coping strategies such as using problem solving or seeking help and distraction seem to generate control over the experiences. In contrast, more passive coping strategies such as going along with and indulging in the content of hallucinations, isolating oneself, or getting involved in nonspecific activities do not generate more control over the experiences. An added (albeit related) key factor distinguishing clinical from nonclinical populations may be the presence of distress associated with the presence of psychotic experiences such as hallucinations (Garety et al., 2007).

The above-mentioned illustration of the clinical hallucination-prone subject and the nonclinical hallucination-prone subject also permits us to develop yet another important distinction: the one between two different approaches to investigating hallucinations. One involves researchers who are interested in hallucinations as phenomena in themselves, regardless of their clinical character. If clinical and nonclinical samples are compared from this standpoint, a major objective would be to investigate similarities between clinical and nonclinical hallucination-prone subjects to document any shared underlying mechanisms involved in hallucination phenotype expression. In a second approach, researchers may be more interested in the clinical aspects of hallucination-proneness. Here, the major question would be why certain hallucination-prone subjects become clinical cases and why other hallucination-prone subjects do not. From this perspective, if clinical and nonclinical hallucination-prone subjects are compared in the same study, researchers would be interested in examining differences between the two populations to elucidate the unique factors that render hallucination proneness dysfunctional. Furthermore, to better differentiate between these two populations, it would be important not only to identify those factors that are unique to the clinical subject but also to recognize those factors that are particular to the nonclinical subject.

It is worth noting that the latter approach does not directly examine hallucinations because this approach is interested in probing factors that may render hallucination proneness problematic, maladaptive, or distressful to the subject. Therefore, these may have little or nothing to do with factors directly related to hallucination proneness. For example, a traumatic life event may be seen as an important factor distinguishing a clinical from a nonclinical hallucination-prone subject but has no role in hallucination proneness per se. That is, whereas the former approach aims at describing and understanding a fundamentally normal process or phenomenon, the latter approach is interested in examining why and how this normal process becomes dysfunctional. Although both approaches are equally important, the latter approach is dependent on the former. Without a highly developed understanding of the nature of hallucination proneness in broad and representative terms, it appears unfeasible to tease out the conditions and factors that may constitute a maladaptive or problematic expression of hallucination proneness. Unfortunately, however, the former approach has remained the least represented in the scientific literature.

It is also necessary to emphasize the fact that the hallucination phenotype is both a continuous and a distinct entity. The continuous nature of the hallucination phenotype may be clearer when related to examples taken from the epidemiological literature (Johns & van Os, 2001). For instance, both blood pressure and glucose tolerance are continuously distributed characteristics in the general population. Because the clinical decision to treat is a dichotomous one, terms such as *hypertension* and *diabetes* are used to characterize patients whose parameters are above or below arbitrary levels. This clinical perspective, however, cannot be taken as evidence that these conditions exist in nature—they are simply extremes of a continuous characteristic. In a similar vein, the hallucination phenotype also may be viewed as a continuously distributed characteristic in the general population, and similarly, because the clinical decision to treat is, as for the blood pressure and glucose tolerance example above, dichotomous, this results in the elaboration of sophisticated diagnostic schemes that provide clinicians with the inclusion and exclusion criteria necessary to define a hallucination and to decide whether a clinical hallucination is present or not.

A number of mechanisms that mediate the transition from experiencing a psychotic symptom (such as a hallucination) to becoming a patient with a psychotic disorder may be proposed. Krabbendam, Myin-Germeys, Bak, and van Os (2005) focused on psychological factors and argued that at least two mechanisms seem important: the attribution of the experience by the individual and the level of functional coping that the person mobilizes in the face of stressful experiences (i.e., the psychotic experience). Krabbendam and van Os (2005) argued that (a) a high tendency to worry (e.g., reflected in high Neuroticism scores) increases the risk for development of psychotic symptoms, and (b) a delusional interpretation or a negative emotional state (e.g., depression or distress) in response to hallucinatory experiences predicts the onset of psychotic disorder. The former suggestion is based on Krabbendam et al. (2002), although other studies have found an association between hallucinations and neuroticism or aspects related to neuroticism in both nonclinical samples (Barrett & Etheridge, 1994; Jakes & Hemsley, 1987;

Larøi, DeFruyt, et al., 2005; Young et al., 1987) and clinical samples (Delespaul, deVries, & van Os, 2002; Krabbendam et al., 2002; van Os & Jones, 2001; van Os, Jones, Sham, Bebbington, & Murray, 1998). The second is based on findings from Krabbendam et al. (2004; Krabbendam, Myin-Germeys, Hanssen, et al., 2005).

CONCLUSION

Hallucinations may present themselves in a number of different clinical disorders and therefore lack diagnostic specificity. At least three groups of hallucinations may be distinguished: those observed in psychotic disorders, those seen in neurological disorders, and those seen in the context of substance use. Although these three types of clinical hallucination may share common mechanisms, certain distinguishing characteristics seem nonetheless to dominate in each type regarding their phenomenological characteristics and underlying psychological and biological mechanisms (the two latter issues are dealt with in more detail in ensuing chapters). In addition, the fact that a substantial number of nonclinical individuals also experience hallucinations suggests that hallucinations are not necessarily a sign of a pathological condition. Subsequently, hallucinations should be viewed as lying on a continuum with normality, that is, as a dimensional phenomenon.

In the next chapter, which presents studies examining cognitive–perceptual processes that are implicated in hallucinations, it will become apparent that many of the groups of hallucinators described in this chapter vary in this respect. Whereas so-called "bottom-up" or data-driven perceptual processing is clearly implicated in hallucinations associated with sensory impairment in older people and in hallucinations in conditions of sensory deprivation, top-down processing involving perceptual expectations (e.g., based on prior experience and knowledge) play an integral part in those hallucinations observed in schizophrenia.

CHAPTER HIGHLIGHTS

- Hallucinations may present themselves in a number of different psychiatric and neurological disorders (not only in people with schizophrenia) but may also be present in nonclinical individuals, that is, people without either psychiatric or neurological disorders.
- Specificity of hallucinations to a particular disorder is therefore questionable, and equally questionable is that their presence is necessarily a sign of a pathological condition.

- Hallucinations should not be seen as a categorical phenomenon or as experiences that are qualitatively different from normal phenomena or experiences but rather should be viewed as lying on a continuum with normality; consequently, it should be considered a dimensional phenomenon or entity.
- Studying hallucinations in all these different groups of individuals will provide essential information concerning the etiology of hallucinations, including their development and maintenance.

4

COGNITIVE–PERCEPTUAL PROCESSES: BOTTOM-UP AND TOP-DOWN

Hallucination can be seen as an erroneous perception, or "sensory deception" (Slade & Bentall, 1988), and hence it is understandable that researchers have been investigating the integrity of perceptual functions in people with hallucinations. Basically, two approaches can be distinguished. The first is concerned with *bottom-up* or data-driven perceptual processing, such as deficits in the processing of incoming visual stimuli in early cortical areas (e.g., primary visual cortex). Other examples are hearing impairment and auditory hallucinations associated with sensory impairment in older people or the emergence of hallucinations in conditions of sensory deprivation. The second approach is concerned with *top-down* or conceptual processing in perception. This refers to processes that contribute to perception but do not originate in the external world but in the mind–brain of the perceiver. Examples of such top-down factors are prior knowledge, perceptual expectations, attentional modulation, and mental imagery (which are all interrelated). Cognitive models of perception generally include a top-down component as an influential factor in determining subjective perception (Biederman, 1972; Massaro, 1987). Indeed, acknowledgment of top-down factors as intrinsic to human conscious perception goes back to the pioneering work of Helmholtz (1894/1924), who coined the term *unconscious inference* to describe the processes by which the perceptual system uses inductive inference to derive perceptual interpretations from incomplete sensory information (see Proffitt, 1999). Most cognitive theorists see perception as constructive. Gregory (1978) stated that it may be that perception is a "hypothesis" tested by data provided by the senses.

Frith and Dolan (1997), in discussing the relationships among perception, imagery, and hallucination, suggested that normal perception comes out of an interaction between signals to the central nervous system and prior knowledge; in the extremes, on the one hand, perception is based entirely on prior knowledge, and on the other, prior knowledge has no influence on perception. These cases can both lead to hallucinatory experiences, but experiences that are different in quality. Frith and Dolan also pointed out that normal mental imagery can be completely dependent on prior knowledge, but self-awareness of such imagery's origin (i.e., knowing that it comes from one's own mind rather than from the outside world) differentiates this from hallucinatory experience.

The first situation (percept entirely determined by prior knowledge) could occur in schizophrenia, in which patients perceive sounds or objects that are not triggered at all by sensory input. As an example of the latter situation (percept fails to be appropriately modified by prior knowledge), Frith and Dolan (1997) cited functional experiential hallucinosis. They referred to a patient who recounted how she heard excerpts from television programs, including voices and background music, whenever she started her washing machine.

IMAGERY AND PERCEPTION: FIVE POSSIBILITIES

Horowitz (1975) defined hallucinations as "images based on immediately internal sources of information, which are appraised as if they came from immediately external sources of information" (p. 176). Starting from that definition, Horowitz proposed that "relative intensification of internal sources of information" (p. 176) lies at the basis of hallucinations. Such intensification can occur under divergent circumstances, according to Horowitz, which include the following:

1. relative reduction of external input with no relative lowering of activity of the representational system;
2. increase in activity of the representational system without increase in availability of external signals;
3. augmentation of internal input due to arousal of ideas and feelings secondary to drive states;
4. reduction of usual or "homeostatic" levels of inhibition over the internal inputs; and

5. alteration of the transition between "matrices," permitting internal inputs to gain more representation on matrices oriented to, and more often associated with, perception. (Horowitz, 1975, p. 177)

In the following sections, we will see that there is evidence for the first item on the list above from studies in people with sensory impairment, and in chapter 7 we will see that neuroimaging studies have reported evidence for the second item from activation patterns during hallucinations in schizophrenia patients. The other possibilities suggested by Horowitz (1975) can be found in certain contemporary approaches. The role of emotion and motivation that has been acknowledged by several authors (e.g., B. Smith et al., 2006) is consistent with the third item. Furthermore, recent models regarding the interplay between sensory impairment (bottom-up) and attentional modulation (top-down) and regarding the role of neurotransmitters also bear similarities to several of the mechanisms mentioned by Horowitz.

SENSORY DEFICITS

There is ample empirical evidence from neurology and psychology for the assertion that perceptual deficits may be associated with hallucinations. As described in chapter 3, this volume, hallucinations have been reported in normal people during sensory deprivation. With regard to experimental induction of sensory deprivation in healthy subjects (e.g., by being confined to a darkened and soundproof room for several hours), Slade and Bentall (1988) cautioned that these experiences mainly concern simple sensations such as light flashes or clicks and tones, and only a minority (some 15%) of participants report complex, meaningful visual or auditory hallucinations. In addition, suggestion may play an important role in these kinds of reports.

Other studies have focused on sensory impairment. For example, acquired deafness in old age has been associated with the emergence of hallucinations. Thewissen et al. (2005) investigated the onset of positive psychotic experiences (delusions and hallucinations) prospectively in a general population sample. Of the 109 subjects with deafness or hearing impairment (DHI) at baseline, 11 (10.1%) displayed psychotic experiences at Time 2 versus 137 (2.9%) of the non-DHI subjects. The large effect size for this difference was only slightly attenuated after adjustment for baseline psychotic experiences and a range of other confounders. These results confirm previous findings of an association between hearing impairments and psychosis and show that this association can also be found prospectively in a nonclinical population.

Sensory Impairment and Hallucinations in Neurological Conditions

With regard to neurological conditions, brain injury, Charles Bonnet syndrome, and Guillan–Barré syndrome are explicitly associated with hallucinations in the context of sensory impairment. Hallucinations have been described in several cases of brain injury. Visual hallucinations can occur after damage to the thalamus (Noda, Mizoguchi, & Yamamoto, 1993), parietal cortex (Critchley, 1951; Rousseaux, Debrock, Cabaret, & Steinling, 1994), or early visual cortex (Kölmel, 1985; Wunderlich et al., 2000).

Hallucinations arising from various forms of sensory impairment have been termed *release* hallucinations. This refers to a putative mechanism by which lesions to sensory cortical areas or to sensory pathways cause loss of inhibition in other cortical areas, resulting in the release of cortical activity there and in the experience of hallucinations (Manford & Andermann, 1998; L. J. West, 1975). Another explanation has been proposed by the cerebral irritation model, which holds that hallucinations in patients with lesions to sensory cortical areas may result from irritation of intact or partly damaged sensory cortical areas by pathological or regenerational processes.

Schizophrenia and Speech

The evidence for an association between sensory impairment and hallucinations in schizophrenia is mixed. On the one hand, it is important to note that patients with schizophrenia as a group show sensory abnormalities. These are present both in the auditory and visual modalities (David, Malmberg, Lewis, Brandt, & Allbeck, 1995). Other modalities have been less well studied. Furthermore, sensory deficits in schizophrenia may be more pronounced for the language domain. Stevens, Donegan, Anderson, Goldman-Rakic, and Wexler (2000) studied 30 patients with schizophrenia and 32 control subjects who were matched for comparable tone discrimination, so there were no apparent differences in basic auditory acuity. The participants were assessed on verbal serial position tasks on the one hand and on tone serial position tasks on the other. Remarkably, patients performed poorly on all four verbal tasks but performed comparably to controls when tones served as stimuli.

Hoffman, Rapaport, Mazure, and Quinlan (1999) argued that schizophrenia patients with hallucinations are characterized by speech perception deficits. Patients with hallucinations made more errors than patients without hallucinations when required to repeat degraded speech (a spoken sentence with "speaker babble" imposed on it). In a comprehensive study of auditory sensory deficits in schizophrenia, and a possible association with hallucinations, McKay, Headlam, and Copolov (2000) also observed sensory deficits mainly in tasks involving speech stimuli. In this study, three groups of subjects participated: 22 patients with psychosis and a recent history of auditory hallucinations, 16 patients with psychosis and no history of auditory hallucinations, and 22 normal subjects. Of nine auditory assessments, patients with and without hallucinations only differed on one subtest: Patients with hallucinations performed worse on a test for monaural filtered speech delivered to the left ear (there was no difference for the right ear). As a group, the patients differed from the controls on right-ear presentation in a dichotic speech test, whereas only the hallucinating group differed from the control group on left-ear presentation for the same test. This may reflect auditory dysfunction in the right hemisphere or in the interhemispheric pathways associated with hallucinations.

Other studies have also reported a reduced right-ear advantage (REA) during dichotic listening in patients with hallucinations (Bruder et al., 1995; Green, Hugdahl, & Mitchell, 1994; Levitan, Ward, & Catts, 1999; Løberg, Jørgensen, & Hugdahl, 2004). Normal subjects have shown an REA in dichotic listening tests, which reflects the dominance of the left hemisphere for speech processing (Tervaniemi & Hugdahl, 2003). Conn and Posey (2000) reported a reduced REA in college students who reported auditory hallucinations compared with students who did not. This implies that the reduced REA in hallucinating schizophrenia patients cannot be attributed solely to psychiatric symptoms in general or to other confounding factors such as hospitalization or medication but is specifically associated with the occurrence of hallucinations. Two different mechanisms could account for the reduced REA associated with hallucinations, as has been suggested by Green et al. (1994). First, it is possible that auditory hallucinations arise from activity in speech regions in the brain that is similar to activity induced by real speech input, resulting in reduced ability to process stimuli from the right ear (because the processing resources are already "occupied"). The second possibility is that a left hemispheric brain impairment causes the reduced REA. We discuss structural and functional neuroanatomical evidence for both possibilities in chapter 7, this volume.

In other studies, positive biases (i.e., false positives) have been observed in people who experience hallucinations in reporting the detection of stimuli. Bentall and Slade (1985a) reported that hallucinating patients erroneously indicated a word to be present in a burst of white noise. The ability to discriminate between the presence or absence of stimuli has been termed *reality discrimination* or *reality testing* (Bentall & Slade, 1985a), and studies into this phenomenon are further discussed in chapter 5.

In opposition to the speech perception deficit models, one could even argue that patients with auditory–verbal hallucinations should more readily detect words under conditions of perceptual uncertainty and thus perform better rather than worse compared with nonhallucinating patients. Indeed, this hypothesis has been put forward by Dolgov and McBeath (2005) on the basis of signal detection theory. They contended that the larger proportion of false alarms made by hallucination-prone people under certain perceptual conditions implies a shift in *decision criterion* (the point at which a person decides he or she perceives something). Yet, the number of misses (or instances in which a stimulus is not picked up) will then also decrease. In other words, these subjects thus benefit from an increased attentional acuity in the perception of veridical stimuli because of a willingness to err more on the side of false positives than on the side of false negatives. Vercammen, de Haan, and Aleman (in press) reported evidence that seems to favor this hypothesis, using a task in which subjects were asked to discriminate hardly discernible spoken words that were presented in white noise. Hallucinating patients with schizophrenia were found to have a higher sensitivity for auditory–verbal material compared with nonhallucinating patients, although they did not differ from normal controls. However, they were the only group that showed a significant response bias (i.e., affirmed having heard a word that was not actually presented). Notably, hallucinators and nonhallucinators did not differ in their sensitivity for detecting tones. The finding is consistent with the suggestion that hallucinators in the schizophrenia spectrum are prone to focus excessive attention on auditory–verbal stimuli (Beck & Rector, 2003).

Perception and Attention Deficit Model

Collerton, Perry, and McKeith (2005) have proposed a perception and attention deficit (PAD) model of complex visual hallucinations like those that may occur in neurodegenerative disorders such as Alzheimer's disease and dementia with Lewy bodies. Collerton et al. noted that in complex visual hallucinations, the hallucinatory images generally occur in the focus of the visual field and are seen against the background of the existing visual scene. An example would be seeing a (nonexistent) dog in the corner of the (existent) room. According to the PAD model, both sensory impairment and attentional abnormalities are needed for hallucinations to arise. More specifically, Collerton et al. proposed that a combination of impaired attentional binding and poor sensory activation of a correct proto-object, in conjunction with a relatively intact scene representation, biases perception to allow the intrusion of a hallucinatory proto-object into a scene perception. *Proto-objects* refers to holistic or part-based abstracted object representations that are segmented from visual information and act as candidates for further processing but are at such an early processing stage that they have not yet entered conscious awareness. Such proto-objects are in multiple competition for further processing: The interplay of top-down and bottom-up biasing information will eventually determine which proto-object will "win" and enter conscious awareness. Cholinergic dysfunction may result in a failure to properly integrate sensory information (bottom-up) and prior expectations (top-down).

Collerton et al. (2005) also linked dysfunction of specific neural systems to the different components of their model: Impaired attentional binding would be due to abnormal lateral frontal activity, poor sensory activation of a correct proto-object would be due to abnormal ventral visual stream activity, and intrusion of a hallucinatory proto-object would be mediated by increased temporal versus frontal activity. A criticism of the PAD model could be the fact that many patients in neurology and psychiatry present with perceptual and attentional dysfunction without experiencing hallucinations. Another point of concern is the lack of sufficient detail regarding the key phenomenon of the proto-object (Halliday, 2005): If the properties of proto-objects are not well defined, it will be difficult to map hallucinations onto these undefined properties. Halliday also drew attention to the fact that the PAD model is similar to an integrative model published in the same year by Diederich, Goetz, and Stebbins (2005). These authors suggested that visual hallucinations should be considered a dysregulation of the gating and filtering of external perception and internal image production. Contributive elements and anatomical links for their model include poor primary vision, reduced activation of primary visual cortex, aberrant activation of associative visual and frontal cortex, lack of suppression or spontaneous emergence of internally generated imagery through the ponto–geniculo–occipital system, intrusion of rapid eye movement dreaming imagery into wakefulness, erratic changes of the brainstem filtering capacities through fluctuating vigilance, and medication-related overactivation of mesolimbic systems. Not all of these have to be present, and different combinations will lead to differences in phenomenology.

TOP-DOWN PROCESSING

Mental Imagery

In the 19th century, Francis Galton (1883/1943) wrote that mental imagery exists as a continuum in the population, ranging from a total absence of mental images (subjectively) to imagery of great intensity and vividness, ending in pure hallucination. He collected responses to questions about vividness of mental imagery among 100 of his male acquaintances, which varied from "brilliant, distinct, never blotchy" to "My powers are zero. To my consciousness there is almost no association of memory with objective visual impressions." Galton concluded that remarkable variations exist in the strength and quality of mental imagery faculties.

Mental imagery can be defined as the introspective persistence of a perceptual experience, including one constructed from components drawn from long-term memory, in the absence of direct sensory instigation of that experience (Intons-Peterson, 1992). Richardson (1999) proposed that mental images serve as relatively faithful models of a perceptual object, event, or scene from which it may be possible to "read off" relevant visual or auditory information. According to Richardson, the key notion here is that mental images possess emergent properties that could not readily be deduced simply from abstract descriptions of the object or event in question. He gave an example of asking about the number of windows in one's house. To answer this question, people typically report "reading off" the information from mental images depicting different views of the outside of the house or different rooms within the house. In other words, visual mental imagery is "seeing with the mind's eye," and auditory mental imagery is "hearing with the mind's ear."

Early studies into the role of imagery in hallucinations were concerned with the question of whether the occurrence of hallucinations is related to a preference for one particular imagery modality (e.g., auditory imagery in schizophrenic patients) as opposed to another (e.g., visual imagery). Cohen (1938) asked patients with schizophrenia which images came to their mind in reaction to 130 words and phrases that were read to them. For example, one of the questions was, "What sort of image do you have when I say 'pipe' to you?" A stenographer recorded everything the participants said. The data of 19 patients were compared with those obtained from 19 normal individuals of the same general social and educational background as the patients. The main finding was that schizophrenic patients reported fewer visual and auditory images and more somatosensory images.

Seitz and Molholm (1947) tested the mental imagery of 40 patients with schizophrenia (20 with auditory hallucinations and 20 without hallucinations), 10 patients who had recovered from an alcoholic hallucinosis, and 114 normal subjects using the same method as Cohen (1938). Patients with hallucinations were found to report fewer instances of auditory imagery than the other groups. Seitz and Molholm (1947) concluded, "Not only do these findings disprove the old theory that auditory hallucinations are exaggerations of predominating auditory imagery, but they suggest the new concept that one of the factors responsible for auditory hallucinations is relatively deficient auditory imagery" (p. 480). Roman and Landis (1945) investigated preferred imagery modality in 20 patients with schizophrenia who all experienced auditory hallucinations (2 patients also had visual hallucinations); they did not include a control group. They used a structured interview asking about specific instances of mental imagery (e.g., "Get a mental picture of your bedroom at home" or "Try to imagine the sounds of high heels on a hard surface"). There was no relationship between auditory hallucinations and preference for either auditory or visual imagery.

Mintz and Alpert (1972) claimed to have measured vividness of imagery in hallucinating and nonhallucinating subjects, but their paradigm can be better seen as perceptual suggestion and is discussed below in the section on attentional modulation. A number of studies have used the Betts Questionnaire Upon Mental Imagery (QMI; Betts, 1909) to investigate vividness of imagery in hallucinating subjects (Brett & Starker, 1977; Catts, Armstrong, Norcross, & McConaghy, 1980; Starker & Jolin, 1982). In this test, respondents are asked to think of visual and auditory events such as "the sight of the sun as it is sinking below the horizon" or "the sound of the mewing of a cat" and asked to rate the vividness of the evoked mental image on a 7-point scale ranging from *perfectly clear and as vivid as the actual experience* to *no image present at all, you only know that you are thinking of the object*. The original Betts QMI contains 150 items covering seven different sensory modalities, with 40 items concerning visual imagery and 20 items concerning auditory imagery. Most researchers have used a shorter version of the test. Brett and Starker (1977) used an adapted version based on the Betts QMI consisting of 18 items (all concerning auditory imagery). They included 6 items in each of three categories: inanimate (e.g., rain falling on a roof), neutral interpersonal (e.g., someone singing "White Christmas"), and emotional interpersonal (e.g., a man crying). Overall, no significant differences were observed in vividness of imagery ratings between patients with schizophrenia with and without hallucinations. However, hallucinating patients reported significantly lower vividness scores for the emotional interpersonal items.

In a subsequent study, Starker and Jolin (1982) used the same self-report imagery measure to compare three groups of patients with schizophrenia: one group with hallucinations ($n = 36$), one group with a history of hallucinations but without present hallucinations ($n = 22$), and one group of patients who had never hallucinated ($n = 9$). No significant differences among the groups emerged. The authors also included a questionnaire concerning daydreaming as a measure of spontaneous imagery–fantasy. Again, the groups did not differ in their answers. Slade (1976) also reported few differences between hallucinating and nonhallucinating schizophrenic patients on the Betts QMI, although overall the patients reported more vivid imagery than healthy control subjects. The patient groups were small (only 8 patients in each) but carefully matched to differ only on hallucinations. Two other studies also failed to find differences between hallucinating and nonhallucinating patients on ratings of imagery vividness (Catts et al., 1980; Chandiramani & Varma, 1987).

In summary, the studies that investigated the imagery hypothesis by using self-report measures have been inconsistent in their results, but most point to a lack of an association between self-reported imagery vividness and hallucinations in schizophrenia. Curiously, visual imagery vividness as measured with the Betts QMI scale has been reported to be more vivid in hallucination-prone subjects than in the normal population in three different studies (Aleman, Böcker, & de Haan, 1999, 2001; Barrett & Etheridge, 1992). It is remarkable that the visual but not auditory imagery scale showed the effects, whereas the hallucinatory experiences largely concerned the auditory modality. The unsatisfactory psychometric properties of the Betts QMI scale (Richardson, 1999) might contribute to this discrepancy. More recently, it has been suggested that increased vividness of subjective, self-reported mental imagery may be a trait characteristic of schizophrenia in general (i.e., not specifically associated with hallucinations; Sack, van de Ven, Etschenberg, Schatz, & Linden, 2005). This finding is consistent with the report by Slade (1976).

Behavioral Measures of Imagery

The fact that none of the above-mentioned studies included objective behavioral measures may account for the inconsistency in results. Slade and Bentall (1988) drew attention to the fact that explaining hallucinatory experiences with a phenomenologically highly similar event—subjectively rated imagery vividness—borders on circularity. Correlations between imagery scales and hallucination scales may be due, in part, to the same method variance. In addition, there are other problems associated with self-reports of imagery vividness that have to do with the introspective nature of such a measure. Patients with schizophrenia may be impaired in their ability to judge private mental events. Furthermore, demand characteristics, social desirability, response tendency, and different conceptions of vividness and of the rating scale may all pose a threat to a reliable interpretation of the results.

Richardson (1999) distinguished between imagery as a phenomenal experience (measured by self-report questionnaires) and imagery as an internal representation (measured by performance on objective tests). As suggested by Aleman, Nieuwenstein, Böcker, and de Haan (2001), both approaches may have their own merits: Indices of subjective imagery vividness may be especially useful in enhancing psychological insight into the individual, whereas behavioral indices may serve to reflect more general information-processing characteristics underlying liability to hallucinations. However, it is not easy to think of a method to measure vividness of mental imagery behaviorally.

A possible approach could be the one first described by Aleman et al. (1999; cf. Aleman, Nieuwenstein, Böcker, & de Haan, 2000; Böcker, Hijman, Kahn, & de Haan, 2000), in which performance is compared on a perception and on an imagery condition of the same behavioral task. An example would be the sound comparison task, in which three common sounds are presented close to each other and subjects have to indicate which one is the odd one out in terms of acoustic characteristics (Aleman, Böcker, Hijman, de Haan, & Kahn, 2003; Böcker et al., 2000). In the perceptual condition, the sounds were really presented by playing the corresponding sound files on a computer, whereas in the imagery condition, the names of the sounds were read from cards. An example of the sounds would be a crying baby, a laughing baby, and a mewing cat, in which the laughing baby was considered the deviant item in terms of sound characteristics. In a similar vein, 20 other triads of items were presented. According to M. K. Johnson and Raye (1981), percepts, which originate from externally presented stimuli, are characterized by more detailed sensory, contextual, and semantic information than internally generated images. Kosslyn, Sukel, and Bly (1999) have presented evidence suggesting that mental images are less rich in perceptual details than "real" percepts and that as a consequence, images are more difficult to perform mental operations on. The hypothesis that imagery and perception are more alike (and therefore harder to discern from each other) because of increased sensory characteristics of mental images in individuals who experience hallucinations thus predicts that these subjects will show smaller performance differences between a perception and an imagery condition of the same task. It is interesting to note that it has also been argued that hallucinating patients may suffer from an imagery deficit rather than a general increase in vividness. For example, Horowitz (1975) hypothesized that hallucinating patients have less vivid mental images, which leads them to attribute occasional vivid images to an external source. However, in both instances of imagery theory, a vivid mental image ultimately gives rise to the hallucinatory experience. Before we discuss empirical studies of imagery and hallucinations, it is of interest to mention that neuroimaging studies are consistent with activation that would be predicted by the imagery hypothesis: Both auditory hallucinations and auditory imagery appear to activate auditory association areas (Dierks et al., 1999; Zatorre & Halpern, 2005). The same holds for visual hallucinations and visual imagery (ffytche & Howard, 1999; Kosslyn et al., 1999). More detailed discussion of neuroimaging findings are presented in chapter 7.

Using the method of comparing imagery and perception conditions of a task that was identical in other respects, Böcker et al. (2000) compared hallucinating and nonhallucinating patients on two measures of auditory and two measures of visual imagery and perception. No differences were found between both groups when performance on imagery measures relative to perception performance was compared. However, after performing within-group comparisons, the authors observed more vivid auditory than visual imagery in patients who hallucinated in the auditory modality. Evans, McGuire, and David (2000) also reported a lack of differences between hallucinating and nonhallucinating patients with schizophrenia on a number of auditory imagery measures. However, these authors did not include perception conditions or measures in another nonhallucination modality. In a case study of a continuously hallucinating schizophrenia patient, Aleman, Böcker, Hijman, de Haan, and Kahn (2002) reported evidence for stronger mental imagery relative to perception in two auditory imagery versus perception tasks but not in two visual imagery versus perception tasks relative to 5 control patients without hallucinations. This was in line with the theoretical prediction, as the patient only hallucinated in the auditory modality (he heard a voice in his ears). However, in the largest study using performance measures of mental imagery, Aleman et al. (2003) again failed to observe differences between patients with hallucinations ($n = 21$) and patients without hallucinations ($n = 26$). Performance was compared on multiple measures of auditory and visual mental imagery. In contrast to the case study, patients in the hallucinations group did not hallucinate during testing (they reported having experienced hallucinations in the week prior to testing). Thus, the possibility must be considered that an imbalance between mental imagery and perception is only present during the actual hallucinatory state, and hence is not a trait characteristic of people with a strong disposition toward hallucination. It goes without saying that this is a preliminary conclusion and that additional research into this issue is warranted. Specifically, more research is needed exploring the interaction between imagery and perception or on the way imagery can modulate perception. We turn to this in the next section.

Attentional Modulation: Perceptual Expectations

Expecting that you are about to see or hear something primes the perceptual system and actually lowers thresholds for perception. Such expectations can be conscious (e.g., explicit task instructions that you are going to hear something) or implicit and nonconscious (e.g., by being conditioned to expect hearing certain noises in certain environments without being aware of that). In a fascinating study, Barber and Calverley (1964) reported that hallucinatory experiences can be easily elicited in normal subjects by means of brief instruction. Specifically, the authors asked 78 female secretarial students to close their eyes and hear the record "White Christmas" being played. No record was actually played. As many as 49% of the subjects subsequently affirmed that they had heard the record clearly, and 5% stated that they also believed that the record had actually been played. Young, Bentall, Slade, and Dewey (1987) replicated and extended this finding by reporting that hallucination-prone individuals are more responsive to auditory suggestions than people without such proneness. However, the groups did not differ on two scales of general suggestibility. Such general suggestibility scales are designed to assess the tendency of individuals to comply with the expectations of an interrogator or with suggestive statements (e.g., to experience thirst). Thus, hallucinators are not just more responsive to any instruction or expectation but seem particularly to respond stronger to perceptual suggestions.

Merckelbach and van de ven (2001) investigated the role of fantasy proneness in a sample of 44 undergraduate students. The students were asked to listen to white noise and instructed to press a button when they believed they were hearing a recording of Bing Crosby's "White Christmas" without this record actually being presented. Fourteen participants (32%) pressed the button at least once. These participants had higher scores on fantasy proneness and the Launay–Slade Hallucination Scale (LSHS) compared with participants without hallucinatory reports, but logistic regression analysis suggested fantasy proneness to be the strongest predictor.

On the basis of a different effect, Haddock, Slade, and Bentall (1995) concluded that "the auditory judgments of hallucinators are highly influenced by beliefs and expectations" (p. 301). In their study, Haddock et al. investigated the role of suggestion in eliciting the verbal transformation effect in patients with schizophrenia with and without hallucinations. *Verbal transformation effect* refers to the tendency to perceive illusory transformations of repeatedly presented words, for example, hearing the word *tress* repeated over and over induces hearing transformations like *stress*, *dress*, or *press* in most people. In one condition, the participants were told that the word that was repeated over and over again *might* change to other words after a while (the no-suggestion condition), whereas in the suggestion condition participants were told that the word *would* change to other words. Results showed that in both groups, more transformations were reported in the suggestion condition. However, this effect was stronger for participants who had experienced hallucinations for more than 6 months compared with the control group of participants who had not experienced hallucinations in the past 5 years. In addition, hallucinators reported more weakly associated transformations, such as *Christmas*, *Jason*, *blood*, and *cat* (from the presented word *tress*).

The finding is consistent with research in hallucination-prone subjects from the normal population (Bullen, Hemsley, & Dixon, 1987), in which a positive correlation was observed between the number of transformations experienced and disposition toward hallucination as measured by the LSHS. In a study of susceptibility to auditory conditioning, Kot and Serper (2002) noted that experimental auditory hallucinations have been elicited in the laboratory after repeated pairings of a tone (unconditioned stimulus) with a light (conditioned stimulus) until the presentation of the light alone resulted in subjects hearing the tone. They hypothesized that hallucinating patients would more readily acquire and be more resistant to extinguish a conditioned hallucination than nonhallucinating psychotic patients. Therefore, they compared 15 schizophrenic patients with hallucinations with 15 patients without hallucinations using a sensory conditioning paradigm involving lights and tones. They observed that hallucinating patients acquired and maintained sensory-conditioned hallucinations more quickly than their nonhallucinating counterparts. However, Kot and Serper pointed out that suggestibility may play an important role in this enhanced susceptibility to auditory conditioning in hallucinating patients.

Using a more objective task of top-down effects on perception, Aleman et al. (2003) measured the effect of imagining a tone (e.g., with a high pitch) on the subsequent detection of that tone in white noise. The burst of white noise could contain the target (imagined) tone, a different tone (with a low pitch), or no tone at all. There is ample evidence that people detect the tone they are imagining better than other tones (Farah & Smith, 1983). This is an attentional effect that could be termed *imagery gain*. If you imagine a tone, you will hear it more readily than if you do not imagine it. Although Aleman et al. did not observe significant differences between patients with and without hallucinations on this task, within the group of hallucinators there was a strong correlation between severity of hallucinations and imagery gain. In other words, imagery affected perception more in patients with severe hallucinations than in patients with mild hallucinations.

Theoretical Models of Top-Down Involvement

It has been suggested that alterations in information processing in which the cognitive–perceptual system assigns a decisive priority to top-down factors in determining the final percept, at the expense of bottom-up information, may contribute to the genesis of hallucinations (Behrendt, 1998; Grossberg, 2000). Under certain circumstances, top-down factors may subsequently "override" bottom-up information in determining the final percept. Grossberg's (2000) account started from the thesis that top-down mechanisms play an important role in perception in general, and he detailed neurophysiologically plausible mechanisms for such modulation within adaptive resonance theory. However, although such top-down expectations can modulate, sensitize, or prime the processing of bottom-up information, they cannot by themselves cause suprathreshold activation of their target cells. Nevertheless, according to Grossberg, a volitional signal can be phasically turned on that can alter this balance to favor top-down excitation, which can create conscious experiences in the absence of bottom-up information. In this way, conscious mental imagery can arise. Grossberg then proposed a mechanism by which this phasic signal becomes chronically hyperactive, through which top-down sensory expectations can generate conscious experiences (through the activation of mental images) that are not under volitional control of the subject—in other words, hallucinations.

Behrendt and Young (2004) formulated a theory of hallucinations in which hallucinations are viewed as "underconstrained perceptions" (cf. Behrendt, 1998). In fact, they integrated the sensory impairment approach with the top-down approach. Their theory can be seen as an elaboration of proposals by Llinas and Pare (1991) regarding conscious perception in wakefulness on the one hand and dream imagery on the other. More specifically, Llinas and Pare suggested that conscious perception is subserved by intrinsic activity in thalamocortical circuits that is constrained or modulated by sensory input. They considered the primary difference between conscious perception and dream imagery to be found in the weight given to sensory input, which is a large weight in conscious perception, and hence sensory factors largely determine the final percept, whereas this weight is negligible in dream imagery. Behrendt and Young likewise asserted that hallucinations can be regarded as underconstrained perceptions that arise when the impact of sensory input on thalamocortical circuits is reduced. In short, if sensory constraints (i.e., bottom-up processing of incoming information) are weak, for example, because of sensory impairment, attentional mechanisms (i.e., top-down influences) may become the dominant modulatory influence on thalamocortical oscillatory activity that gives rise to conscious percepts—in this case, hallucinations.

As evidence for such mechanisms, Behrendt and Young (2004) cited neuroimaging studies that have revealed modulation of brain activity in primary and secondary cortical areas by top-down attention (O'Leary et al., 1996; Shulman et al., 1997). A strength of their model is that it also includes a role for hyperarousal. They pointed out that central cholinergic activation during psychological stress and anxiety can excessively facilitate thalamocortical gamma oscillations and thereby perceptual productivity. Some arguments put forward by Behrendt and Young in support of their model are less convincing, however—for example, their case for sensory impairment in schizophrenia on the basis of the robust finding of lack of suppression of the P50 brain wave amplitude in response to the second of paired auditory stimuli or the reduced auditory acuity that has been reported in schizophrenia patients (Mathew, Gruzelier, & Liddle, 1993). The problem here is that these findings are not specific to hallucinations but have also consistently been documented in patients without hallucinations (Heinrichs, 2001).

It is important to note that Hoffman's account regarding a deficient speech perception system giving rise to schizophrenic hallucinations also incorporates elements of a top-down approach. Hoffman, Rapaport, et al. (1999) pointed to the fact that syntactical and semantic expectations are crucial in speech perception because of the significant degree of acoustic ambiguity in perceiving everyday speech. This ambiguity is due, among other things, to background noise, large interindividual differences in articulation, and the "pasting" of phonemes (also called *blurring*; refers to a lack of pauses between words and omitting certain phonemes or merging them together). Hoffman, Rapaport, et al.'s hypothesis is that hallucinations arise from an impairment in verbal working memory, which leads to pronounced linguistic expectations that could generate spontaneous perceptual outputs. It is clear from this formulation ("pronounced linguistic expectations") that this hypothesis gives top-down influences a decisive role.

Absorption and Self-Focused Attention

Absorption, which can be defined as the devotion of thought to inner experiences, is a construct denoting several facets of subjective experience that are closely related to hallucinatory experiences. For example, the Absorption scale (Tellegen, 1982) was devised to assess synesthesia, *eideticism* (extraordinary recall of vivid visual images), daydreaming, and high imaginative involvement, in addition to altered states of consciousness and anomalistic subjective experience and belief. Glicksohn, Steinbach, and Elimalach-Malmilyan (1999) hypothesized that the absorption personality trait can serve as a predisposing factor for hallucinatory experience. Consistent with this, several investigations have found large correlations between questionnaires about absorption and hallucination scales. Indeed, in factor analyses, they appear to load on the same factor (Glicksohn & Barrett, 2003). A more parsimonious explanation would be that these phenomena are so closely related that they can be considered to form a single dimension. Besides the phenomenological similarities, both may converge in an openness to experience and a strong focus on internal mental experience. Hallucinatory disposition has been reported to be correlated with the personality trait of openness to experience (Larøi, DeFruyt, van Os, Aleman, & Van der Linden, 2005).

Morrison and Haddock (1997) asked schizophrenic patients with and without hallucinations, in addition to a normal control group, to complete the Private Self-Consciousness subscale of the Self-Consciousness Scale. They found that patients experiencing auditory hallucinations exhibited significantly higher levels of self-focus than those not experiencing hallucinations, although they did not differ from normal subjects. Moreover, level of self-focus predicted whether subjects experienced hallucinations. Consistent with this finding, Allen et al. (2005) analyzed data from a questionnaire survey in a student population ($N = 327$) and observed self-focus to be associated with hallucinatory predisposition. Jones, Griffiths, and Humphris (2000) hypothesized that the high occurrence of hallucinatory experiences in patients who have been admitted to an intensive care unit (ICU) may have to do with the almost obligatory increase in self-focused attention induced by the setting. The physical constraints and social isolation experienced by ICU patients and the life-threatening nature of the illness may increase the experience of hypnagogic hallucinations. Attentional shift during hypnagogic images from external stimuli (which are very limited when one is confined to a bed in an ICU) to internally generated images would explain why ICU patients have such poor recall of external ICU events but can clearly remember hallucinations and nightmares.

Neural Network Model

Hoffman and McGlashan (2006) developed a neural network simulation to test different hypotheses regarding the neurocognitive basis of hallucinations (cf. Hoffman & McGlashan, 1997). Their model specifically concerns speech hallucinations as typically reported in people with schizophrenia and is based on two widely endorsed hypotheses regarding the neurobiological basis of schizophrenia: (a) suggestions in the literature that schizophrenia may arise from overzealous *pruning of synapses* (refers to the natural elimination of unnecessary synapses) that are an extension of normal developmental pruning during adolescence, and (b) the evidence regarding alterations in the dopaminergic neuromodulatory systems in schizophrenia. To further assess and compare these two hypotheses, Hoffman and McGlashan (2006) developed a computer simulation of some aspects of speech perception using a recurrent, backpropagation model of working memory. This system was found to produce spontaneous percepts simulating hallucinated speech when the working memory component either was excessively pruned or when neuronal responses were modulated to simulate a hyperdopaminergic system. When they compared performance of the network with that of actual hallucinating patients and normal controls while *tracking* (repeating while simultaneously listening to) speech that was phonetically degraded, they found that the neural network simulation producing the best match to speech tracking performance of human hallucinators was an overpruned system with compensatory hypodopaminergic adjustments. Thus, the authors suggested that a curtailed connectivity in working memory systems may play a major role in top-down reshaping of receptive language neurocircuitry. Dopaminergic alterations may reflect secondary compensatory adjustments.

SUMMARY

There is evidence for a role of both sensory impairment and perceptual expectations (through attentional modulation or mental imagery) in hallucinations. There is no convincing evidence of abnormalities in mental imagery ability in people who experience hallucinations. This does not imply that activation of mental images may not be central to hallucinations. For example, it has been suggested that pronounced perceptual expectations could generate spontaneous perceptual outputs by overactivating sensory aspects of mental images. There is evidence for an association between sensory deficits and hallucinations, although not all people with hallucinations have sensory deficits, and not all people with sensory deficits have hallucinations. Several models have been proposed that focus on a failure to integrate sensory information (bottom-up) and prior expectations (top-down) as mechanisms that may lead to the emergence of hallucinations. Although such models certainly have explanatory power, more empirical studies are needed to test them. Such studies should also further investigate the relationship between cognitive–perceptual processes (discussed in this chapter) and metacognitive processes that have been suggested to play a role in hallucinations (Bentall, 1990). An example of such processes is *reality monitoring*, or the process of determining whether the activation of a mental representation was triggered by an external stimulus or, alternatively, was internally generated. We turn to such processes in the next chapter.

CHAPTER HIGHLIGHTS

- Sensory impairment has been associated with hallucinations, specifically in neurological conditions (e.g., dementia with Lewy bodies) and acquired blindness or deafness. In schizophrenia, the link between sensory impairment and hallucinations is less firm.

- There is no strong evidence in support of the hypothesis of increased vividness of mental imagery in subjects who are prone to hallucinations. The research that has been reported over the past decades has been limited mainly to subjective self-reports, the validity of which remains uncertain.
- Although mental imagery ability does not seem deficient in patients with hallucinations, a role for top-down factors (focused attention, perceptual expectations) has been suggested in generating spontaneous perceptual outputs by overactivating sensory aspects of mental images.

5

METACOGNITIVE PROCESSES: REALITY MONITORING AND METACOGNITIVE BELIEFS

In general, *metacognition* refers to "thinking about thinking" or "cognition about cognition"—in other words, to beliefs and attitudes held about cognition (Flavell, 1979; Flavell & Ross, 1981). Such beliefs and attitudes may be implicit, that is, the subject is not necessarily consciously aware of them. Most recent models of hallucinations assume that hallucinations are related to a particular metacognitive process, namely, the misattribution of private events. These private events may include a number of types and modalities, such as inner images, inner speech, voices, intrusive thoughts, vivid daydreams, and bodily sensations. Different approaches have attempted to explain this misattribution, with the most prominent of these in the literature relating hallucinations to a misattribution of inner speech, problems in source monitoring, and relations between hallucinations and beliefs. We describe these approaches in this chapter, along with some of the studies that have examined them. For more detailed information, see Ditman and Kuperberg (2005); Larøi and Woodward (2007); Nieznański (2005); and Seal, Aleman, and McGuire (2004).

MISATTRIBUTION OF INNER SPEECH

There is a certain consensus in the literature that auditory hallucinations occur when the individual misattributes inner speech (an example of a private event) to a source that is external or alien to the self (Bentall, 1990; Frith, 1992; Hoffman, 1986). The term *inner speech* refers to the internal dialogue one uses to regulate one's own behavior (Bentall, 2000). This may include commenting to oneself about what is happening or issuing instructions to oneself about what to do.

The development of inner speech in children was first described by Lev Vygotsky (1962) and Alexander Luria (1981). According to them, inner speech is something that occurs in the child at a later stage (i.e., after about the age of 3). Children first learn to respond to instructions from others (e.g., parents). After age 3, they respond to instructions from others by speaking out loud to themselves (also known as *private speech*). Later, children learn to internalize these instructions and perform them silently (as adults do), resulting in inner speech. However, even in adulthood, this speech is not always done internally (Bentall, 2003). For example, under conditions of stress or solitude or when performing a particularly demanding task people often speak out loud to themselves. Thus, inner speech can be seen as a dialogue with oneself that can occur privately or publicly, depending on the age of the subject or situational factors. Leudar, Thomas, McNally, and Glinski (1997) noted from their interviews with people who heard voices that the most common form of auditory hallucination (i.e., a voice or voices issuing instructions) mirrors the most common form of inner speech (i.e., a stream of instructions to the self).

Inner speech in adulthood, even when silent, is accompanied by subvocalization or electrical activation of the speech muscles (McGuigan, 1978). A number of early studies have shown that auditory hallucinations are often accompanied by subvocalization. The first studies that demonstrated a link between inner speech and auditory hallucinations involved electromyographic (EMG) measures of subvocalization in hallucinating patients. For example, L. N. Gould (1948) measured passive lip and chin EMG activity in a large group of psychiatric patients and found increased activity in 83% of the hallucinating patients, yet this was the case in only 10% of the nonhallucinating patients. One year later, L. N. Gould (1949) demonstrated that it was possible, using a sensitive microphone, to record subvocal speech from a patient who was hallucinating. This technique was later replicated by P. Green and Preston (1981), who showed that the content of the recorded speech matched the content of their patient's auditory hallucinations. Subsequent studies by L. N. Gould (1950) and others (M. F. Green & Kinsbourne, 1990; Inouye & Shimizu, 1970; McGuigan, 1966) established that the onset of electromyographically recorded subvocalization coincided with the onset of auditory hallucinations. Furthermore, they found that increased electrical activity was not concurrently observable from control muscles in other parts of the body.

Some behavioral studies have provided (indirect) evidence that hallucinations may involve a misattribution of inner speech. These studies are based on the assumption that if hallucinations are the consequence of subvocal speech, then it should be possible to suppress them by occupying the speech musculature in some way (i.e., directly or through verbal tasks). For instance, Bick and Kinsbourne (1987) found that holding the mouth wide open reduced auditory hallucinations in 14 out of 18 patients with schizophrenia, whereas other maneuvers such as making a fist had no effect. In a subsequent study of 17 patients, M. F. Green and Kinsbourne (1989) failed to replicate this result but did find that humming significantly reduced the time spent hallucinating.

Some studies revealed that verbal tasks that block subvocalization also inhibit the occurrence of auditory hallucinations (Gallagher, Dinin, & Baker, 1994; Margo, Hemsley, & Slade, 1981). Margo et al. (1981) investigated the impact of different types of stimulation on hallucinations. In this study, a group of schizophrenic patients with auditory hallucinations sat in a soundproofed room and listened to various kinds of sounds. The experiment included a control condition (no earphones), a sensory-restriction condition (the participants wore headphones through which no sound was played), and other conditions in which participants heard interesting speech, boring speech, speech in a foreign language, pop music, meaningless blips, and white noise. Immediately following each condition, the earphones were removed and the patient reported on his or her auditory hallucinatory experiences. These were rated on three dimensions: duration, loudness, and clarity. The main finding was that patients' auditory hallucinations became worse during both the sensory-restriction (i.e., significant increases in the loudness, duration, and clarity of the auditory hallucinations) and white noise (i.e., significant increases in the loudness and duration of the auditory hallucinations) conditions. In contrast, the auditory hallucinations became less troublesome when the patients were listening to interesting speech.

In addition, Margo et al. (1981) found that asking patients to read aloud also seemed to suppress their auditory hallucinations, and this condition produced the largest decrease in auditory hallucinations. Some years later, using a similar experimental paradigm, Gallagher et al. (1994) replicated these findings. In particular, they found that the experimental conditions that included speech (i.e., reading aloud, interesting speech, boring speech, pop music) had the most beneficial effect on the reported duration of auditory hallucinations, whereas in conditions that did not have speech (i.e., sensory restriction and white noise), the reported duration of auditory hallucinations increased.

Finally, neuroimaging studies have also shown that auditory hallucinations coincide with the activation of those areas in the brain responsible for the production and perception of speech, which in most people is located in the left hemisphere (for more detail, see chap. 6, this volume). Thus, the observations from behavioral, electrophysiological, and neuroimaging studies all provide strong evidence that inner speech may occur simultaneously with auditory hallucinations and, therefore, that hallucinations reflect the individual's mistaken judgments about the source or location of their inner speech.

This account of the misattribution of inner speech goes some way toward explaining the impact of various factors known to influence hallucinations. In particular, the idea that some sort of misattribution or judgment is involved about the source of internal experiences has been particularly fruitful. This approach, nonetheless, contains certain limitations. For example, a considerable number of neuroimaging studies either have not found auditory hallucinations to be associated with brain activation in language production areas or have only found this to be the case for a subgroup of patients with hallucinations (Copolov et al., 2003; Lennox, Park, Jones, & Morris, 1999; Lennox, Park, Medley, Morris, & Jones, 2000; Shergill, Brammer, Williams, Murray, & McGuire, 2000; Shergill et al., 2001; Silbersweig et al., 1995; Van de Ven et al., 2005).

Even though studies have shown that inner speech generally co-occurs with auditory hallucinations, this is not always the case (L. N. Gould, 1948), leaving the inner speech account futile in such cases. Inner speech may be present without the patient reporting any auditory hallucinations (L. N. Gould, 1948). Here, the inner speech account does not provide any explanations as to why certain types of inner speech would lead to hallucinations whereas others would not. Furthermore, nonhallucinating patients also experience inner speech yet do not misattribute these experiences as hallucinations. An inner speech account also cannot explain why auditory hallucinations are mostly in the second or third person. If misattribution of inner speech is involved in hallucinations, then one would expect predominantly first-person auditory hallucinations. In addition, a case study by David and Lucas (1993) failed to confirm predictions based on an inner speech account; the authors failed to find interference with phonological loop functioning using a dual-task paradigm in a continuously hallucinating patient. Finally, Hoffman and Varanko (2006) reported on 2 patients who described visual hallucinations of speechlike lip and mouth movements fused with simultaneous auditory–verbal hallucinations superimposed on perceptions of faces of actual persons in their immediate environment. They argued that such fused, multimodal verbal hallucinations are unlikely to be due to inner speech mislabeled as nonself but instead suggest top-down reshaping of activation in visual processing brain centers by pathogenically active receptive language neurocircuitry.

Finally, and perhaps most important, an explanation for why these patients misattribute inner speech as an auditory hallucination is not provided by this approach. In particular, inner speech observations do not provide information concerning the cognitive processes responsible for this misattribution.

In contrast, recent cognitive models of hallucinations have provided a number of propositions regarding these processes. An important distinction is the one proposed by Bentall (1995, 1996) between cognitive deficits and cognitive biases. According to Bentall, cognitive deficits occur when there are disruptions of specific cognitive functions. This may include, for example, problems with working memory, inhibition, or attention. Cognitive deficits are usually assessed using emotionally neutral test materials and are most likely due to neurobiological abnormalities. On the other hand, cognitive biases are present when some forms of information are processed preferentially in comparison with others. These cognitive anomalies can be best assessed using emotionally and personally salient materials. In other words, cognitive biases involve the processing of information according to content. Examples of cognitive biases include the preferential recall of negative information in patients with depression or obsessive–compulsive patients' better recall of "pathology-pertinent" words (e.g., words such as *contamination*, *wash*, *dirty*, *clean*).

Some authors have argued that the misattribution of internally generated information to external sources observed in hallucinators reflects some kind of stable cognitive deficit (David, 1994; Frith, 1987; Garety, Kuipers, Fowler, Freeman, & Bebbington, 2001; Hemsley, 1993; Hoffman, 1986). These authors have offered bottom-up explanations—in other words, they locate a defect in the structure or mechanism of the system. Others have postulated misattribution of internal cognitive events to an external source to be influenced by both cognitive deficits and cognitive biases (or top-down explanations; Bentall, 1990; Morrison, Haddock, & Tarrier, 1995). Here, it is supposed that both bottom up-factors (e.g., disturbances in cognitive processes as a result of cognitive deficits) and top-down factors (such as cognitive bias factors) are both responsible for hallucinations.

COGNITIVE DEFICIT MODELS OF HALLUCINATIONS

One important cognitive deficit model of hallucinations was put forward by Ralph Hoffman and colleagues (Hoffman, 1986; Hoffman & Rapaport, 1994). They suggested a link between incoherent speech and auditory hallucinations. These authors proposed that schizophrenic speech appears incoherent because words and phrases that are unrelated to the theme of the conversation are inserted randomly into the patient's speech. Furthermore, because these words and phrases are unrelated to what the patient intended to talk about, they are perceived as alien even though they stem from the patient. According to Hoffman and colleagues, these alien phrases are the basis of auditory hallucinations.

Although rarely stated clearly in the literature, this approach seems to suggest that deficits to two cognitive functions are responsible for the appearance of auditory hallucinations, namely, inhibition and discourse planning. *Inhibition* refers to the idea that patients with schizophrenia are overly sensitive to the apparition of competing ideas and stimuli, and *discourse planning* refers to a difficulty in planning what a patient intends to say. In brief, the consequence of the former deficit is that schizophrenic patients are frequently faced with irrelevant intrusive ideas and thoughts during conversations, whereas the latter deficit leads to a large discrepancy between what is said or thought and what the patient intended to say or think. It is important to note that in more recent papers, Hoffman and colleagues have emphasized the role of speech perception deficits rather than erroneous discourse planning (cf. Hoffman, Rapaport, Mazure, & Quinlan, 1999; also see chap. 4, this volume).

Christopher Frith (1987, 1992) proposed another influential cognitive deficit model of hallucinations. According to his neuropsychological model of schizophrenia, alien control symptoms (which include auditory hallucinations) result from a failure to properly monitor intentions to act, or self-monitor. According to the theory, impaired self-monitoring can lead to the misattribution of internally generated actions or intentions as having external origins. In particular, a self-monitoring deficit might cause thoughts or actions to become isolated from the sense of will normally associated with them. In the case of hallucinations, this would result in the interpretation of internally generated voices as external voices. Thus, in keeping with the example of inner speech, Frith argued that the problem is not that inner speech is occurring (as this occurs in normal mental processes) but rather that patients with hallucinations are failing to recognize that this activity is self-initiated. Consequently, this self-generated activity is misattributed as being generated by an external agent and therefore interpreted as being a hallucination.

Frith's proposition is largely based on Feinberg's (1978) assumption that self-monitoring deficits in schizophrenia reflect dysfunction of the efference copy–corollary discharge mechanism (for a detailed explanation, see Ford & Mathalon, 2005). In brief, each action a person makes (e.g., speech) is presumed to be accompanied by an efference copy of the action that sends a corollary discharge signal to the sensory cortex, thus signaling to the person that impending sensations are self-initiated or self-generated. During talking, for example, the plan to speak (originating in the frontal lobes) sends an efference copy of the planned sounds to the auditory cortex, where it becomes a corollary discharge. Simultaneously (or milliseconds later), talking is initiated, and the speech sounds arrive at the auditory cortex as the auditory reafferent. In normal speech experience, the corollary discharge matches the auditory reafferent, and the sensory experience is then canceled or reduced in its impact. However, in the case of schizophrenic patients, it is presumed that an efference copy of an intended action (speech, in the case of auditory hallucinations) does not produce a corollary discharge of the expected experience, and the individual may fail to distinguish between his or her own thoughts and externally generated voices, resulting in auditory hallucinations (or passivity experiences).

A series of studies have directly examined Frith's proposal of a self-monitoring deficit in hallucinations. Johns and McGuire (1999) studied verbal self-monitoring function in schizophrenic patients with auditory hallucinations, schizophrenic patients without hallucinations, and normal controls. For the reality monitoring task, participants were asked to read out single words (complimentary, derogatory, or neutral adjectives) presented on a computer screen. The derogatory words consisted of adjectives that were applicable to people and reflected the typically personal, derogatory content of auditory hallucinations in schizophrenia (Nayani & David, 1996). Construction of the stimuli consisted of giving a list of 160 adjectives to 40 normal volunteers who were asked to rate each adjective on a scale from –3 to 3 as to how negative, neutral, or positive they thought it was when used to describe someone. The adjectives were then ranked with respect to mean ratings of emotional valence, and 108 were selected to make up positive, negative, and neutral groups. Finally, these groups of adjectives were matched for word frequency, word length, and number of syllables. The experimental procedure consisted of asking subjects to speak into a microphone that was connected to an amplifier and an acoustic-effects unit, which allowed the experimenters to alter the pitch of the speech. Their speech was instantaneously fed back to them through headphones as they read out the words. After articulating each word, participants were required to identify, by pressing a button, the source of the speech they had heard as either "self," "someone else," or "unsure." The effects of moderate distortion (i.e., pitch lowered by three semitones) and severe distortion (i.e., pitch lowered by six semitones) on response choice were examined in relation to reading aloud normally (i.e., no distortion).

Results revealed that even though the pitch had been changed by only a few semitones, patients in both groups had difficulty recognizing their own speech; that is, they were either unsure about its source or misattributed it to someone else. Furthermore, the hallucinators were particularly prone to concluding that their distorted voice belonged to someone else as opposed to simply being unsure. Finally, the hallucinators were more likely to make errors when the words they read were derogatory rather than neutral or complimentary. These results showed that patients with hallucinations are not only uncertain about the source of their own speech when it was distorted but that they also positively misidentified it as belonging to someone else. Furthermore, Johns and McGuire (1999) argued that the tendency to make errors when articulating negative emotional material suggests that the typically derogatory content of auditory hallucinations might reflect a bias whereby the patient is particularly likely to attribute unpleasant thoughts about him- or herself to somebody else.

Using the same participants, albeit a slightly different methodology,[1] Johns et al. (2001) reported similar findings. That is, patients with schizophrenia made more errors than control subjects with feedback of their own voice (distorted and nondistorted) but not for the alien voice. Impaired verbal self-monitoring was evident in both hallucinating and nonhallucinating groups, but hallucinating subjects were more likely to misattribute their own distorted voice to another speaker. Johns, Gregg, Allen, and McGuire (2006), in a study that used a similar methodology, found misattribution of own distorted speech to an alien source was in greater schizophrenic patients who were currently experiencing hallucinations. In contrast, patients who had previously experienced hallucinations but who were hallucination free (for at least a month) did not make more external misattributions than controls. According to the authors, these findings suggest that external misattributions may be more related to current symptoms (state-related) than to a trait vulnerability. Another recent study, however, failed to find evidence of more verbal self-monitoring errors in people with psychotic symptoms (Versmissen et al., 2007).

Whether defective verbal self-monitoring alone can account for the presence of auditory hallucinations has been questioned (Allen et al., 2004), suggesting that additional cognitive processes (such as an externalizing bias) may also be involved. In Allen et al.'s (2004) study, schizophrenic patients with hallucinations and delusions, schizophrenic patients not experiencing hallucinations and delusions, and normal controls recorded their voices. After a delay, they were asked to identify the source (i.e., their voice or another voice) of prerecorded speech (distorted or nondistorted). Because participants were simply required to indicate when they recognized their own voice after a delay, online reality testing of speech was not examined. The results revealed that when listening to distorted words, patients with hallucinations and delusions were more likely than the two other groups to misidentify their own speech as alien (i.e., spoken by somebody else). Furthermore, across the combined patient groups, the tendency to misidentify self-generated speech as alien was positively correlated with current severity of hallucinations but not with ratings of delusions or positive symptoms in general. These findings were partially confirmed in a study (Allen, Freeman, Johns, & McGuire, 2006) that included nonclinical participants using the same experimental task as in Allen et al. (2004). In this study, although the severity of delusional ideation was associated with the tendency to make external misattributions about the source of distorted speech, there was no significant association with hallucination-proneness, although there was a statistical trend

---

[1]Two new conditions were added in this study: reading aloud with alien feedback (someone else's voice) and reading aloud with distorted alien feedback.

($p = .09$). Finally, it is important to add that because the effect was observed after a delay, this is at odds with Frith's (1987, 1992) hypothesis of deficient corollary discharge (which is supposedly an online mechanism) and therefore provides evidence of Bentall's (1990) model of an externalizing bias in hallucinations (this model is described in more detail below).

Cognitive deficit models of hallucinations, however, contain several drawbacks. To begin with, a number of them only explain auditory hallucinations, resulting in their inability to account for other types of hallucinations. For example, visual, olfactory, or gustatory hallucinations cannot be integrated into Hoffman's (1986; Hoffman & Rapaport, 1994) account because it is based on language processing. In addition, Hoffman's model assumes an association between incoherent speech and hallucinations, yet studies do not report evidence of such an association (e.g., Liddle, 1987). That is, schizophrenic patients with auditory hallucinations are not more or less likely to be incoherent than any other schizophrenic patient.

Furthermore, many of the cognitive deficit models tend to explain categories of symptoms and not hallucinations. For example, Frith's account mainly refers to so-called "alien" control symptoms, which include auditory hallucinations, but also *passivity experiences* (experiencing one's will as replaced by that of some other force or agency) such as *thought insertion* (experiencing thoughts coming into one's mind from an outside source) and *delusions of control* (experiencing one's actions as being controlled by an outside force). Consequently, studies investigating this model typically include patients with positive symptoms (e.g., Stirling, Hellewell, & Ndlovu, 2001), passivity experiences (e.g., Blakemore, Smith, Steel, Johnstone, & Frith, 2000; Frith & Done, 1989; Stirling, Hellewell, & Quraishi, 1998), or various Schneiderian symptoms (e.g., Mlakar, Jensterle, & Frith, 1994). Some of the self-monitoring studies described above have found that misattributions are associated not only with hallucinations but also with delusions (Allen et al., 2004, 2006). The cognitive neuropsychological model proposed by Frith, and the studies examining it, are thus not specifically concerned with the phenomena of hallucinations. Although there is evidence that dysfunction of the efference copy–corollary discharge mechanism may be a fundamental deficit in schizophrenia, studies have not been able to demonstrate that this dysfunction is clearly and specifically related to the experience of auditory hallucinations (Ford & Mathalon, 2005).

In addition, cognitive deficit models cannot account for the cultural and historical variations in the form, content, and prevalence of hallucinatory experiences. If hallucinations are related to cognitive deficits, then their prevalence and characteristics should be similar across cultures and epochs. Yet, as revealed in chapter 2, this volume, numerous studies have demonstrated that this is not the case. Cognitive deficit models also do not provide explanations for the influence of external factors such as stress and emotion on hallucination formation. Studies suggest, however, that emotion or stress may play an important part in triggering hallucinations (for a review, see chap. 3, this volume).

MODELS IMPLICATING BOTH COGNITIVE DEFICIT AND BIAS FACTORS

A number of different models integrating both cognitive deficit and bias variables can be identified in the literature (e.g., Beck & Rector, 2003; Bentall, 1990; Chadwick & Birchwood, 1994; Morrison et al., 1995). Two of the most prominent are the cognitive models proposed by Bentall (1990) and Morrison et al. (1995).

Reality Monitoring and Hallucinations: Richard Bentall's (1990) Hallucinations Model

Richard Bentall (1990) proposed an influential cognitive model in which hallucinations are explained by an impairment in the ability to discriminate between real and imagined events, otherwise known as *reality monitoring*. In particular, Bentall argued that hallucinating subjects might have a specific bias toward attributing their thoughts to an external source. This stance is in accordance with the general supposition made by several cognitive theorists that hallucinations are private events misattributed to a source that is external or alien to the self. One important and unique aspect of Bentall's contribution to the cognitive understanding of hallucinations, however, is that a large part of the model is based on an experimental approach to the question at hand. In particular, his model is inspired by the experimental work of M. K. Johnson, Hashtroudi, and Lindsay (1993) with nonclinical subjects on an ability termed *source monitoring*.

Source monitoring refers to the set of metacognitive processes involved in making attributions as to the origins of memories, knowledge, and beliefs (M. K. Johnson et al., 1993). This ability may involve either identifying an internal source (e.g., thoughts) or an external source (e.g., perceived events). Work on source monitoring is based on the idea that people do not have a priori knowledge about whether perceived events are internal to themselves and generated in their minds or are external and generated by agencies other than the self.

In particular, M. K. Johnson et al. (1993) argued that source monitoring decisions may be based on heuristic[2] (or relatively automatic) judgment processes on the one hand or on more strategic (or controlled) judgment processes on the other hand. Johnson et al. suggested that the former type of source monitoring decisions are made on the basis of qualitative characteris-

---

[2]The term *heuristic* in this context refers to judgments based on experience-derived knowledge (e.g., schemas). One may also describe heuristic judgment processes as *educated guesswork* or *rule of thumb*.

tics of memories, such as the amount or type of perceptual information (e.g., color, shape), contextual information (spatial and temporal), semantic detail, or affective information (emotional reactions). On the other hand, source monitoring decisions may be based on more strategic processes or more extended reasoning such as retrieving additional information (e.g., information about the cognitive operations put into effect during encoding of the event) or discovering inconsistencies with one's general knowledge and beliefs about themselves and the world.

In particular, the experimental work on source monitoring in normal subjects has shown that people use a variety of heuristic or strategic cues when discriminating between memories of self-generated thoughts and memories of real events. In general, memories originating in perception (real events) typically have more perceptual information (e.g., color, sound, vividness, details) and contextual time and place information. For instance, a memory that is rich in contextual information about time and location may help a person determine whether the event really occurred. Consequently, memories that lack this type of information are less likely to be attributed as originating in perception. In contrast, memories originating in imagination (self-generated) typically have more accessible information about cognitive operations—that is, those perceptual and selective processes that took place when the memory was established.

One example of this is that people are more likely to recognize a recalled event as a self-generated thought if they recall the cognitive effort associated with generating the thought. Subsequently, for memories in which information about cognitive operations (e.g., cognitive effort) are lacking or are less accessible to the subject, these events are less likely to be attributed to an internal source (i.e., self-generated). Bentall (2003) used lack of information concerning cognitive operations to explain why Paul McCartney was in such doubt as to the origin of his song "Yesterday." Because the song was so effortlessly written (it practically "came to him" one morning when lying in bed), he could not possibly accept it as being his own (thinking that it was an old jazz tune) and relentlessly began to search his record collection to find the "true" source of the melody.

M. K. Johnson et al. (1993) argued that the coherence and plausibility of the memory trace may influence a person's source monitoring judgments. In other words, if people recall themselves performing acts that violate natural laws or that conflict with what they know about themselves or the world, they know that what they are remembering is almost certainly a fantasy or a dream. For example, a memory of having played tennis with Stephan Edberg one summer many years ago as an adolescent is likely to be a self-generated fantasy if the subject recalls that she or he is a poor tennis player, did not start to play tennis until late adulthood, and has never met Stephan Edberg. Furthermore, if there are few perceptual details regarding this event (weather conditions, sounds, details about the surroundings, etc.), the hypothesis that the event was self-generated is further strengthened. These observations suggest that discriminating between self-generated events and externally generated events is best thought of as a skill and, like all skills, is likely to fail under certain circumstances. Studies using source monitoring tasks essentially examine the extent and nature of hallucinators' inability to perform this skill (Bentall, 2003).

The source monitoring perspective has a number of advantages in the context of hallucinations. One general advantage is that it provides researchers with a sophisticated and well-documented experimental paradigm that is entrenched within an equally sophisticated and well-documented theoretical framework. It is important, however, to underline that the goal of research carried out from this approach is not simply to conclude that hallucinations are related to a specific source monitoring deficit, such as a reality monitoring error (e.g., mistaking internal events as external events). Coming to such a conclusion would simply provide evidence of an experimental analogy, definition, or tautology of a hallucination. Few would deny that hallucinations involve mistaking an internal event for something else. The advantage with utilizing a source monitoring framework is that it provides researchers with the possibility of examining why a reality monitoring error occurs. In other words, a reality monitoring error in hallucinators is seen as the result of a long chain of processes. It is up to researchers, equipped with the source monitoring paradigm, to identify the contributing factors leading to this misattribution.

Bentall (2000, 2003) provided a number of more specific advantages of the source monitoring framework in the context of hallucinations, including this framework's ability to integrate the influence of culture, external stimulation, and the impact of stress and emotional arousal on hallucinations. The suggestion that source monitoring judgments are influenced by the inherent plausibility of perceived events helps to explain the role of culture in shaping hallucinatory experiences. Bentall went on to explain that an individual who grows up to adulthood in a society that recognizes the existence of ghosts or that values spiritual experiences is more likely to attribute reality to the image of a deceased relative compared with a person who reaches maturity in a materialistic, scientifically oriented society.

The impact of external stimulation on hallucinations can also be understood in terms of the source monitoring hypothesis. In conditions in which one's perception of one's surroundings is degraded, one is likely to adopt more liberal or "weak" criteria for assuming that perceived events are real and is therefore more likely to misattribute internally generated cognitive events (e.g., thoughts) to an external source. For instance, internal cognitive events are more likely to be misattributed as voices in conditions in which there is very little external stimulation (e.g., when alone at night) or when external stimulation is chaotic and unpatterned (e.g., in the middle of a noisy crowd).

The impact of stress and emotional arousal on hallucinations can be understood on the basis of the source monitoring paradigm if it is assumed that the cognitive operations involved in source monitoring, like other cognitive operations, are disrupted by emotional arousal. M. K. Johnson, Nolde, and Leonardis (1996) suggested that the emotional charge of material may disrupt normal encoding processes that bind source-specifying cues to the memory, resulting in increased source memory errors. Furthermore, this negative effect of emotional arousal may be "induced" when subjects are asked to focus on their own feelings (a so-called "self-focus" condition) during the study phase, resulting in reduced source monitoring accuracy.

Going beyond the simplistic assumption of a general source monitoring deficit, Bentall (1990) proposed that hallucinations are explained by an impairment in a specific aspect of source monitoring, namely the ability to discriminate between external (real) and internal (imagined) events (M. K. Johnson et al., 1993; M. K. Johnson, Raye, Foley, & Foley, 1981) or reality monitoring. Bentall further argued that hallucinating subjects might have a specific bias toward attributing their thoughts to an external source. A number of studies have attempted to assess source monitoring judgments in patients with hallucinations and in nonclinical, hallucination-prone subjects. In terms of the type of source monitoring ability that was assessed in the study, studies examining reality testing (or the ability to discriminate, online, between self-generated events and external stimuli) are distinguished from those investigating reality monitoring (i.e., the discrimination between memories of internal and external events) in hallucinators. These two types of tasks differ in terms of the delay between stimuli presentation (study phase) and response (recognition). That is, reality testing tasks usually involve tasks with no (or a minimal) delay between these two experimental phases. Reality monitoring tasks, in contrast, require some sort of delay between study and recognition phases.

Note that the term *verbal self-monitoring* is also used in the literature to denote a process similar to reality testing in that both reality testing and verbal self-monitoring (verbal self-monitoring studies have been described earlier in this section) involve the online ability to discriminate self-generated or one's own speech in contrast to external stimuli or another's speech. Although reality testing and verbal self-monitoring denote similar mechanisms, it is important to underline that the two terms come from two different (albeit comparable) theoretical paradigms. As mentioned above, reality testing essentially comes from the source monitoring framework (M. K. Johnson et al., 1993) and furthermore, in the context of hallucinations, is used in Bentall's (1990) model of hallucinations. In contrast, the theoretical background for self-monitoring (explained earlier in this chapter) is based on the idea that (auditory) hallucinations (and indeed other positive symptoms in schizophrenia) are the result of a breakdown in the systems monitoring one's intention to make an action (Blakemore & Frith, 2003; Blakemore, Wolpert, & Frith, 2002; Frith, 1992).

In particular, to distinguish between self-generated and externally generated actions, one relies on an internal monitor. However, if information about one's goals or plans fails to reach the internal monitor, then the resulting actions of those willed intentions can be experienced as unintended. When this occurs, inner speech is misinterpreted as alien or as coming from another's voice (i.e., resulting in a hallucination) if the sense of intention does not accompany the experience of "hearing" it. It is important, however, to note that Bentall's (1990) account possesses certain similarities with this model. In particular, both models suggest that hallucinations are the result of deficits to a particular metacognitive skill, and both propose that the deficient metacognitive skill implicated in hallucinations is related to problems in discriminating between self-generated events and events that are not generated by the subject. The two differ, however, in the term used to describe this skill. Bentall used the term *source monitoring* to describe this metacognitive skill, whereas Frith and collaborators used the term *self-monitoring*.

Both reality testing and reality monitoring are important and relevant in the context of hallucinations. For example, a hallucinator may ask him- or herself if a given internal event is self-generated either at the time of the event or some time after the event has occurred. Furthermore, reality testing and monitoring abilities are involved in both the development and maintenance of hallucinations. In other words, hallucinations may first appear as due to a reality testing or reality monitoring deficit. Likewise, either reality testing or reality monitoring skills may be implicated in the maintenance of hallucinations. In sum, there is no a priori reason to believe one skill to be more important than the other in hallucinations in general, or in terms of hallucination genesis and maintenance in particular.

Reality Testing

In the first study of its kind, Bentall and Slade (1985a) examined the relations between reality testing and auditory hallucinations in hallucination-prone subjects and in hallucinating schizophrenic patients. To test the subjects' reality testing abilities, Bentall and Slade (1985a) constructed a task based on signal detection theory (SDT). SDT is a theory of perception that proposes that the detection of an external stimulus (or signal) is a function of two factors. The first factor, perceptual sensitivity, refers to the general efficiency of the perceptual system. The second factor, response bias, refers to the individual's private criteria for deciding that a perceived event is an actual stimulus. On the basis of SDT, four types of judgments can be identified: *hits* (a signal is correctly detected), *misses* (a signal is present yet is judged to be absent), *correct rejections* (a signal is absent and is correctly judged to be absent), and *false alarms* (a signal is judged to be present when it is not). The last type of judgment (false alarms) is the experimental equivalent to hallucinations (Bentall, 2000, 2003). Thus, SDT represents a method for determining whether hallucinations are the product of perceptual problems or response biases.

Two groups of nonclinical subjects (hallucination-prone subjects and nonhallucination-prone subjects) were selected based on scores on the Launay–Slade Hallucination Scale (LSHS; this scale is described in the Appendix). The clinical subjects consisted of schizophrenic patients who were all currently hallucinating at the time of the study and nonhallucinating schizophrenic patients. The experimental task consisted of presenting a 1-second warning tone followed by 1 second of silence, then 5 seconds of white noise, and finally 8 seconds of silence during which subjects were required to record their response. The word *who* was randomly presented on half of the trials, whereas no word was presented on the other half of trials. The subjects' task was to detect the trials in which they heard the voice saying "who" by responding on a 5-point scoring scale (ranging from "I am sure I did not hear the voice" to "I am sure I heard the voice"). On the basis of the participants' responses, the authors then obtained separate measures for sensitivity and bias. Hallucinators and nonhallucinators, whether clinical or nonclinical, did not differ on sensitivity. In contrast, hallucinators differed from nonhallucinators in terms of mean bias scores, whereby subjects with hallucinations showed a significant bias to detect the *who* when it was not presented compared with subjects without hallucinations. Thus, hallucinators are more willing to believe that a stimulus was present, given a poor signal-to-noise ratio and a reasonable expectation that a stimulus might be presented.

Baker and Morrison (1998) wished to replicate and extend the findings of Morrison and Haddock (1997; this latter study included both types of task; it is described in detail later in this chapter under the heading "Reality Testing and Reality Monitoring"). Baker and Morrision included groups of schizophrenic patients with auditory hallucinations, nonhallucinating schizophrenic patients, and nonpsychiatric control subjects. The reality testing task used in this study was similar to the ones used in other studies (cf. Ensum & Morrison, 2003; Morrison & Haddock, 1997). Stimuli for the reality testing task involved a 15-item word list consisting of words rated by schizophrenic patients for emotional salience. The list was made up of 5 emotionally salient positive words, 5 emotionally salient negative words, and 5 neutral words. The experimenter read aloud the words from the 15-item word list, and participants were asked to provide associates after each word. Immediately after responding to each word, participants were asked to rate their responses for internality ("How much was the word that came to your mind your own?"), control ("How much control did you have over the word that came to your mind?"), and "wantedness" ("How much did you want to think of that word rather than another one?") using 0–100 visual analog scales.

Results indicated that the hallucinating patients scored significantly lower on internality, control, and wantedness than the other two groups, indicating that they had lower perceived levels of internality, control, and wantedness for self-generated words. There were also significant main effects. Baker and Morrison (1998) concluded that these findings support the hypothesis that patients experiencing hallucinations have a bias toward misattributing self-generated words to an external source. The cognitive bias toward external misattribution was magnified for emotionally salient stimuli (both positive and negative) for all three experimental groups, indicating that the cognitive processes involved in this misattribution can be understood within a framework of normal functioning. It is important to note, however, that when Baker and Morrison referred to evidence of a misattribution of self-generated items to an external source, this is essentially their interpretation of the findings. In practical terms, there is no direct evidence of an externalization bias but rather a significant decrease in the internality and wantedness ratings made by the participants. Baker and Morrison were therefore interpreting these significantly decreased rates as evidence of an external attributional bias (note that this issue also applies in two studies that we detail later in this chapter, namely, Ensum & Morrison, 2003, and Morrison & Haddock, 1997).

Ensum and Morrison (2003) examined relations among reality testing function, emotionality of stimuli, and self-focused attention. They recruited 30 patients with a diagnosis of schizophrenia spectrum disorder (schizophrenia, schizoaffective disorder, schizophreniform disorder), all of whom reported hearing voices within the week prior to participation. The experimental paradigm consisted of two parts: attentional focus (with internal and external focus conditions) and a reality testing task. Attentional focus was manipulated by presenting subjects with one of three sets of 20 words. Subjects were instructed to incorporate as many of these words as possible into a short story. One of the 20-word sets included words that were intended to facilitate the production of self-referent stories (i.e., 5 of the words were *I*, *me*, *my*, *myself*, and *alone*). This set of words thus encouraged an internal focus of attention (internal focus condition). In the other 20-word sets, the self-referent words were substituted for 5 other-referent words (*he* or *she*, *him* or *her*, *his* or *hers*, *himself* or *herself*, and *together*). These word sets were intended to direct the attention of participants externally (external focus condition). The remaining 15 words were there to provide help for participants stuck in the production of their narrative and were identical for each set.

Immediately following each attentional manipulation, reality testing performance was assessed (the reality testing task was very similar to the one used in Baker & Morrison, 1998), and immediately following the reality testing task, participants' levels of self-focused attention were measured using the modified Private Self-Consciousness Scale (Sedikides, 1992) as a manipulation check. To maximize and maintain the impact of attentional focus, throughout the reality testing tasks, participants were encouraged to concentrate as much as possible on either their thoughts and feelings (internal focus condition) or the voice of the researcher in terms of its accent, pitch, tone, and volume (external focus condition).

Results revealed that participants' ratings of both internality and control of their responses to the word association task were lower in the internal focus condition than the external focus condition. Furthermore, it was found that ratings of internality and control were lower for responses to both positive and negative stimuli compared with responses to neutral stimuli, and the magnitude of these differences was amplified in the internal focus condition compared with the external focus condition. The finding that hallucinators' tendency to misattribute internally generated information to external sources is sensitive to changes in their levels of self-focused attention is interpreted by Ensum and Morrison (2003) as consistent with accounts arguing for the implication of top-down or cognitive bias factors in hallucinations (e.g., Bentall, 1990; Morrison et al., 1995).

Reality Monitoring

One of the earliest attempts to examine reality monitoring in hallucinations was reported by Heilbrun (1980) and involved assessing subjects' ability to recognize their own thoughts. Heilbrun included a group of psychiatric inpatients (17 schizophrenics and 3 nonschizophrenics) who were further divided into patients with a history of hallucinations and nonhallucinating patients. Subjects were told that their opinions on several topics would be sought and that they were to answer briefly (i.e., about 1 minute per response) into a tape recorder after deciding on their opinions. Subjects were then asked to give their opinion to the five following questions (in their standard order): (a) "What are some of the important things to look for in a friend?"; (b) "What do you think about politicians' honesty?"; (c) "What do you think about keeping the differences between what men and women do?"; (d) "In what ways can religion play an important part in today's world?"; and (e) "To what extent is money a good indication of success in life?" Important to note is that subjects were not told that they would be tested later (this would take place 1 week later).

Three of the statements provided by each subject were used to prepare an individualized recognition task requiring the recognition of his or her own expressed thoughts. A multiple-choice format (each time with four choices) was used that required subjects to identify actual elements of their own thoughts. Subjects' ability to recognize the lexical characteristics of their own expressed thought was assessed by having them choose among four 10-word lists that included varying proportions of words actually used by the patients in response to a particular question. One list included 10 of 10, whereas the remaining three lists included 7, 4, and 1 relevant words, respectively. The ability to recognize the semantic properties of subjects' expressed thought was assessed by having the participants choose among four alternative meanings conveyed by his or her response to a second question. One alternative was the actual meaning, and the remaining three represented decreasingly adequate approximations of the correct meaning. The third part of the recognition task was designed to evaluate the subject's recognition of the syntactical characteristics of his or her expressed thoughts. The best response for each subject was to choose his or her verbatim reply. For the other choices, varying approximations of the actual style of the patient's original answer were constructed. In addition to the thought recognition task, all patients also completed various control tests, including a measure of verbal memory, a measure of patients' stability of opinion (i.e., the extent to which patients' expressed opinions did not change over time, in this case over the 1-week delay), and a measure of patients' communication skills (consisting of rating the extent to which patients' responses were comprehensible and relevant).

The mean thought recognition scores for the two groups were compared using nonparametric analysis. Results revealed that the hallucinating patients were significantly more likely to display poor recognition of the characteristics of their own expressed thoughts compared with the nonhallucinating group. According to Heilbrun (1980), these results help explain how hallucinators mislabel their own lexical thoughts as having an external source when experiencing auditory hallucinations. That is, in that hallucinators seem less capable of recognizing the characteristics of their own thinking, they will be at a disadvantage in situations in which a discrimination between an external voice and a personal thought is required.

Although Heilbrun (1980) demonstrated that hallucinators had difficulties recognizing the characteristics of their own thinking, this is only indirect evidence of a reality monitoring deficit. In particular, no clear distinction was made between internally generated and externally generated events in the task used in this study. In contrast, Bentall, Baker, and Havers (1991) included a task explicitly constructed to examine reality monitoring. They also wished to manipulate a variable that has been shown to play an important role in reality monitoring, namely, cognitive effort (M. K. Johnson et al., 1993). In particular, Bentall et al. examined whether hallucinators, compared with nonhallucinators, are able to use cognitive effort as a cue when discriminating between internally generated and externally generated events. This study compared three experimental groups (psychiatric patients suffering from auditory hallucinations, psychiatric patients suffering from delusions but without hallucinations, and normal controls) on a reality monitoring task. Subjects were presented a list of clues (a category and a letter; e.g., "Think of a type of dwelling beginning with H") mixed with paired associates (a category and an exemplar; e.g., "A country–Norway"). Subjects were told to answer each clue and to repeat each associate. A week later, the experimenter read a list of words consisting of subjects' answers to the clues, the associates produced by the experimenter, and new items not previously presented. Subjects had to classify the words as "mine," "given," or "new."

This task used self-generated events requiring both high ("Think of a fruit beginning with *T*") and low ("Think of a type of dwelling beginning with *H*") cognitive effort. This distinction between high and low cognitive effort events was included to assess whether hallucinating subjects were able to use cognitive effort to help discriminate between internal and external events, as has been shown in studies with normal subjects (M. K. Johnson et al., 1993). Source attributions were recorded for each type of item (i.e., low cognitive effort self-generated, low cognitive effort experimenter-generated, high cognitive effort self-generated, high cognitive effort experimenter-generated, and new words). Following the procedure of M. K. Johnson et al. (1981), the proportion of each item type attributed to each source was calculated.

Mean recognition accuracies (i.e., proportion of items correctly attributed to source) for low and high cognitive effort items for each group were compared. This comparison revealed that both psychiatric groups had poorer performances than the control group, recognition was easier for all subjects for the high cognitive effort items, and recognition was better for self-generated items for all subjects. There was also a significant interaction between source and cognitive effort, revealing that self-generated items were more likely to be correctly attributed to their source if they required cognitive effort. In contrast, little difference was observed in the correct identification of the low and high cognitive effort associates (i.e., experimenter-generated).

Group comparisons were also carried out that focused on the type of errors made by subjects, in particular, those errors that involved attributing self-generated items to the experimenter (i.e., mistaking their own answers to clues for associates read out to them). Although there was a tendency for the patients with hallucinations to make more errors of this type overall, the main group effect just failed to reach significance ($p = .063$). The high versus low cognitive main effect was significant, and the interaction also reached significance. This revealed that both normal controls and patients without hallucinations, but not the patients with hallucinations, made fewer self-to-experimenter misattributions on the low cognitive effort items than on the high cognitive effort items, and the patients with hallucinations made significantly more self-to-experimenter misattributions on the high cognitive effort items compared with normal controls and patients without hallucinations. That is, hallucinating subjects attributed more self-generated high cognitive effort words to the experimenter than both the normal controls and the psychiatric patients without hallucinations, but no significant group differences for low cognitive effort words were found. The authors interpreted these findings as being consistent with the hypothesis that hallucinations are self-generated events misattributed to an external source. Furthermore, the results also suggest that hallucinators fail to use cognitive effort as a cue when determining the source of their experiences.

In another study including a typical reality monitoring task, Seal, Crowe, and Cheung (1997) observed that performance on this task was related to verbal IQ and verbal memory. Twenty-one patients with schizophrenia (10 with auditory hallucinations, 11 without hallucinations) and a group of normal controls ($n = 15$) were included in this study. The source monitoring task measured the subject's accuracy in recalling the source of a word over two different levels of cognitive and affective difficulty. The material consisted of four categories of words (fruit, European countries, household furniture, and strong feelings) each containing 12 examples of a category. The fruit and household furniture items were considered to contain words that demand little cognitive or emotional effort. However, examples of European countries were theorized by the authors to demand more cognitive effort to generate for Australian subjects than types of fruit. Similarly, examples of "strong feelings you have felt" were considered to demand more emotional effort to generate than fruit or furniture.

Subjects were required to produce four examples for each of the categories. The experimenter then provided the next four most common examples of these categories. After a delay, a list of 48 items (16 subject-generated, 16 experimenter-generated, and 16 novel but category-appropriate words) was read out loud by the experimenter in random order. Subjects were told that they would be read some of the items that had been produced earlier (by the subject or experimenter) and some that had not been mentioned in the testing period. They were asked to make an attribution of the source of the word: "mine (I said it)," "yours (you said it)," and "new (I did not hear it before)." In addition to the source monitoring task, patients also completed the National Adult Reading Test (Nelson, 1982) to determine premorbid IQ and a short form of the Logical Memory subsection of the Wechsler Memory Scale—Revised (Wechsler, 1987) to assess verbal memory.

First, Seal et al. (1997) observed that normal controls obtained higher scores for verbal IQ (National Adult Reading Test scores) than did both groups of patients with schizophrenia. There was also a significant main effect between the clinical groups for length of current hospitalization. To investigate the extent that these differences may have had on the performance on the reality monitoring task, the authors performed correlational analyses relating the reality monitoring performance with the key demographic variables. This showed that performance on the task was moderately related to performance on the verbal IQ and verbal memory measures. Seal et al. then controlled for the confounding covariates (i.e., verbal IQ, verbal memory) for the subsequent analyses. In terms of overall source memory task performance (i.e., overall accuracy scores and proportion of items correctly attributed to its source), group comparisons revealed that the control group demonstrated a significantly higher level of accuracy than did the two schizophrenic groups (the latter two groups' scores were highly similar). Significant main effects for source of item were apparent for both the cognitive and affective items, indicating that subjects were more accurate at attributing self-generated material to its source than experimenter-generated or novel material. In terms of source memory performance for self-generated items, analyses revealed that the normal control group made a consistently low level of self-to-experimenter misattribution errors across levels of cognitive effort and item type, for both cognitive and affective items, which was interpreted by the authors as being a ceiling effect. There were no significant differences between the groups with respect to the number of self-to-experimenter misattribution errors for either the cognitive and affective items. In addition, tests for simple main effects revealed that none of the groups varied significantly in the proportion of self-to-experimenter errors made across the two levels of cognitive effort.

Seal et al. (1997) then compared two statistical procedures (analysis of variance vs. analysis of covariance) to investigate the relative influences of the covariates on group differences more precisely. When analyses of variance were performed on the same above-mentioned means (i.e., without adjustment for the covariates), source memory task performances were significant for three of the four analyses. That is, significant group differences were found for overall accuracy for cognitive items, for overall accuracy for affective items, for self-to-experimenter misattributions for affective items, but not for self-to-experimenter misattributions for cognitive items. The authors interpreted these findings as suggesting that the inconsistent findings previously noted on source monitoring tasks in schizophrenic patients may be due to a failure to identify and control for important covariates, such as verbal memory and intelligence.

Brébion et al. (2000) conducted another study of reality monitoring in hallucinations. They examined source monitoring functioning in a group of 40 patients with schizophrenia and 40 nonclinical controls. Each patient was evaluated in terms of the presence of positive and negative symptoms. Material for the reality monitoring task consisted of words from eight categories: fruits, sports, furniture, animals, states of the United States, cereals, transport, and famous monuments. Two examples from each category were selected. One of these examples was either produced verbally (by the experimenter) or visually (as a picture). For each category, subjects were required to produce a third example of their own. Distractors were made up of three other examples of each of the eight categories (one supplementary item was available for each category, for use in cases when the item produced by the subject was also one of the distractors). The experimenter first indicated the name of the category (e.g., *fruits*), then produced verbally an example of that category (e.g., *plum*), followed by a visual presentation of a second example (e.g., a picture of grapes), and finally the subject was required to provide a third example of that category. This procedure was repeated for the eight categories. Important to note is that subjects were not warned that they would be required afterward to remember the produced items. After a delay, the experimenter read out loud the list of items from a recognition list that included the produced target items (i.e., those produced by the experimenter verbally or visually and by the subject) mixed with distractors. For each item, participants were required to indicate whether it was one of the previously produced items or a new one. If they thought the item had been presented previously, they were required to remember whether its source of production was the experimenter, themselves, or a picture.

Four categories of source attribution errors for recognized target items were used. Self misattributions consisted of the items produced by another source (either the experimenter or the picture) but remembered as produced by the subject. Nonself misattributions included items produced by the subject but remembered as produced by another source (either the experimenter or the picture). Verbal misattributions consisted of the items presented by the subject but remembered as spoken (either by the experimenter or by the subject). Finally, picture misattributions were the items spoken (either by the experimenter or by the subject) but remembered as pictures. On the basis of these four categories of variables, two types of response bias were assessed: tendency toward nonself misattribution of self-produced items and tendency toward picture misattribution of spoken items.

Results showed that hallucinations were significantly related with an increased tendency toward false alarms, reflecting the belief that nonevents (nontarget words) have really occurred. Furthermore, when hallucinators and normal controls were compared, analyses revealed a significant effect of group, showing that hallucinators made more misattributions compared with normal controls. There was also a significant interaction between group and type of misattribution (self vs. nonself), indicating that hallucinators made significantly more nonself than self misattributions. When nonhallucinators and normal control subjects were compared, only a significant group effect was found (indicating that patients without hallucinations made more misattributions of both types) but no interaction between group and type of misattribution. However, when hallucinators and nonhallucinators were compared, this did not result in a significant effect of subgroup, showing that both subgroups were equivalent in the overall number of misattributions. Furthermore, although hallucinators made more nonself misattributions than did nonhallucinators, this did not reach significance as indicated by the lack of a significant interaction between subgroup and type of misattribution. In sum, hallucinating patients revealed a cognitive bias of misattributing items they had produced themselves to nonself or external source (i.e., words or pictures produced by the experimenter).

Evidence of disturbances in reality monitoring in a group of nonclinical participants prone toward hallucinations was reported in Larøi, Van der Linden, and Marczewski (2004). Participants were administered a reality monitoring task that consisted of presenting words. After each word, subjects were asked to say the first word that came to mind. Words varied in terms of emotional valence and cognitive effort. High cognitive effort words consisted of those words requiring longer latency times to associate a word, and low cognitive effort words consisted of those requiring shorter latency times to associate a word. Following a delay, words were presented consisting of those already presented by the experimenter or the subject (old) and those never presented before (new). For each word, subjects were required to identify if the word was old or new. If the word was identified as old, subjects were required to identify the source of the word (subject or experimenter). Results showed that hallucination-prone subjects had significantly more source discrimination errors than nonhallucination-prone subjects for self-generated items. In other words, hallucination-prone subjects tended to misattribute items that they had produced themselves to the experimenter. This pattern was especially marked with emotionally charged material and with words that required more cognitive effort. In addition, hallucination-prone subjects scored significantly higher on a scale assessing metacognitive beliefs compared with nonhallucination-prone subjects. Finally, scores on a scale assessing metacognitive beliefs were positively associated with source discrimination errors.

Reality Testing and Reality Monitoring

Both reality testing and reality monitoring tasks have been included in some studies (Böcker, Hijman, Kahn, & de Haan, 2000; Rankin & O'Carroll, 1995). For instance, Rankin and O'Carroll (1995) examined reality testing and reality monitoring abilities in a group of nonclinical subjects with hallucination-proneness. There were several reasons for carrying out this study. One was to examine relations between reality monitoring and reality testing skills in the context of hallucinations. The reason for including a reality testing task in the study was to replicate the findings of Bentall and Slade (1985a). Rankin and O'Carroll also wished to assess reality monitoring ability in a more appropriate manner than had previously been done in the context of hallucinations. They argued that previous studies (e.g., Bentall et al., 1991) typically included reality monitoring tasks that require subjects to discriminate between memories of words they had spoken and words they had heard. However, they argued, the cognitive models of hallucinations (e.g., Bentall, 1990) assume that hallucinators mistake internal, private, or imaginary words with words they have heard in public. When subjects speak a word out loud (as is done in typical reality monitoring tasks), the word is no longer qualitatively similar (in contextual and associative cognitive operations) to a word that they have heard in public and qualitatively different from an internal, private, or imagined word. Therefore, they suggested that a more appropriate reality monitoring task would be one that requires subjects to discriminate between memories of words they had imagined and words they had heard.

Two groups of subjects (hallucination-prone and non-hallucination-prone) were selected from a group of 250 nonclinical participants based on their scores on the LSHS (the scale is described in the Appendix). The reality monitoring task consisted of repeatedly presenting paired associates (e.g., vehicle–car). Some of the paired associates had been previously read to the subject, whereas other paired associates had been previously read and the subject had been later asked to imagine them. The number of times that the items were presented and tested (e.g., "Which word goes with vehicle?") was carefully manipulated so that, for example, some of the associates were presented many times but tested few times, whereas others were presented on only a few trials but tested on many. Subjects were asked to listen to each paired associate that was read out by the experimenter and to try to remember them. The task consisted of five auditory study trials and five tests. On each of the study trials, there was a list of 12 associates. Each of the five study trials was followed by a test asking the subjects to remember 10 of the associates. After the presentation and testing of the paired associates, cues of the paired associates (e.g., "Do you remember which word was associated with table?") were presented, and participants were asked to answer "yes" if they recalled which word was associated with the cue (i.e., without actually saying the word) or "no" if they could not remember which word had been associated with the cue. They were then asked to say how many times they thought they had been presented with each item. The reality testing task consisted of the same procedure used in Bentall and Slade (1985a), which was described earlier in this chapter.

Results from the reality monitoring task revealed that hallucination-prone subjects did not differ significantly from non-hallucination-prone subjects on their frequency estimates for words that they had heard but had not been required to imagine. In contrast, results revealed that, as M. H. Johnson and Magaro (1987) had previously found, participants gave inflated frequency estimates for words that had been most tested, indicating that they were mistaking occasions on which they had recalled the words for occasions on which the words had been presented. This effect was most evident in participants who scored high on the LSHS (see the Appendix), indicating that these people were most prone to misattributing their mental events (the times they recalled the words) for events in the world (presentations). That is, self-generated events (i.e., imagined words) were significantly more often considered as externally generated (i.e., presented by the experimenter) in hallucinators compared with nonhallucinators. Results from the reality testing task showed that there was no significant difference between hallucination-prone and non-hallucination-prone subjects in terms of mean sensitivity scores. In contrast, the two groups differed in terms of mean bias scores, in which hallucination-prone subjects showed a significant bias to detect the word *who* when it was not presented compared with non-hallucination-prone subjects. These findings essentially replicated those reported in Bentall and Slade (1985a), showing a greater tendency of the hallucinating group to detect the signal when it was not actually presented.

The observed externalizing bias in hallucinators was further investigated by Morrison and Haddock (1997). One particular innovation in this study was the examination of the influence of the emotional content of stimuli on source monitoring performance in hallucinators (based on the literature suggesting that emotion and stress play an important part in the occurrence of auditory hallucinations). In addition, the authors included a reality testing task (whereas most of the previous studies had only included reality monitoring tasks) to assess source monitoring for self-generated events that are naturally occurring (i.e., spontaneous). According to Morrison and Haddock, it is this spontaneous misattribution that is hypothesized to account for the occurrence of auditory hallucinations. They examined the reality testing and reality monitoring abilities of clinical subjects with hallucinations compared with clinical and normal controls. Fifteen schizophrenic patients with auditory hallucinations, 15 schizophrenic patients without hallucinations, and 15 normal controls were included in the study. Material for the reality testing and reality monitoring tasks consisted of three sets of words: eight positive words, eight negative words, and eight neutral words. The experimenter presented the eight negative, positive, and neutral words verbally to the subjects in randomized order, one at a time. For the reality testing task, subjects were asked to provide associates for each word ("Think of the first word that comes to mind when I say . . ."). Immediately after responding to each word, participants were asked to rate their responses for internality, control, and involuntariness using 0–100 visual analog scales. On completion of the reality testing task and after a short delay, subjects were given the reality monitoring task: They were asked to decide whether particular words had been given by the experimenter or had been self-generated by themselves.

Results for the reality testing task indicated that the hallucinating patients scored significantly lower on internality than the other two groups, indicating that they had lower perceived levels of internality for self-generated words. There was also a significant main effect of word type, revealing that this difference was accounted for by the higher internality scores for the neutral words compared with both positive and negative words. For the reality monitoring task, there was a significant main effect for source, which was accounted for by more errors being made for self-generated items wrongly attributed to the experimenter. In addition, there was a main effect for valence, which was accounted for by more errors being made for emotional material. The only interaction that reached significance was that between source and valence, indicating that more errors were made for positive material for errors wrongly attributed to the experimenter and more errors being made for negative material wrongly attributed to self. Morrison and Haddock (1997) concluded that these findings support the hypothesis that patients experiencing hallucinations have an external attributional bias for their immediate thoughts (i.e., based on results from the reality testing task) but not for memories of those thoughts (i.e., based on findings from the reality monitoring task).

Summary

Despite varying methodologies, the above-mentioned studies (and others not examined in detail) seem to provide evidence for Bentall's (1990) notion that hallucinators are impaired in their ability to discriminate between real and imagined events and reveal a specific bias toward attributing their thoughts to an external source. In particular, this externalizing bias seems related, at least in part, to both an inadequate use of cognitive effort cues (e.g., Bentall et al., 1991; Larøi, Van der Linden, & Marczewski, 2004) and the emotional salience of stimuli (Baker & Morrison, 1998; Ensum & Morrison, 2003; Larøi, Van der Linden, & Marczewski, 2004; Morrison & Haddock, 1997) on source monitoring tasks. These latter findings reveal that the emotional salience of stimuli may have a disruptive effect on source monitoring performance. In particular, the emotional charge of material may disrupt normal encoding processes that bind source-specifying cues to the memory (M. K. Johnson et al., 1996), resulting in increased source memory errors. This interpretation is in accordance with studies that reveal that focusing on one's own feelings during the study phase reduces reality monitoring accuracy (M. K. Johnson et al., 1996). Also, it may be that the disrupted effect of emotionally charged stimuli is even greater in hallucinators; studies have provided evidence for increased emotional arousal in both hallucination-prone subjects (van't Wout, Aleman, Kessels, Larøi, & Kahn, 2004) and schizophrenic patients with hallucinations (Delespaul, deVries, & van Os, 2002).

However, it is important to note that a number of studies have failed to show an association between hallucinations and a tendency to misremember an internally generated event as originating from an external source (for a review of these studies, see Larøi & Woodward, 2007). Some authors have suggested that for at least some of these studies, this may be due to a number of methodological issues (for a detailed discussion, see Ditman & Kuperberg, 2005; Larøi & Woodward, 2007; Nieznański, 2005; Seal et al., 2004).

Another important limit of many of these reality monitoring studies is that they have not captured the phenomenological complexity of hallucinations in their experimental design. For instance, on the basis of a study by Stephane, Thuras, Nasrallah, and Georgopoulos (2003; described in detail in chap. 2, this volume), two important phenomenological dimensions in hallucinations appear: (a) the *self-generated/nonself-generated* dimension and (b) the *inner/outer* dimension. The first dimension refers to the perceived or subjective origin of a given cognitive event. For example, a cognitive event that is perceived as produced by the person him- or herself is considered a self-generated event, but a cognitive event that is perceived as generated not by the person, but by an external agent, is characterized as a nonself-generated event. The second dimension refers to the localization of the cognitive event in space. When an event is located in inner space, this is referred to as an inner event. In contrast, when an event is located in outer space, that is, outside of the subject, this is referred to as an outer event. However, most source monitoring studies ask participants to produce a word out loud when generating an event from the internal source. One problem with this methodology is that although the event is self-generated, it contains both inner and outer localization qualities. Specifically, the generation of the word is indeed an inner event, but the production of the word also leads to stimulation of sensory organs, thereby adding outer localization qualities. Thus, a purely inner, self-generated event that seems a basic requirement for the study of alienation is rarely used (see Böcker et al., 2000, for an exception). Instead, there is typically a mixture of inner and outer qualities that characterizes a self-generated event.

The importance of recognizing the limitations of the aforementioned experimental designs is accentuated by phenomenological studies of hallucinations, which show that patients do not necessarily externalize their hallucinations (although this may occur). Indeed, studies have revealed that subjects may perceive their hallucinations as occurring "on the outside" (i.e., externalizing) but may also perceive them as occurring "in their head"—both within and outside the self, and some find it difficult to make this distinction when reporting hallucinations (this aspect was detailed in chap. 2, this volume). In other words, a hallucination does not necessarily have to be attributed to an external object to be a hallucination. Therefore, whether hallucinations are externalized or internalized may be no more important than whether they are experienced as "me"/self-generated or "not me"/non-self-generated.

Support for the contention (based on phenomenological studies) that hallucination-prone individuals do not necessarily externalize their hallucinations was suggested by Larøi, Collignon, and Van der Linden (2005). In this study, the relative influences of several internal encoding conditions on reality monitoring functioning were examined. Sixty-five normal subjects were administered an action source monitoring task and were each asked to (a) perform the action, (b) watch the experimenter perform the action, (c) imagine herself or himself performing the action, (d) imagine the experimenter performing the action, or (e) listen to the experimenter say the action verbally. Following a delay, actions were presented consisting of those already presented in one of the five conditions (old) and those never before presented (new). For each action, subjects were required to identify if the action was old or new. If the action was identified as old, subjects were required to identify the source of the action (i.e., one of the five conditions). Subjects were grouped (hallucination-prone and nonhallucination-prone) according to their scores on the LSHS (see the Appendix).

The results revealed that within the internal conditions, hallucination-prone subjects confused the two internal sources (a specific internal–

internal source discrimination error). That is, for imagined actions in which the subjects performed the action, hallucination-prone subjects erroneously attributed these to an imagined action performed by the experimenter. These results suggest that the inability to adequately attribute the detailed origin of an internal cognitive event may be seen as an important cognitive difficulty in hallucinations. Also, lack of an externalizing effect, coupled with the fact that the source monitoring errors that significantly differentiated the two groups remained confined within the two internal encoding conditions, may be related to phenomenological characteristics of hallucinations. In particular, phenomenological studies report that hallucinations do not necessarily have to be attributed to an external object for them to be a hallucination. Indeed, they may remain internal–perceptual experiences that subjects simply characterize as having an alien or nonself quality to them (i.e., not experienced as belonging to them) but not necessarily externalized. In this context, the "imagine-myself actions" can be viewed as relatively more personal and less alien compared with the "imagine-experimenter actions." If a feeling that internally generated stimuli originate from alien or nonself sources occurs in hallucination-prone subjects, then this may explain why the imagine-myself actions were attributed to the imagine-experimenter modality and not the imagine-myself modality. For more detailed information concerning similar limits to source monitoring studies in the context of hallucinations and their theoretical implications, consult Larøi and Woodward (2007) and Larøi (2006).

Hallucinations and Beliefs: Anthony Morrison's Hallucination Model

Another important cognitive model of hallucinations is presented in Anthony Morrison and colleagues' work. In general, Morrison is in agreement with the supposition that hallucinations are internal cognitive events that are misattributed to an external source. His explanation for this misattribution, however, is based on the fact that hallucinations are in some way linked to normal intrusive thoughts and that because of motivational factors, these intrusive thoughts become externalized by the individual (Morrison et al., 1995).

Because the genesis of hallucinations is seen as a reaction to intrusive experiences, an important aspect of Morrison's model concerns research showing similarities between intrusive thoughts and hallucinations. Like hallucinations, intrusions are also often experienced as ego dystonic and uncontrollable; share similarities in terms of form, content, and triggers (e.g., stressful events); and are usually accompanied by subjective discomfort (Morrison, 2001; Morrison et al., 1995).

Support for the importance of intrusive thoughts in the context of hallucinations has come from a study by Morrison and Baker (2000) that examined the cognitive intrusions of psychotic patients compared with nonpatients.

In this study, a group of 15 schizophrenic patients with hallucinations, 15 schizophrenic patients without hallucinations, and 15 nonpsychiatric control subjects were asked to complete a questionnaire examining the frequency of intrusive thoughts (i.e., distressing thoughts) and their reactions to them. Results revealed that patients who experienced auditory hallucinations had more intrusive thoughts than did the group of schizophrenic patients without hallucinations and the nonpsychiatric control group. This was the case for both types of intrusive thoughts examined, namely, anxiety-related and depression-related cognitive intrusions. Furthermore, patients experiencing auditory hallucinations perceived both anxiety-related and depression-related intrusive thoughts as more worrying and more difficult to remove and disapproved of such intrusions more than the two other groups. The authors argued that these findings support the suggestion of Morrison et al. (1995) that intrusive thoughts are involved in the development of auditory hallucinations. Furthermore, these findings are consistent with the view that such intrusions are disapproved of by patients experiencing auditory hallucinations (Morrison et al., 1995).

Morrison et al. (1995) argued that the need to attribute intrusive thoughts to an external force is due to motivational factors. The presence of certain intrusive thoughts may lead to negative affect in the subject in the form of anxiety (Bentall, 1990) or cognitive dissonance (Morrison et al., 1995). According to cognitive dissonance theory (Festinger, 1957), dissonance occurs when two cognitions (e.g., thoughts, beliefs, and feelings the person is aware of) contradict each other, resulting in an uncomfortable state from which an individual is motivated to escape. Morrison et al. argued that to reduce levels of negative affect, the subject chooses to externalize the intrusive thought, resulting in hallucinations. In particular, Morrison (1998, 2001; Morrison et al., 1995) posited the important role that metacognitive beliefs may play in this misattribution process.

Metacognitive beliefs can be defined as beliefs concerning one's own mental processes. This may include, for example, beliefs that mental events should be controllable, that thoughts are dangerous or harmful, or that intrusive thoughts are acceptable and beneficial. When the occurrence of intrusive thoughts does not comply with the subject's metacognitive beliefs, an aversive state of arousal results (cognitive dissonance), which the subject tries to escape by externalizing the intrusive thoughts (resulting in hallucinatory experiences), thus maintaining consistency in his or her belief system (Morrison et al., 1995). For example, if a person believes that all thoughts should be intended but the same person also experiences intrusive thoughts, the attribution of such thoughts to an external agent or source may be negatively reinforced by preventing the occurrence of cognitive dissonance because personal responsibility is removed.

Morrison's (1998, 2001; Morrison et al., 1995) cognitive account of the development of hallucinations has a number of advantages. For instance, both pleasant and unpleasant hallucinations can be explained within this model. Thus, regardless of whether intrusive thoughts are perceived as being pleasant or unpleasant, if they do not correspond with the subject's (metacognitive) belief system, they will nonetheless result in negative affect because of the level of cognitive dissonance they create. Another advantage of this model is that it is easy to interpret the presence of hallucinations from other modalities within the model. For example, visual hallucinations may reflect the misattribution of (undesired) intrusive images. Finally, this cognitive account of hallucinations also has clinical implications (see chap. 8, this volume, for more information concerning these clinical implications).

A number of studies have found evidence for an association between metacognitive beliefs and the presence of hallucinations in both clinical samples (Baker & Morrison, 1998; García-Montes, Pérez-Álvarez, Balbuena, Garcelàn, & Cangas, 2006; Lobban, Haddock, Kinderman, & Wells, 2002; Morrison & Wells, 2003) and nonclinical samples (Cangas, Errasti, García-Montes, Álvarez, & Ruiz, 2006; S. R. Jones & Fernyhough, 2006; Larøi, Collignon, & Van der Linden, 2005; Larøi, Van der Linden, & Marczewski, 2004; Larøi & Van der Linden, 2005a; Morrison & Petersen, 2003; Morrison, Wells, & Nothard, 2000, 2002). Some of these studies are described in detail below.

Studies Including Clinical Participants

Baker and Morrison (1998) examined relations between metacognitions and hallucinations. They included 15 schizophrenic patients with hallucinations, 15 schizophrenic patients without hallucinations, and 15 normal controls. All of the participants completed the reality testing task used in Morrison and Haddock (1997; described earlier in this chapter). In addition, all of the participants also completed the Meta-Cognitions Questionnaire (MCQ; Cartwright-Hatton & Wells, 1997) to assess metacognitive beliefs. In brief, the MCQ is a self-report measure that assesses individual differences in positive and negative beliefs about worry and intrusive thoughts, metacognitive monitoring, and judgments of cognitive efficiency. It consists of five subscales: (a) positive beliefs about worry (beliefs that worry helps one to solve problems and avoid unpleasant situations); (b) negative beliefs about the uncontrollability of thoughts and corresponding danger (beliefs that worry is uncontrollable, that one must control one's worrying, and that worrying is dangerous); (c) cognitive confidence (concerns about one's cognitive efficiency); (d) negative beliefs about thoughts in general and in particular relating to superstition, punishment, and responsibility (fears of outcomes that might result from having certain thoughts and the acceptance of responsibility for having such thoughts); and (e) cognitive self-consciousness (the tendency to monitor and focus on one's thinking processes). Baker and Morrison found that schizophrenic patients with hallucinations scored higher (indicating a higher frequency of metacognitive beliefs) than both nonhallucinating patients and normal controls on two subscales of the MCQ: negative beliefs about the uncontrollability of thoughts and corresponding danger and positive beliefs about worry. Furthermore, ratings of, on the one hand, controllability and wantedness and, on the other hand, negative beliefs about the uncontrollability of thoughts and corresponding danger were associated with source monitoring attributions.

Baker and Morrison (1998) interpreted these findings as providing support for Morrison et al.'s (1995) account that implicates cognitive dissonance in the experience of auditory hallucinations, in particular, the role of both positive and negative metacognitive beliefs in creating a cognitive dissonance. In this study, positive beliefs included such beliefs as "worrying helps me to get things sorted out in my mind," whereas negative beliefs included such beliefs as "worrying could make me go mad." According to Morrison et al. (1995), the presence of both positive and negative metacognitive beliefs (concerning intrusive thoughts, hallucinatory experiences, worry, etc.) leads to cognitive dissonance because they are incompatible with each other. That is, it is supposed that a subject who deems these experiences to be both positive (or adaptive, constructive, beneficial, etc.) and negative (or maladaptive, unconstructive, distressful, etc.) will experience an aversive state of arousal (cognitive dissonance) because of this presence of two incompatible or conflicting ideas or thoughts. As the hallucinators in Baker and Morrison's study reported holding both positive and negative metacognitive beliefs, according to the authors, it would appear that the likelihood of cognitive dissonance would be increased in these subjects.

To test the hypothesis that metacognitions are a general vulnerability factor for psychological disorder, Morrison and Wells (2003) administered the MCQ to a group of schizophrenic patients with auditory hallucinations, a group of schizophrenic patients who were currently experiencing persecutory delusions (but with no history of auditory hallucinations in the past year), a group of panic disorder patients, and a normal control group. All of the participants completed the MCQ. The results showed that the schizophrenic patients with auditory hallucinations tended to exhibit higher levels of dysfunctional metacognitive beliefs than the other patient groups and the nonpatient controls.

García-Montes et al. (2006) compared five different groups: current hallucinators with schizophrenia, never-hallucinated schizophrenic patients, recovered hallucinators (no report of hallucinatory experiences of any kind in the past 6 months), obsessive–compulsive disorder (OCD) patients, and a nonclinical group. They then compared these groups in terms of their metacognitive beliefs and found evidence of a certain parallelism between the current hallucinators and the patients with OCD. That is, both the current hallucinators and OCD groups revealed significantly higher scores on negative beliefs about uncontrollability and danger of thoughts compared with the nonclinical group. Also, both current hallucinators and OCD patients appeared to have more firmly rooted superstition and responsibility beliefs than the clinical control group and the nonclinical group. However, these two groups differed in terms of cognitive self-consciousness: OCD patients presented a significantly higher score compared with all the other groups.

Studies Including Nonclinical Participants

In a large group of hallucination-prone subjects, Morrison et al. (2000) replicated the finding of an association between the presence of hallucinations and metacognitive beliefs. One hundred and five nonclinical subjects completed the LSHS (see the Appendix) and the MCQ. In addition, visual analog scales rated on a scale of 0 to 100 were used to assess subjects' positive and negative beliefs about unusual perceptual experiences (one measure for each). Positive beliefs were assessed with the item "Unusual experiences, such as those mentioned in the previous questionnaire, are beneficial and help me cope," and negative beliefs were assessed with the item "Unusual experiences, such as those mentioned in the previous questionnaire, are potentially dangerous and interfere with my life." (For both items, "previous questionnaire" refers to the LSHS that all subjects had completed before.) Participants indicated their responses by placing a mark on a 10-centimeter line with the endpoints *not at all* and *could not be more so*.

Subjects were then divided into two groups (high and low hallucination proneness) based on a median split on the total hallucination score. Multivariate analysis of variance was conducted using the subscales of the MCQ as the dependent variables and using high or low predisposition to hallucinations as the grouping factor. An overall significant difference was found between the metacognitive beliefs of participants high or low in their predisposition to hallucinations. That is, hallucination-prone subjects scored significantly higher on the MCQ (indicating a higher frequency of metacognitive beliefs) compared with the nonprone subjects. Furthermore, these two groups differed significantly in terms of three MCQ subscales (cognitive self-consciousness; negative beliefs about the uncontrollability of thoughts and corresponding danger; negative beliefs about thoughts in general and in particular relating to superstition, punishment, and responsibility). Finally, on the basis of multiple regression analysis, positive beliefs about hallucinatory experiences were found to be the best predictor of predisposition to hallucination. According to the authors, the observed combination of positive beliefs (i.e., positive beliefs about hallucinatory experiences) and negative beliefs (i.e., negative beliefs about the uncontrollability of thoughts and corresponding danger; negative beliefs about thoughts in general and in particular relating to superstition, punishment, and responsibility) present in the hallucination-prone subjects offers support for the view that cognitive dissonance may be involved in the development of hallucinations.

On the basis of the idea that it may be the co-occurrence of both positive and negative metacognitive beliefs that elicits cognitive dissonance in hallucinators (Morrison et al., 1995), certain studies have examined the specific roles of positive and negative metacognitive beliefs in hallucinations (Morrison et al., 2000, 2002). Morrison et al. (2000) performed multiple regression analysis with auditory and visual hallucination-proneness as dependent variables. Results revealed that positive beliefs about unusual experiences were the best predictors of both auditory and visual hallucinations. Also using regression analysis, Morrison et al. (2002) found that positive beliefs were the best predictors of proneness toward auditory hallucinations. On the other hand, both negative beliefs about uncontrollability and danger and positive beliefs about worry were found to be significant predictors of proneness toward visual hallucinations. Finally, in Larøi and Van der Linden (2005a), multiple regression analysis revealed that positive and negative beliefs were good predictors of proneness toward hallucinations.

Some studies (Larøi, Collignon, & Van der Linden, 2005; Larøi, Van der Linden, & Marczewski, 2004) have found that metacognitive beliefs in nonclinical hallucination-prone subjects were related to various cognitive processes as measured by experimental tasks, such as source monitoring (described earlier in the chapter). As discussed earlier, in Larøi et al.'s (2004) study, hallucination-prone subjects scored significantly higher on a scale assessing metacognitive beliefs compared with non-hallucination-prone subjects. Furthermore, scores on a scale assessing metacognitive beliefs were positively associated with source discrimination errors. Similarly, in Larøi et al. (2005), hallucination-prone subjects obtained significantly higher scores on a measure of metacognitive beliefs, compared with nonprone subjects. Relations between metacognitive beliefs and source monitoring errors were also studied, which revealed a significant association between specific metacognitive beliefs (cognitive consciousness and positive worry beliefs) and the internal–internal discrimination error observed in hallucination-prone subjects.

Finally, results from one recent study including nonclinical participants suggest that metacognitive beliefs in themselves are not enough to predict hallucination-proneness (S. R. Jones & Fernyhough, 2006). In particular, the authors argued that the production of unwanted intrusive thoughts (viewed by the authors as representing the "raw material" of hallucinations) is due (among other undefined factors) to the use of thought suppression (perhaps either as another type of metacognitive belief inherent in individuals or as a type of safety behavior used by individuals to ease or reduce the danger of having intrusive thoughts). That is, both the presence of certain metacognitive beliefs (in particular, cognitive self-consciousness and, albeit perhaps to a lesser degree, low confidence in memory and beliefs about the uncontrollability of thoughts) and the use of thought suppression (if both co-occur) will together be better predictors of the development of hallucinations. One study, although it did not examine such processes in the context of the presence of hallucinations, seems to support this interpretation (García-Montes, Pérez-Álvarez, & Fidalgo, 2003).

Summary

A number of studies seem to provide evidence of Morrison et al.'s (1995) hypothesis that hallucinations are related to the metacognitive beliefs held by hallucination-prone individuals. In particular, findings suggest that this association is relatively specific for hallucinations (Morrison & Wells, 2003), although studies have found evidence of the association between metacognitive beliefs and other psychotic symptoms such as delusions (Larøi & Van der Linden, 2005a), and there is evidence that this association is, at least to a certain degree, also found in other clinical groups such as patients with OCD (García-Montes et al., 2006). Furthermore, there is some support that it is the co-occurrence of both positive and negative metacognitive beliefs that predicts greater proneness to hallucinations (Baker & Morrison, 1998; Larøi & Van der Linden, 2005a; Morrison et al., 2000, 2002) and that certain cognitive processes such as source monitoring misattributions are related to metacognitive beliefs in hallucination-prone individuals (Baker & Morrison, 1998; Larøi, Collignon, & Van der Linden, 2005; Larøi, Van der Linden, & Marczewski, 2004). Finally, one recent study indicates that processes related to thought suppression, in addition to metacognitive beliefs, may also play an important role in the development of hallucinations (S. R. Jones & Fernyhough, 2006).

THE ROLES OF CONTEXTUAL MEMORY AND INHIBITION

Waters, Badcock, Michie, and Maybery (2006) proposed a cognitive model of auditory hallucinations in schizophrenia whereby hallucinations are considered as auditory representations derived from the unintentional activation of memories and other irrelevant current mental associations. According to Waters et al., at least two (co-occurring) deficits seem to be responsible for this, namely, inhibition and context memory. Deficits in intentional inhibition will result in auditory mental representations that intrude into consciousness in a manner that is beyond the control of the individual. Furthermore, these involuntary and intrusive events are not recognized because of a deficit in contextual memory that particularly affects the ability to associate (or bind) contextual cues together. This model further hypothesizes that nonhallucinating individuals may show either deficit but that it is only in hallucinating patients (with schizophrenia) in whom both deficits are present.

In terms of inhibition, Waters, Badcock, Maybery, and Michie (2003) administered the Hayling Sentence Completion Test (HSCT) and the Inhibition of Currently Irrelevant Memories Task (ICIM) to a group of patients with schizophrenia and a group of normal controls. In the HSCT, participants are to provide single-word completions to sentences. In the critical inhibition condition, the completion is required to be unrelated to the preceding sentence. Two types of error are recorded: Category A errors, in which the supplied word completed the sentence in a plausible fashion, and Category B errors, in which the response is semantically connected to the sentence but did not represent the most plausible completion. The ICIM (adapted from Schnider & Ptak, 1999) involves the presentation of a series of animal pictures from which participants must detect those pictures that are repeated (targets) within a single run. Targets then become distractors in subsequent runs. For each subsequent run, participants are instructed to forget that they had already seen the pictures and to indicate picture reoccurrences only within that run. A total of four runs was administered. The number of false positives to these distractors (or false alarms) in the last three runs reflects the ability to suppress memories that are no longer relevant. Waters et al. found that the patient group and the control group differed significantly in terms of the HSCT (for both types of errors) and in terms of the number of false alarms (higher in the patient group) on the last three runs of the ICIM. Correlational analyses revealed a significant relation between the number of Type A errors (but not Type B errors) and auditory hallucination severity. There was also a significant correlation between the number of false alarms on the ICIM and auditory hallucination severity. In contrast, no significant correlations were obtained between any of the inhibition measures and negative, general, or positive (where the auditory hallucination ratings were subtracted) symptom ratings.

Badcock, Waters, Maybery, and Michie (2005) compared three groups in terms of inhibition efficiency: schizophrenic patients currently experiencing auditory hallucinations, schizophrenic patients who had not experienced auditory hallucinations within the last 4 weeks, and a normal control group. The ICIM (described above) was used. Results revealed that the three groups differed significantly in terms of the number of false alarms for the last three runs: Current hallucinators made significantly more false alarms than healthy controls, and the patients without hallucinations made significantly fewer false alarms than the current hallucinators and were not significantly different from healthy controls. These two studies, therefore, seem to suggest that hallucinations in schizophrenia patients are related to an inability to suppress recently activated memory traces. Similarly, albeit in a study comparing nonclinical hallucination-prone and nonhallucination-prone participants, Paulik, Badcock, and Maybery (2007) found that hallucination-prone participants also had difficulties intentionally inhibiting strongly activated memory traces (on the basis of performances on the ICIM).

Concerning context memory, in an initial study, Waters, Maybery, Badcock, and Michie (2004) found evidence of deficits in retrieving contextual information and in binding different components of a memory together in patients with schizophrenia compared with normal controls. Participants were asked to either watch the experimenter pair two household objects together or pair them themselves. This was done over two sessions, 30 minutes apart. In the recognition test, intact pairs (i.e., those kept in their original combination) and rearranged pairs (new combinations) were presented. Participants then indicated whether each pair was intact or rearranged, and for those judged as intact, they had to indicate who performed the pairing (i.e., the participant or the experimenter) and in which session (first or second). Results revealed that patients with schizophrenia recognized significantly fewer object pairs than controls and were less accurate in recalling the source and temporal context of events. Furthermore, whereas normal subjects tended to retrieve all the features of events, patients with schizophrenia tended to retrieve only individual features in isolation or none at all, suggesting that patients with schizophrenia present difficulties in binding together all the original components of an event.

Waters, Badcock, and Maybery (2006) reanalyzed data on 43 patients with schizophrenia whose results were previously published in Badcock et al. (2005) and Waters et al. (2003, 2004) to examine any specific relations between auditory hallucinations and context memory deficits. They reported that schizophrenic patients with active hallucinations differed significantly from patients without hallucinations and control subjects in terms of judgments of self-monitoring (i.e., who performed the pairing). However, hallucinating and nonhallucinating patients did not differ from each other in terms of temporal accuracy (i.e., which session), but control subjects performed significantly better than both patient groups. Evidence of deficits in contextual memory is in line with other studies that have found significant correlations between auditory hallucinations and context (temporal) memory (Brébion et al., 1999; Brébion, Gorman, Amador, Malaspina, & Sharif, 2002). One recent study has also reported that difficulties in remembering the temporal context are significantly correlated with the presence of auditory hallucinations but not with visual hallucinations (Brébion, David, Jones, Ohlsen, & Pilowsky, 2007).

To test the specificity of this two-deficit model to hallucinations more directly, Waters, Badcock, Michie, and Maybery (2006) reanalyzed data from the above-mentioned studies in terms of the percentage of patients impaired on tasks of both intentional inhibition and contextual memory. They found that the percentage of hallucinating patients having both deficits was significantly higher compared with nonhallucinating patients. In particular, with a criterion of 1 standard deviation, 89.5% of hallucinating patients had both deficits compared with 33.3% of nonhallucinating patients. With a more stringent criterion (i.e., 2 standard deviations), these were 52.6% and 16.7%, respectively. Although not all hallucinating patients had both deficits, and a certain percentage of nonhallucinating patients showed evidence of having both deficits, these studies do seem to suggest that inhibition and contextual memory deficits play an important role in auditory hallucinations.

CONCLUSION

This chapter has shown that metacognitive processes (reality monitoring and metacognitive beliefs) are clearly associated with hallucinations. However, studies examining reality monitoring errors in hallucinations have suggested that they are not sufficient to account for hallucinations and, furthermore, that reality monitoring errors may be nonspecific to hallucinations in that they also occur in other symptoms such as delusions and may even be a general deficit in schizophrenia. Metacognitive beliefs are also clearly involved in hallucinations. However, once again, these beliefs are also associated with other symptoms (e.g., delusions) and other clinical disorders (e.g., OCD). What is clearly needed is a multifactorial account of hallucinations that takes into account a number of factors, including (but not restricted to) reality monitoring errors and metacognitive beliefs, in addition to other factors such as deficits in inhibition and contextual memory. To date, no studies have included these factors in the same study to examine their relative predictability of hallucinations. Furthermore, contextual and emotional factors (e.g., stress, culture) that may influence metacognitive processes involved in hallucinations should also be considered. An externalizing bias could arise as a result of hallucinations and not necessarily as the cause of hallucinations. However, studies revealing externalizing biases on source monitoring tasks in nonclinical subjects (e.g., Larøi, Van der Linden, & Marczewski, 2004; Rankin & O'Carroll, 1995) and in unaffected siblings of patients (e.g., Brunelin, d'Amato, et al., 2007), who presumably do not experience hallucinations frequently, suggest that such an explanation is not very likely. Finally, it is important to underline that any theoretical conception of hallucinations must also be able to integrate the phenomenological diversity of hallucinations (Larøi, 2006; Larøi & Woodward, 2007).

In the next chapter, brain areas involved in hallucinations are reviewed, some of which are implicated in the metacognitive processes described in this chapter.

CHAPTER HIGHLIGHTS

- Metacognition (i.e., thinking about thinking) plays an important role in hallucination development and maintenance.
- Hallucinations may be viewed as misattributions of inner cognitive events. Theoretical models seem to vary in terms of their explanations as to why this misattribution occurs.

- Metacognitive beliefs (i.e., beliefs concerning own mental processes) may influence the manner in which inner cognitive events are anxiety provoking and ultimately if they are perceived as an external or nonself event (i.e., resulting in a hallucinatory experience).
- Other cognitive processes that do not necessarily involve metacognitive processes, such as inhibition and context memory, may also be involved in hallucination development and maintenance.

6

HALLUCINATIONS AND THE BRAIN

What happens in the brain when people see things others do not see or hear voices when nobody is speaking? Which neurotransmitters are involved in such experiences? Which brain areas mediate the experience of a hallucination? We try to answer these questions in this chapter. First, we briefly review findings from early neurological studies. We then describe the role of neurotransmitters in hallucinations. Subsequently, we review structural and functional neuroimaging evidence. Finally, we present a neuroanatomical model.

EARLY NEUROLOGICAL STUDIES: BRAIN STIMULATION

The first groundbreaking observations regarding elicitation of hallucinations by temporal lobe stimulation were reported in the mid-20th century. The Canadian neurologist Wilder Penfield, while conducting surgeries to remove specific types of temporal lobe loci that were causing epilepsy, discovered that his unanesthetized patients (with local pain blockers) could listen and respond to his questions while their temporal lobe was being operated on. Stimulation of the temporal lobe induced several instances of hallucinations of autobiographic memory. For example, one of Penfield's patients heard a specific music selection being performed by an orchestra when a point on the superior surface of the right temporal lobe was stimulated after removal of the anterior half of the lobe (Penfield, 1955). The sound was so clear that the patient believed that there was a phonograph in the operating room. If Penfield withheld the electrode, the patient heard nothing. He found that the patient could not guess what was to happen after the electrode had been withdrawn. The experiences could also be visual. Penfield (1955) wrote, "L.G. saw a man fighting. When the point was re-stimulated he saw a man and a dog walking along a road" (p. 455).

Penfield (1955) called the results of the experience "a new order" of phenomena, which John Hughlings Jackson (an early British neurologist) had recognized in epileptic patients. Jackson (1931) grouped such phenomena as "dreamy state," which encompassed a sensation of déjà vécu, complex visual hallucinations, and sensations of "strangeness." Such dreamy state experiences were restudied by Vignal, Maillard, McGonigal, and Chauvel (2007), who recorded 15 sensations of déjà vécu, 35 complex visual hallucinations, and 5 sensations of strangeness after 40 cortical stimulations in 16 subjects and 15 seizures in 5 subjects. These experiences were primarily evoked by stimulation of the amygdala or hippocampus.

NEUROTRANSMITTERS

Four neurotransmitters have been associated with hallucinations: dopamine, acetylcholine, serotonin, and glutamate.

Dopamine

In schizophrenia, there is evidence that too-high levels of dopamine in the limbic system (amygdala, hippocampus, ventral striatum, cingulate) may play an important role in the emergence of psychotic symptoms such as hallucinations and delusions (Laruelle, 2003). A key component of the mechanism of action of most antipsychotics is the blockade of D2 dopamine receptors. These drugs can effectively reduce hallucinations in approximately 70% of patients with schizophrenia (Johnstone, Owens, & Leary, 1991; cf. chap. 8, this volume). More evidence for the role of dopamine in hallucinations comes from the effects of dopaminergic drugs in healthy people. For example, psychostimulants such as amphetamine have been shown to induce hallucinatory experiences. Harris and Batki (2000) used structured interviews to assess 19 patients seen at a psychiatric emergency service with amphetamine- or cocaine-induced psychotic disorder and concluded that a majority experienced hallucinations.

The occurrence of delusions and hallucinations is rather common (approximately 25% of patients) in Parkinson's disease (Wolters & Berendse,

2001). Drugs with a strong dopaminergic effect, such as L-dopa, which is prescribed for Parkinson's disease, may induce vivid visual hallucinations (Onofrj et al., 2006). Indeed, it is dopaminomimetic agents that are thought to be mainly responsible for hallucinations in Parkinson's disease (Wolters & Berendse, 2001). They induce dopamine hypersensitivity in the frontal and limbic dopamine projection regions and, consequently, either directly or indirectly elicit psychotic signs and symptoms. A Parkinson's disease–related cholinergic deficit in combination with an age-related further loss of cholinergic integrity may also play a role. The fact that hallucinations were also described in Parkinson's disease in the period before the introduction of L-dopa indicates that not only hyperdopaminergic states but also *hypo*dopaminergic states, presumably due to the progressive loss of dopamine projections to the cortex, can induce hallucinations (Aarsland, Larsen, Cummings, & Lake, 1999). This has been confirmed in a study by Onofrj et al. (2006).

Acetylcholine

There is ample evidence for the involvement of cholinergic function in complex visual hallucinations (Manford & Andermann, 1998). As reviewed by Perry and Perry (1995), pharmacological cholinergic manipulations can both induce and treat such hallucinations. Schultes, Hofmann, and Ratsch (1998) noted that acetylcholine might be involved in the majority of plants with identified hallucinogenic chemicals. For example, alteration of consciousness with induction of hallucinations has been described widely since ancient times for members of the Solanaceae family of plants (belladonna, henbane, or datura), which contain scopolamine, atropine, and other closely related tropane alkaloids. Tropane alkaloids are antimuscarinic agents, muscarinic receptors being the postganglionic receptors of acetylcholine in the brain.

Visual hallucinations are a prominent aspect of Lewy body dementia (LBD), in which cholinergic dysfunction has been well documented. Hallucinations may occur in approximately 30% of patients with Alzheimer's disease, whereas they may occur in 60% of patients with LBD. Cholinergic deficits are evident in both LBD and Alzheimer's disease, with reductions in acetylcholine and abnormalities in nicotinic and muscarinic receptor expression in both diseases. Cholinergic deficits are greater in LBD than in Alzheimer's disease, although generally there is less brain atrophy in LBD (Duda, 2004). Harding, Broe, and Halliday (2002) reported a striking association between the distribution of temporal lobe Lewy bodies and well-formed visual hallucinations in patients with LBD. Colloby et al. (2006) observed a significant elevation of muscarinic acetylcholine receptors in the occipital lobe in patients with LBD and Parkinson's disease with dementia. They suggested that this may relate to visual hallucinations and other visual distur-

bances. Evidence for a causal relationship between acetylcholine and hallucinations was found by Perry and Perry (1995).

It is interesting that whereas reductions of cortical acetylcholine are
associated with hallucinations, cholinergic activation of the thalamus during REM sleep has been shown to be associated with the occurrence of dreams.
Such paradoxical effects of muscarinic receptor blockade to induce hallucinations and of REM-sleep-associated cholinergic activation of the thalamus
to induce dreaming have been suggested by Perry and Perry (1995) to be
related to the differential distribution and activity of muscarinic receptor
subtypes or to the differing responses of intrinsic gamma-aminobutyric acid
neurons in the cortex and thalamus.

After reviewing the evidence concerning the role of acetylcholine in
hallucinations, Collerton, Perry, and McKeith (2005) proposed that cortical
cholinergic projections from the basal forebrain rather than those from the
brainstem to the thalamus (as proposed by Behrendt & Young, 2004) are
crucially involved in hallucinations. Perry and Perry (1995) hypothesized
that cortical acetylcholine may play a role in modulating the content of conscious awareness. This extends the concept that cortical acetylcholine enhances neuronal signal-to-noise ratio. More specifically, they suggested that
in the absence of cortical acetylcholine, currently irrelevant intrinsic and
sensory information, which is constantly processed in parallel at the subcon-
scious level, enters conscious awareness.

Serotonin

Serotonin has also been implied in the neurogenesis of hallucinatory
experiences. The main strand of evidence comes from the effects of psychoactive drugs that boost serotonin transmission. The most potent of these is
lysergic acid diethylamide (LSD). LSD-induced hallucinations mainly concern the visual modality and may be limited to forms and patterns such as
gratings, honeycomb, or chessboard designs or spiral figures (Kluver, 1966).
LSD use in certain individuals may result in chronic visual hallucinations, a
Diagnostic and Statistical Manual of Mental Disorders (American Psychiatric
Association, 1994) syndrome known as hallucinogen persisting perception
disorder.

Mescaline and psilocybin, extracted from a cactus and a mushroom,
respectively, have also been reported to induce hallucinations in healthy
people. The same holds for 5-MeO-DMT, which is a psychoactive substance
that can be found in the venom of an American toad, the *Bufo alvarius*. Although toad-licking has been reported to induce psychedelic experiences, it
does not induce hallucinations because 5-MeO-DMT is not active orally
(Lyttle, Goldstein, & Gartz, 1996). The most common mode of administration is smoking after the substance has been dried. It is interesting to note
that a relationship between toads and mushrooms has infiltrated several lan-

guages for centuries. For example, the English word *toadstool* dates back to 1398. The Dutch word *paddestoel* (toad's stool) is nearly identical to the English expression. The Norwegians use the word *paddehatt* (toad's hat), whereas the French say *pain de crapaud* (toad's bread). Apparently, the mind-altered state induced by both the amphibian and fungus was perceived to be similar enough to warrant such verbal expressions. In fact, mescaline, psilocybin, and 5-MeO-DMT can all be seen as LSD-type drugs, hallucinogens that are serotonin 5-HT$_{2A}$ receptor agonists or partial agonists.

The party drug "Ecstasy" also strongly increases serotonin levels in the brain besides having effects on other neurotransmitters such as dopamine. Using transcranial magnetic stimulation, Oliveri and Calvo (2003) measured excitability of the visual cortex in Ecstasy users compared with control subjects by eliciting *phosphenes* (light flashes). They observed that phosphene thresholds were significantly lower in Ecstasy users compared with control subjects, which is indicative of increased excitability of the visual cortex. Lower phosphene thresholds correlated negatively with frequency of Ecstasy use. Frequency of use was positively correlated with the presence of visual hallucinations. The phosphene threshold of subjects with hallucinations was significantly lower than that of subjects without hallucinations. Oliver and Calvo suggested that the increased excitability of the visual cortex due to recreational Ecstasy use is possibly linked with massive serotonin release, followed by serotonin depletion, in this cortical area. A final source of evidence for the involvement of serotonin in hallucinations comes from studies of antidepressant medication, or SSRIs, which increase the availability of serotonin in the synaptic cleft. Hallucinations have been reported as side effects of such SSRIs (Kumagai, Ohnuma, Nagata, & Arai, 2003).

Glutamate

As in the case for serotonin, evidence for a possible role of glutamate in hallucinations comes from pharmacological compounds that have been shown to induce hallucinatory experiences. The two most prominent drugs in this regard are phencyclidine (PCP, or angel dust) and ketamine (an anesthetic), which are both glutamate antagonists. Ketamine, a PCP hydrochloride derivative, is frequently used in experimental studies as a "psychotomimetic" (i.e., to mimic the symptoms of psychosis). Ketamine is a noncompetitive antagonist of the N-methyl-D-aspartate (NMDA) subtype of excitatory amino acid receptor. It is quite successful in doing this because it mimics not only positive features like hallucinations and delusions but also negative features such as emotional blunting or apathia. Fortunately, for healthy subjects participating in such experiments, the effects are transient and short-lived, and no adverse effects are observed on follow-up.

In an interesting study, Krystal et al. (1994) set out to characterize the effects of subanesthetic doses of ketamine hydrochloride in healthy human subjects. In a randomized, double-blind, placebo-controlled study, they asked 19 healthy subjects to complete 3 test days involving 40-minute intravenous administrations of placebo or ketamine hydrochloride (which could be either 0.1 or 0.5 mg/kg). They found that ketamine produced behaviors similar to the positive and negative symptoms of schizophrenia, including perceptual aberrations. Furthermore, ketamine impaired neuropsychological performance in a pattern similar to that seen in schizophrenia and evoked symptoms similar to dissociative states. The authors concluded that NMDA antagonists produce a broad range of symptoms, behaviors, and cognitive deficits that resemble aspects of endogenous psychoses, particularly schizophrenia and dissociative states.

With regard to drug-induced hallucinations, two major classes of hallucinogens have been described: PCP type and LSD type (see section on serotonin). The PCP-type drugs concern glutamate NMDA receptor antagonists, whereas the LSD-type drugs concern serotonin 5-HT$_{2A}$ receptor agonists or partial agonists. Both types have been used in research as psychopharmacological models of psychosis, and more specifically schizophrenia. Because of their different psychotropic profile, it has been suggested that they model different aspects of schizophrenia. Specifically, the PCP type would be more appropriate to model disorganized types of schizophrenia, with hallucinations and delusions, as well as negative symptoms, whereas the LSD type would be more suitable as a model for the paranoid subtype of schizophrenia (Gouzoulis-Mayfrank et al., 2006).

The antiglutamatergic effects of PCP and ketamine are mainly mediated by inhibition of NMDA receptors. This has led to the hypothesis that psychotic symptoms (e.g., in schizophrenia) may in part be attributed to hypofunction of NMDA receptors (Javitt & Zukin, 1991). Vollenweider, Vontobel, Oye, Hell, and Leenders (2000) used positron emission tomography (PET) to determine whether ketamine exerts its psychomimetic effects through modulation of the dopamine system. If ketamine increases subcortical dopamine, this would be measurable as a decrease in the vivo binding of [11C]raclopride to striatal dopamine D2 receptors. Ketamine elicited a psychosis-like syndrome in the 8 volunteers studied by Vollenweider et al., including alterations in mood, cognitive disturbances, hallucinations, and ego disorders. Ketamine decreased [11C]raclopride binding potential significantly, indicating an increase in striatal dopamine concentration. The authors concluded that the glutamatergic NMDA receptor may contribute to psychotic symptom formation via modulation of the dopamine system. It is important to note, however, that although ketamine in most cases induces a range of perceptual distortions, not all studies have consistently reported the induction of hallucinations (Pomarol-Clotet et al., 2006). It should therefore be cautioned that ketamine does not necessarily reproduce the full picture of psychosis or schizophrenia.

Summary

Several neurotransmitters have been implicated in hallucinations: dopamine, acetylcholine, serotonin, and glutamate. Dopamine plays a key role in the hallucinations of schizophrenia, whereas acetylcholine plays a key role in the hallucinations of dementia. Manford and Andermann (1998) noted that two neurotransmitters that appear to be particularly important in visual hallucinations, serotonin and acetylcholine, are concentrated in the visual thalamic nuclei and visual cortex rather than in regions involved in other sensory modalities. It is important to be aware of the fact that the four neurotransmitter systems interact and that effects may be due to modulations of one system over another. Serotonin can influence glutamate transmission by excitation of gamma-aminobutyric acid interneurons. Modulatory effects of serotonin and glutamate on dopamine have also been described. For example, using PET scans in people who had received a psychotomimetic dose of ketamine, Vollenweider et al. (2000) provided evidence of an increased striatal dopamine concentration. Finally, it is important to note that the phenomenology of experimentally induced hallucinations may be different from that of clinical hallucinations in disorders such as schizophrenia and dementia, suggesting the need for additional approaches to the neural basis of hallucinations.

GENETICS OF HALLUCINATIONS

Few studies have addressed the genetics of hallucinations. Malhotra et al. (1998) found an association between hallucinations in neuroleptic-free patients with schizophrenic disorders and the long variant (l/l) in a region of the serotonin transporter gene, 5-HTT. This finding implies that the increased frequency and intensity of hallucinations in these patients might be associated with the functional consequences of higher than average 5-HTT availability. Specifically, such high availability will lead to a decrease of serotonin in the synaptic cleft. Postsynaptic serotonin receptors (also involved in the effects of LSD) will respond with an increase in responsivity and enhanced sensitivity (Lesch, 1998). Other genes associated with serotonin might also be involved in the hallucinatory experience. Ott, Reuter, Hennig, and Vaitl (2005) reported that a variant of the T102C polymorphism (that affects the 5HT2a receptor) was associated with the trait of absorption (see chap. 4, this volume, for the relevance of this trait to hallucinations). There was also a significant interaction between T102C and COMT genotypes in association with absorption scores. COMT codes for an enzyme that is involved with the dopaminergic neurotransmitter system.

Other studies have focused on genes related to dopamine function. A number of studies have reported an association between the CCK-AR gene and hallucinations in schizophrenia (Sanjuán, Toirac, et al., 2004; Wei & Hemmings, 1999) and with hallucinations accompanying delirium tremens (Okubo, Harada, Higuchi, and Matsushita, 2002). Two studies found associations with positive symptoms of schizophrenia, not specifically hallucinations (Tachikawa, Harada, Kawanishi, Okubo, & Suzuki, 2001; Zhang, Zhou, Zhang, & Wei, 2000). The CCK-AR gene codes for the CCK-AR receptor, which is a receptor for cholecystokinin, a neuropeptide that modulates dopamine release in the brain.

Chang et al. (2004) studied 135 patients with Alzheimer's disease and reported that the presence of the ApoE ε4 allele was associated with a 19-fold risk for developing hallucinations. ApoE ε4 has been implicated in atherosclerosis and Alzheimer's disease in general, as well as to impaired cognitive function and reduced neurite outgrowth. Sanjuán et al. (2006) observed an association between polymorphisms of the FOXP2 gene and schizophrenia with auditory hallucinations in a sample of 186 schizophrenia patients and 160 healthy controls. The FOXP2 gene has been implicated in the ability to articulate speech.

NEUROIMAGING

Researchers have tried to answer the question of which brain areas are involved in hallucinations with the use of modern functional neuroimaging techniques, such as PET and functional magnetic resonance imaging (fMRI). PET and single photon emission computed tomography (SPECT) are methods of mapping activity in the living brain by recording the emission of radioactivity from injected chemicals. fMRI is more frequently used because it does not require the injection of radioactive chemicals, allows for more repeated measurements, and has a higher spatial resolution. fMRI is based on the increase in blood flow to the local vasculature that accompanies neural activity in the brain. This results in a corresponding local reduction in deoxyhemoglobin because the increase in blood flow occurs without an increase of similar magnitude in oxygen extraction. Because deoxyhemoglobin is paramagnetic, it alters the magnetic resonance image signal. Studies have also been directed at investigating the structural correlates of hallucinations, that is, whether volume reductions of certain brain areas are associated with hallucinations. We first discuss evidence for structural abnormalities and then describe the functional studies. Figures 6.1 and 6.2 illustrate some of the major brain regions implicated.

Brain Structure and Hallucinations

Structural neuroimaging, using computerized tomography (CT) or magnetic resonance imaging (MRI), is often used clinically to rule out a focal

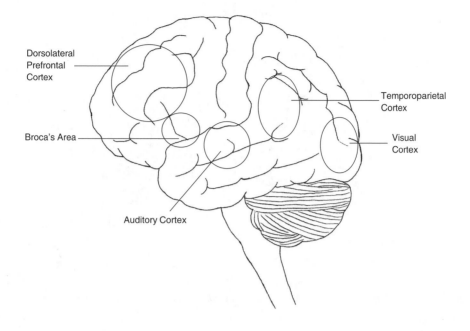

Figure 6.1. Dorsolateral cortex, Broca's area, auditory cortex, temporoparietal cortex, and visual cortex.

lesion such as a tumor or a stroke. Here, no brain activity is measured, but a static image is acquired that can be used to compute volumes of brain structures. This approach has also been used in studies, typically involving only a few patients, of hallucinations after brain injury. In psychiatric groups, however, no gross brain abnormalities can be seen on scans at the individual level. Therefore, scans are generally averaged across groups with and without hallucinations to investigate subtle abnormalities at the group level.

A. P. Weiss and Heckers (1999) summarized the results of studies published up to 1999. Two of these studies concerned Alzheimer's disease (Forstl, Besthorn, Geiger-Kabisch, Sattel, & Schreiter-Gasser, 1993; Howanitz, Bajulaiye, & Losonczy, 1995), one schizophrenia (Barta, Pearlson, Powers, Richards, & Tune, 1990), and the last one older people with idiopathic visual hallucinations (Shedlack, McDonald, Laskowitz, & Krishnan, 1994). The patients with schizophrenia were characterized by volume reductions of the superior temporal gyrus (STG) in addition to larger ventricles. Hallucination severity was inversely correlated with left STG volume. The studies in Alzheimer's patients observed a relationship between hallucinations and enlarged ventricles. A study in schizophrenia patients (Cullberg & Nybäck, 1992), not mentioned in the Weiss and Heckers review, reported a correla-

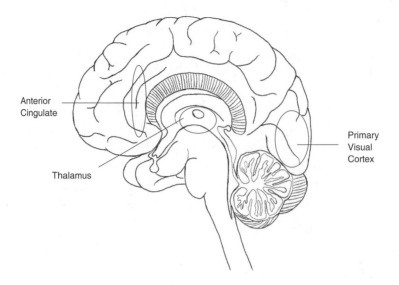

Figure 6.2. Anterior cingulate, thalamus, and primary visual cortex.

tion between persistent auditory hallucinations and width of the third ventricle in patients with schizophrenia. Finally, the older subjects with visual hallucinations were shown to have greater signal hyperintensity in visual pathway white matter tracts (Shedlack et al., 1994). All of these studies concerned small numbers of patients (fewer than 20), which limits the reliability and drawing of firm conclusions. Nevertheless, taking into account the auditory association cortex abnormalities in schizophrenia and the visual pathway abnormalities in idiopathic visual hallucinations, Weiss and Heckers (1999) cautiously suggested that abnormalities in the production of hallucinations may be specific to sensory modality. Research published after their review supports this assertion as discussed in the remainder of this section.

With regard to auditory hallucinations and the STG, several studies have reported a relationship. For instance, Flaum, Andreasen, Swayze, O'Leary, and Alliger (1994) and Rajarethinam, DeQuardo, Nalepa, and Tandon (2000) replicated the finding of Barta et al. (1990) of an inverse correlation between STG volume and auditory hallucinations in patients with schizophrenia. However, in their review of the literature, Stephane, Barton, and Boutros (2001) cautioned that several studies have also been published that failed to find a relationship between STG volume and hallucinations (e.g., Cowell, Kostianovsky, Gur, Turetsky, & Gur, 1996; Havermans et al., 1999). Stewart and Brennan (2005) reported a case study of a neurological patient who developed auditory hallucinations secondary to right temporal lobe damage and resection of right temporal gyri. For example, some months after the resection, when he was in the passenger seat while his wife was driving the car, the patient heard "a deep male voice" telling him to grab the steering wheel and crash the car. On another occasion, he was upset after a disagreement with somebody and reported hearing a voice saying, "Do not take that abuse from anyone; go and sort it out." When he did not act on this, the voice asked, "Why are you not doing what I said?" (Stewart & Brennan, 2005).

Whereas most other studies report volume decreases, Shin et al. (2005) reported increased gray and white matter volumes in 17 hallucinating patients versus 8 nonhallucinating patients. Larger temporal gray and white matter and frontal gray matter volumes were found in hallucinating patients. The authors suggested that increased volumes may be due to patient characteristics because their study included unmedicated first-episode patients. One other study also reported increased total brain volumes in patients with auditory hallucinations compared with patients without (Rossell et al., 2001). Such findings may be consistent with theories of increased connectivity between cerebral regions in hallucinating patients, which are discussed later in this chapter.

Finally, Sumich et al. (2005) assessed positive and negative symptomatology in 25 first-episode patients and its relationship with gray matter volumes in the temporal lobe. The study used linear regression to establish associations between symptom dimensions and stereological measurements of Heschl's gyrus and the planum temporale. Decreased volume in left Heschl's gyrus was associated with hallucinations, whereas increased volume in the left planum temporale was associated with delusions.

In summary, although the results from structural MRI studies are not entirely unequivocal, the vast majority of findings strongly suggest that reduced gray matter volumes in the temporal lobe are associated with auditory hallucinations. In particular, gray matter reductions are seen in the left STG, including the primary auditory cortex. Volume reductions in the prefrontal and cerebellar cortices have also been reported and may be associated with impairments in the monitoring or awareness and volition of internal speech. One study reports increased gray and white matter volumes in the left temporal lobe (Shin et al., 2005). As this study included only first-episode patients in the hallucinating group, this finding may reflect the structural alterations associated with the early phase of schizophrenia.

Two other studies concerning regional abnormalities in brain structure related to hallucinations were designed to answer different questions. First, an MRI study by Shapleske, Rossell, Simmons, David, and Woodruff (2001) addressed whether auditory hallucinations in schizophrenia are the consequence of abnormal cerebral lateralization. Reduced cerebral lateralization of language in schizophrenia has been documented in a substantial number of studies (Sommer, Ramsey, & Kahn, 2001) and has been suggested to underlie hallucinations. Shapleske et al. compared structural brain asymmetry of the planum temporale and sylvian fissure of patients with no history of hallucinations (30 patients) and patients with a strong definitive history of auditory verbal hallucinations (44 patients) in addition to 32 matched normal control subjects. They failed to find differences between the groups on these measures. The only significant finding was a modest correlation between leftward asymmetry of the sylvian fissure and hallucinations within the prominent hallucinator group.

In a second study using MRI, Gaser, Nenadic, Volz, Buchel, and Sauer (2004) evaluated 85 patients with schizophrenia, of whom 29 experienced hallucinations. They found severity of hallucinations to be correlated with volume loss in the left transverse temporal gyrus of Heschl (i.e., primary auditory cortex) and left (inferior) supramarginal gyrus (speech perception area) as well as right dorsolateral prefrontal cortex. The authors suggested that the volume reduction in left hemisphere auditory and speech perception areas may lead to a failure to inhibit and attribute internal speech, as proposed in the verbal self-monitoring hypothesis (McGuire et al., 1995). In addition, the volume loss in the right prefrontal cortex is of interest given the role that has been ascribed to frontotemporal interactions in volitional auditory perception (Frith & Dolan, 1997; Silbersweig & Stern, 1998). That is, impairments in this network could erase the volitional signature of subjective perceptual awareness arising from frontotemporal interactions and thus explain why hallucinations are experienced as involuntary. It is interesting that the right prefrontal area described by Gaser et al. (2004) partially concerns the region homotopic to Broca's area (i.e., the right hemisphere counterpart of Broca's area). Homotopic brain regions are connected to each other by inhibitory callosal tracts. Impairment of one region may thus lead to hyperactivation of the homotopic region. Because the authors applied a novel automated whole-brain morphometric technique in a large group of patients using high-resolution scans, this study might have been more sensitive than previous studies. Their method assesses differences at the voxel level over the entire brain and minimizes user bias because there are no predefined regions that are "drawn" manually by researchers. Another recent MRI study applied a slightly different method, voxel-based morphometry, to study gray matter volume differences between patients with schizophrenia and healthy controls (Neckelmann et al., 2006). Areas of gray matter volume reduction that correlated with hallucinations were found in the left STG, in addition to thalamus and cerebellum. This was a very small study, however, including only 12 patients.

Using magnetic resonance diffusion tensor imaging, Hubl et al. (2004) investigated the integrity of white matter tracts in the brains of schizophrenic patients with and without hallucinations (a healthy comparison group was also included). Diffusion tensor imaging assesses the directionality of water diffusion (anisotropy), which is restricted by boundaries such as white matter fibers. Reduced anisotropy implies a loss of white matter integrity. Hubl et al. found significantly higher anisotropy values in patients with hallucinations compared with both control groups in the lateral temporoparietal section of a major fiber tract known as the arcuate fasciculus. This tract connects language production areas (e.g., Broca's area) with auditory processing and language perception areas. The authors speculated that during inner speech, the apparently stronger connectivity between such areas in patients with hallucinations may lead to dysfunctional coactivation of regions related to the acoustical processing of external stimuli.

Brain Activity During Hallucinations

Functional imaging studies of hallucinations can be divided in two types. First, several studies have attempted to directly measure brain activity occurring during the experience of hallucinations. These studies can be called *activation* studies. Second, a number of studies have presented patients with an auditory stimulation task (involving sounds or speech) while they were experiencing hallucinations. Other studies have compared patients with and without hallucinations on cognitive tasks presumed to measure cognitive processes underlying the disposition to hallucinations. For example, one could test the hypothesis that patients who are prone to hallucinations will show different activation during speech monitoring than patients without this disposition. We discuss evidence from both types of studies but emphasize studies involving schizophrenia patients because most studies have been concerned with this group. However, we also pay attention to imaging studies of visual hallucinations in neurological conditions.

Activation Studies

Some heuristic information comes from studies that measured regional cerebral blood flow (rCBF) during a resting state and then correlated this with clinical features. Gur et al. (1995) observed a positive correlation between the presence of positive symptoms (hallucinations and delusions) and superior temporal lobe metabolism in a group of 42 drug-free schizophrenia patients. Lahti et al. (2006) similarly studied two schizophrenia patient groups of 32 and 23 drug-free subjects, respectively, using PET. Positive symptoms (which included hallucinations) correlated positively with activation in the anterior cingulate cortex and negatively with the hippocampus–parahippocampus. A limitation of these studies is that no direct relationship between brain activity and the occurrence of hallucinations during scanning was investigated. Such studies have also been reported, however, and are reviewed below. In general, patients in these studies were using antipsychotic medication at the time of scanning.

McGuire, Shah, and Murray (1993) scanned 13 patients with SPECT in an episode of their illness during which they experienced hallucinations. They were scanned again on a second occasion when the hallucinations were absent. Compared with the second measurement, hallucination-related activity was observed in language-related areas, especially Broca's area (involved in speech production), although to a lesser extent activity was also found in the anterior cingulate (involved in attentional processes) and in the left temporal cortex (auditory perception and memory processes). In a comparable design, Suzucki, Yuasa, Minabe, Murata, and Kurachi (1993) observed an increase in regional blood flow in the left temporal lobe (auditory association cortex) in 5 hallucinating patients. Silbersweig et al. (1995) reported activation of subcortical structures (bilateral thalamus, right putamen, and caudate), bilateral parahippocampal gyrus, right anterior cingulate, and left orbitofrontal cortex in 5 patients during auditory hallucinations. It is of interest to note the extensive activation of brain regions involved in the experience and regulation of emotion (parahippocampal gyri, cingulate, orbitofrontal cortex). These authors suggested that activity in deep brain structures may generate or modulate hallucinations, whereas particular cortical regions that are activated in individual patients may affect the specific perceptual content of the hallucinations. One of the patients studied by Silbersweig et al. also hallucinated in the visual modality. For these hallucinations, activation was observed in visual areas (lingual, fusiform, and occipital gyri) and in the superior and middle temporal cortex. In the only extensive study of brain activation during visual hallucinations, ffytche et al. (1998) also observed activity in extrastriate visual cortex (ventral occipital lobe). They studied 8 patients with Charles Bonnet syndrome with complex visual hallucinations of color, faces, textures, and objects. Besides activation of visual cortex, the authors observed that the content of the hallucinations reflected the functional specializations of the activated regions. Thus, in patients who hallucinated in color, activity was found in the color center, V4, whereas in the only patient who hallucinated in black and white, the activity was outside this region.

Lennox, Park, Jones, and Morris (1999) imaged a hallucinating schizophrenic patient with fMRI. This patient hallucinated with consequent intervals: For approximately 26 seconds he heard a "voice," followed by a comparable period in which hallucinations were absent. As was the case in the Silbersweig et al. (1995) study, the patient indicated with a key press when he heard the voice, which enabled a within-subject comparison between hallucinatory periods and hallucination-free periods. The results revealed strong activity in the right middle temporal gyrus. In the same way, using the button-press method, Dierks et al. (1999) managed to scan 3 patients with fMRI. Besides recording brain activity during hallucination periods, they also measured brain activity in response to acoustic stimulation (speech in one condition and a tone in another condition). They observed hallucination-related activity in Broca's area, in the temporal gyri, and in the primary auditory cortex (Heschl's gyrus). A striking observation of this study was that the highest correlation of the fMRI signal time course with acoustic stimulation was observed in the transverse gyrus of Heschl, at the same location as the focus of activation during hallucinations. Because inner speech in normal people is not associated with activity in primary auditory cortex (Aleman et al., 2005; McGuire et al., 1996), it could be suggested that it is the abnormal occurrence of activity in primary cortex that lends such inner speech the quality of a real, external sound and hence leads hallucinating patients to infer a nonself perceptual source (Dierks et al., 1999; Frith, 1999). On the other hand, selective attention toward perceiving an expected auditory stimulus can by itself increase activation of primary auditory cortex (Jäncke, Mirzazade, & Shah, 1999), which is consistent with the top-down perceptual expectation account described in chapter 4, this volume.

A study that deserves particular interest was reported by Szechtman, Woody, Bowers, and Nahmias (1998), who compared brain activation using PET scans in highly hypnotizable subjects during different experimental conditions: hearing, imagining, and hallucinating. Eight of these subjects were able to hallucinate under hypnosis (these were termed hallucinators), whereas 6 subjects lacked this ability (control group). A region in the right anterior cingulate cortex was activated in the group of hallucinators when they heard an auditory stimulus and when they hallucinated hearing it, but not when they merely imagined hearing it. The same experimental conditions did not yield such activation in the control group. Szechtman et al. suggested that the anterior cingulate activation "tags" an auditory event as originating from the external world. Thus, in hallucinations, such activation may reflect a mismatch between externally directed attention and internally generated events. They pointed out that the anterior cingulate is thought to be part of an anterior attentional system and is extensively connected with the prefrontal cortex and the auditory association cortex. They also proposed that involvement of rostral anterior cingulate cortex (which has been implicated in modulating affect) may imply that the attention of hallucinators is more affect-laden than that of nonhallucinators, and they speculated that when attention is more affect-laden, self-generation of the expected auditory event is more likely to occur. The findings and interpretation of this study are of considerable interest. A major problem, however, is that no anterior cingulate activation was observed in the hearing versus baseline condition for the nonhallucinators. If anterior cingulate activation tags an auditory event as originating from the external world, one would expect such activation also in the control group.

The activation of primary sensory cortex during hallucinations as reported by Dierks et al. (1999) has not been consistently replicated. In a case study of a woman with schizophrenia who experienced continuous auditory–verbal hallucinations that disappeared when she listened to loud external speech, Bentaleb, Beauregard, Liddle, and Stip (2002) reported activation of left primary auditory cortex in addition to right temporal cortex when the hallucination condition was compared with a condition in which external speech was presented. Lennox, Park, Medley, Morris, and Jones (2000) studied 4 patients with schizophrenia who experienced episodes of hallucination while in the scanner that were compared with periods of rest in the same individuals. Group analysis demonstrated shared areas of activation in right and left STG, left inferior parietal cortex, and left middle frontal gyrus.

Shergill, Brammer, Williams, Murray, and McGuire (2000) used a novel fMRI method to measure brain activity during hallucinations in 6 patients with schizophrenia. They tried to overcome the limitations of the button-press method, in which observed brain activity may be modulated by scanner noise and hallucination-related self-reports (which invoke a metacognitive monitoring of hallucinations). In this random sampling method, a large number of individual scans is acquired at unpredictable intervals in each subject while he or she is intermittently hallucinating. Immediately after each scan, subjects report whether they had been hallucinating at that instant. Neural activity is then compared for the scans when patients are and are not experiencing hallucinations. The results revealed a distributed network of cortical and subcortical activity associated with auditory hallucinations: inferior frontal/insular, anterior cingulate, temporal cortex bilaterally, right thalamus and inferior colliculus, and left hippocampus and parahippocampal cortex. No activation was observed in the primary auditory cortex.

In the most recent neuroimaging study of hallucinations, van de Ven et al. (2005) studied 6 hallucinating schizophrenia patients using fMRI. They applied a data-driven analysis method known as spatial independent component analysis, which does not rely on a predefined model of brain activity. Such analysis methods are capable of separating relevant spatial networks from activity patterns related to other sources such as head movement. The authors observed auditory cortex activity (including Heschl's gyrus) during hallucinations of 3 patients. Thus, not all patients activated primary auditory cortex during auditory hallucinations.

Several authors have asserted that auditory–verbal hallucinations may arise from aberrant activation in the right hemisphere (Olin, 1999). This hypothesis goes back to the influential and controversial book by Julian Jaynes (1976), *The Origin of Consciousness in the Breakdown of the Bicameral Mind*. According to Jaynes, human beings lacked conscious awareness until 1000 BC. In ancient times human behavior was controlled by a "bicameral mind": The left hemisphere was the site for speech, whereas the right hemisphere mediated supernatural voices of gods and demons (i.e., hallucinations). Workings of such a bicameral mind would still be reflected in mental disorders such as schizophrenia. This theory is rather speculative, or as Asaad and Shapiro (1987) put it, "Julian Jaynes' hypothesis makes for interesting reading and stimulates much thought in the receptive reader. It does not, however, adequately explain one of the central mysteries of madness: hallucinations" (p. 5). Nevertheless, the hypothesis of a right hemisphere source for hallucinations deserves investigation, because it is certainly possible that aberrant right hemisphere activation could be misinterpreted by a left hemisphere conscious verbal system (Gazzaniga, 1995), giving rise to verbal hallucinations. However, a quantitative examination of neuroimaging studies of hallucinations found a predominance of left hemisphere activation, and thus failed to support Jaynes's hypothesis of distinct roles of both hemispheres in language versus hallucinations (Aleman, 2001; Sommer, Aleman, & Kahn, 2003). Studies published thereafter (and reviewed above) do not imply a special role for the right hemisphere, although two fMRI studies have suggested a role for reduced language lateralization due to a more bilateral activation (Sommer et al., 2001; E. M. Weiss et al., 2006).

In addition to group studies of patients, a number of interesting case studies contribute to the literature. These studies also suggest that hallucinations in a given modality involve areas that normally process sensory information in that modality. Furthermore, these studies have investigated the degree of modality-specific neural correlates of nonauditory hallucinations. For instance, Izumi, Terao, Ishino, and Nakamura (2002) found evidence (based on SPECT) of differing patterns of rCBF during musical hallucinations (increased rCBF in the bilateral lower frontal area and the bilateral basal ganglia) versus verbal hallucinations (increased rCBF in the left lower temporal area, right lower frontal area, and left basal ganglia) in a 51-year-old patient who had experienced a bilateral hearing impairment but who did not suffer from any psychiatric disorders and whose neurological examinations were all normal. Shergill et al. (2001) studied a patient with both auditory and somatic hallucinations and used neuroimaging (fMRI) to identify differences in brain activation underlying both. This analysis revealed that somatic hallucinations were primarily associated with activation in areas classically associated with tactile processing (e.g., primary somatosensory cortex, posterior parietal cortex, thalamus), whereas auditory hallucinations were primarily associated with activation in a distinct set of brain areas, particularly the right temporal cortex. Kasai, Asada, Yumoto, Takeya, and Matsuda (1999) reported right auditory cortex dysfunction (based on SPECT) during musical hallucinations in a cognitively intact 88-year-old woman. Finally, Mori, Ikeda, Fukuhara, Sugawara, et al. (2006) observed increased rCBF (based on SPECT) in left temporal regions and in the left angular gyrus during musical hallucinations in a patient with Alzheimer's disease when compared with a group of controls matched for sex, age, and cognitive function.

In summary, neuroimaging studies reveal a distributed network of cortical and subcortical areas involved in the experience of hallucinations. Although the exact role of these areas is not clear yet, it could be hypothesized that hallucinations are triggered by activity in subcortical areas, which in turn project to modality-specific association cortex, thereby leading to a conscious perceptual experience. Inappropriate anterior cingulate activation reflects a source monitoring error and erroneously tags internally generated imagery as originating from an external source. The lack of activation in dorsolateral regions is responsible for the accompanying feeling of involuntariness. With respect to auditory hallucinations, some studies observe activity in language-production areas during auditory hallucinations, some studies observe activity in the primary auditory cortex, but all studies report activity in the temporal lobe, more specifically in the middle or superior gyri. For visual hallucinations, activity is observed in secondary visual cortex.

Cognitive Studies

Cognitive neuroimaging studies are those studies that have intended to uncover specific cognitive processing abnormalities or biases associated with the disposition to hallucinate. The simplest studies just present sensory stimuli in the same modality as the hallucinations in patients with hallucinations. The rationale behind these "interference" studies is that a lower activation in perceptual areas in response to external stimulation during periods of hallucination compared with periods without hallucination would suggest that hallucinations and the processing of external auditory stimuli compete for common neurophysiological mechanisms.

Studies by David et al. (1996) and Woodruff et al. (1997) provide evidence that sensory areas may be occupied during the experience of hallucination. These investigators found that auditory association cortex (STG) is less responsive to external auditory stimulation during hallucinations compared with in the absence of hallucinations. They interpreted this as indicative of physiological competition for a common neural substrate by the hallucinations. This finding was confirmed in a study by Plaze et al. (2006) involving 15 patients with schizophrenia with daily auditory hallucinations for at least 3 months prior to the study. The patients were studied with fMRI while they listened to sentences or to silence. Severity of hallucinations correlated negatively with activation in the left STG in the speech minus silence condition, suggesting that auditory hallucinations compete with normal speech for processing sites within the temporal cortex in patients with schizophrenia.

For visual hallucinations, an identical finding has been reported (Howard et al., 1995) with respect to visual cortex and a reduced activation to visual stimuli. Indeed, in their study of visual hallucinations in patients with Charles Bonnet syndrome, ffytche et al. (1998) observed that a tonic increase in activity in the ventral occipital lobe, associated with the occurrence of visual hallucinations, decreased the response to external visual stimulation.

These studies support the notion that hallucinations are not just externalized thoughts but have sensory qualities as they involve processing in perceptual brain areas. Other studies have investigated the hypothesis of defective verbal self-monitoring in schizophrenia patients with auditory–verbal hallucinations. McGuire et al. (1996) studied the neural correlates of inner speech and verbal imagery in schizophrenia patients with and without hallucinations. In the inner speech task, subjects were asked to imagine speaking certain sentences. In the imagery task, they were asked to imagine sentences spoken in another person's voice, which, according to the authors, entails the monitoring of inner speech. For the verbal imagery task, hallucinators showed reduced activation in the left middle temporal gyrus and the rostral supplementary motor area, regions that were strongly activated by both normal subjects and nonhallucinators. The authors concluded that a predisposition to verbal hallucinations in schizophrenia is associated with a failure to activate areas implicated in the normal monitoring of inner speech. In a similar study, Shergill et al. (2003) compared 8 schizophrenia patients with a prominent history of auditory hallucinations with 8 healthy control subjects on a task in which the rate of inner speech was manipulated. When the rate of inner speech generation was increased (by a tempo indication), the patients with schizophrenia showed a relatively attenuated response in the right temporal, parietal, parahippocampal, and cerebellar cortex. Although this study lacked a nonhallucinating patient control group, this result also confirms attenuated engagement of the brain areas implicated in verbal self-monitoring in hallucination-prone patients.

Allen et al. (2005) studied the neural correlates of misattribution of self-generated speech. Although their study was limited to healthy participants, the results are of interest because performance on this task has been shown to be different for patients with and without hallucinations (the latter more easily misattribute self-generated speech to an external source; see chap. 5, this volume). In the fMRI study reported by Allen et al., misattribution of self-generated speech was associated with reduced engagement of the cingulate and prefrontal cortices. The misattribution was triggered by distorting the acoustic quality of words participants had spoken themselves. Thus, this study confirms the role of the anterior cingulate in speech monitoring.

Another fMRI study in healthy subjects that may have implications for the neural basis of cognitive processes that might be involved in hallucinations was reported by Aleman et al. (2005), who investigated whether speech perception areas would activate to inner speech in a performance-based task. The results showed that making metrical stress judgments of visually presented words activates speech perception areas in the left superior temporal sulcus. Subjects were asked to imagine hearing somebody else reading the word out loud. Speech perception areas did not activate in a control condition in which subjects were asked to make semantic judgments of the same visually presented words. This study suggests that auditory–verbal imagery relies in part on phonological processing, involving not only speech production processes but also receptive processes. Aberrant overactivation of the latter could account for the perceptual characteristics of voice hallucinations.

Because hallucinations in psychiatric disorders frequently have strong emotional connotations, it is of interest to investigate activation of emotional brain systems in patients with hallucinations. Sanjuán et al. (2007) reported a study in which brain activation was measured with fMRI in reaction to emotional words spoken by an actor in an emotional tone of voice. The words were based on patients' reports of words they frequently heard.

Activation in response to emotional words was compared with activation for neutral words in 11 patients with schizophrenia and persistent hallucinations. Compared with 10 healthy subjects, the patients showed stronger activation of prefrontal areas, temporal cortex, insula, cingulate, and amygdala. The latter finding is consistent with proposals that hyperactivation of the amygdala may be associated with the affective components of positive symptoms of schizophrenia (Aleman & Kahn, 2005).

Electroencephalographic Studies

The number of electroencephalographic (EEG) studies that have examined electrophysiological correlates of hallucinations is limited. The studies used different methods and obtained different results. Stevens and Livermore (1982) reported power spectra derived from scalp EEGs of schizophrenic patients recorded by telemetry during free behavior on their psychiatric wards. Power spectra from patients' EEG epochs coincident with hallucinations were compared with spectra derived during periods of relatively normal behavior, during performance of specific tasks, and spectra from control subjects. Ramp spectra, characterized by a smooth decline in power from lowest to highest frequencies, appeared in spectra from schizophrenic patients during catatonic episodes, hallucinatory periods, and visual checking. According to the authors, such spectra have previously been found in conjunction with subcortical spike activity of epilepsy and were not found in any control subject.

Sritharan et al. (2005) studied the change in EEG alpha-band coherence between auditory hallucination and nonhallucination states in 7 schizophrenia patients. Whereas there was no significant change in the coherence between Broca's and Wernicke's areas, there was a significant increase in coherence between left and right superior temporal cortices during hallucinations. According to these authors, the increased coherence between the auditory cortices is consistent with the earlier behavioral finding of dysfunction of the interhemispheric pathways between auditory association areas (McKay, Headlam, & Copolov, 2000).

Finally, Lee et al. (2006) used quantitative EEG and low resolution electromagnetic tomography imaging of 25 schizophrenia patients with persistent auditory hallucinations who were compared with 23 patients who were at least 2 years hallucination free. They reported significantly increased beta activity in the left inferior parietal lobule and the left prefrontal cortex. The authors concluded that auditory hallucinations may reflect increased beta frequency oscillations with neural generators localized in speech-related areas.

Using cognitive tasks involving speech production and perception, Heinks-Maldonado et al. (2007) suggested that in their healthy subjects, EEG synchrony preceding speech reflects the action of a forward model system, which dampens auditory responsiveness to self-generated speech. However, this dampening was deficient in schizophrenia patients with hallucinations. Their account is consistent with the theory that was proposed by Frith (1992; see chap. 5, this volume). Hubl, Koenig, Strik, Garcia, and Dierks (2007) investigated the responsiveness of the auditory cortex during hallucinations in patients with schizophrenia by using EEG, specifically the N100 evoked potential in response to auditory stimulation. During hallucinations the N100 amplitudes were smaller, presumably because of a reduced left temporal responsivity. Hubl et al. concluded that their finding indicates competition between auditory stimuli and hallucinations for physiological resources in the primary auditory cortex. Thus, abnormal activation of the primary auditory cortex may thus be a constituent of auditory hallucinations. This result is consistent with several findings from fMRI and PET studies mentioned above.

Toward an Integration of Functional Neuroanatomical Findings

On the basis of the findings discussed above, we propose that a network of brain areas contribute to the hallucinatory experience. Specifically, we propose that this concerns several alterations in activation and functional connectivity of a network of brain regions whose interplay subserves the integral process of conscious perception. Hyperactivation of the secondary sensory cortex (i.e., associative perceptual areas) is central to this network. We concur with Manford and Andermann (1998), who concluded from their review of the neurobiology of complex visual hallucinations that the capacity for generating hallucinations is in the association cortex and that it is released by restricted lesions, a loss of cortico–cortical inputs, and/or alteration of activity via the reticular activating system. The secondary sensory cortex is crucial for perception of objects (Haxby et al., 1994), whereas the primary perceptual cortex is concerned with processing of more low-level aspects of a percept, such as line orientations in the case of primary visual cortex (Tootell et al., 1998) or tones in the case of primary auditory cortex (Formisano et al., 2003).

Compared with the nonhallucinating brain, the hallucinating brain is characterized by stronger input from subcortical centers (especially the thalamus), reduced control by the dorsolateral prefrontal cortex, aberrant activation from emotional attention centers (amygdala, ventral anterior cingulate), and attenuated activation of the dorsal anterior cingulate, which is involved in source and error monitoring. This network of areas can apply to hallucinations in any modality. In the case of visual hallucinations, sensory association cortex must be taken to be the secondary visual cortex (Brodmann's area 19) and adjacent object perception areas such as the fusiform gyrus. In the case of auditory hallucinations, sensory association cortex must be taken to be the secondary auditory area (Brodmann's area 42) and adjacent auditory perception areas such as posterior superior temporal sulcus. The only addition for a specific type of hallucination concerns speech hallucinations as typically reported by schizophrenia patients. For these hallucinations, a hypercoupling between language production areas (Broca's area) and language reception areas (Wernicke's area) could be postulated (see Hoffman et al., 2007).

Summary

For auditory hallucinations, structural as well as functional studies point to a pivotal role for the temporal lobe. For visual hallucinations, activity is observed in the secondary visual cortex. However, it is important to keep in mind that activation studies reveal a distributed network of cortical and subcortical areas involved in the experience of hallucinations. Although neuroimaging studies have shown on numerous occasions that primary and association auditory areas are involved in auditory hallucinations, it is important to note that a number of neuroimaging studies have not necessarily found auditory hallucinations to be associated with brain activation in language production areas or have only found this to be the case in a subgroup of patients (Copolov et al., 2003; Lennox et al., 1999, 2000; Shergill, Brammer, et al., 2000; Silbersweig et al., 1995; van de Ven et al., 2005).

The role of regions such as the thalamus in top-down attention and of the anterior cingulate, which may be involved in monitoring processes, deserves further scrutiny. Abnormal connectivity between speech production and speech perception regions may contribute to the genesis of auditory verbal hallucinations in schizophrenia.

In the next chapter, we attempt to integrate proposals regarding cognitive processes involved in hallucinations as described in chapters 4 and 5 with neurobiological findings discussed in the current chapter.

CHAPTER HIGHLIGHTS

- Four neurotransmitters have been associated with hallucinations: dopamine, acetylcholine, serotonin, and glutamate. Dopamine is involved in hallucinations in schizophrenia and drug-induced hallucinations in Parkinson's disease, acetylcholine in hallucinations in the dementias, and serotonin and glutamate in a variety of drug-induced hallucinations.
- Studies of structural brain volumes suggest that reduced gray matter volumes in the temporal lobe are associated with auditory hallucinations.
- Functional neuroimaging studies have shown consistently the involvement of associative sensory areas. Moreover, the hallu-

cinating brain may be characterized by stronger input from sub-cortical centers (especially the thalamus), reduced control by the dorsolateral prefrontal cortex, aberrant activation from emotional attention centers (e.g., amygdala), and attenuated activation of the dorsal anterior cingulate, which is involved in source and error monitoring.

7

TOWARD A COMPREHENSIVE MODEL

As the chapters in this book show, although much is known about hallucinations, a comprehensive and empirically validated account remains elusive. In this chapter, we propose a multidimensional and multifactorial model of hallucinations, one that incorporates the identified cognitive and neural alterations. A comprehensive model should address the following important features of hallucinations:

- Internally generated information is not attributed to an internal source (but rather to an external or nonself source).
- Hallucinations appear unbidden; the experiencer has little or no control over them.
- Hallucinations clearly have sensory characteristics; the experiencer has the (initial) conviction that he or she receives information through the senses.
- There is an emotional component to hallucinations in many cases.

THE MODEL

The model we present is not meant to be the final word about hallucinations, but it is intended to enhance understanding of current research findings and to serve as a guide for future research. In particular, the model integrates proposals by Manford and Andermann (1998), Behrendt and Young (2004), Bentall (1990), Grossberg (2000), and Hoffman and McGlashan (2006). Parts of the model are also consistent with hypotheses by Frith (1992) and Collerton, Perry, and McKeith (2005).

In short, although the model presumes an integrated network of cognitive processes that may contribute to perceptual experience, four different routes are proposed that may result in a hallucination: (a) release phenomena due to lesions in sensory pathways or the arousal system (brain stem, thalamus); (b) irritative processes acting on cortical centers that integrate perceptual information; (c) unconstrained activation of the attentional spotlight; and (d) a cognitive route with key roles for affective state, top-down factors, and source/self-monitoring. The first two are physiological routes and account for hallucinations of a primarily neurological origin. We maintain that most hallucinations arise from the third or fourth mechanism (or a combination of these). This is certainly the case for drug-induced hallucinations, psychotic hallucinations, and hallucinatory experiences in normal subjects.

Release Phenomena

It is generally thought that disturbed visual input may cause hallucinations by means of an abnormal release of central processing. For example, complex visual hallucinations have been described as a result of optic nerve lesions, chronic glaucoma, macular disease, and lesions of the occipital cortex. Manford and Andermann (1998) noted, however, that the level at which the release occurs is unclear. The implication of primary and sensory cortices seems straightforward, but it should be noted that changes have also been observed in subcortical brain areas (e.g., lateral geniculate nucleus) in patients with optic nerve lesions. This implies that involvement of the third mechanism of hallucinations (unconstrained activation of attentional spotlight mediated by reticular thalamic nucleus) may well be possible in some types of release hallucinations. With regard to complex visual hallucinations, Manford and Andermann concluded that the capacity for generating hallucinations may be located in the association cortex and that it is released by restricted lesions, a loss of cortico–cortical inputs, and alteration of activity via the reticular activating system. In our model, release hallucinations would therefore arise from damage to the component sensory input or its connecting pathway to sensory experience.

Irritative Processes

Hallucinations caused by spontaneous activation of sensory cortical areas have been primarily described in epilepsy. On the basis of intracranial electroencephalographic (EEG) recordings and direct stimulation experiments, it has been shown that pathological excitation of visual cortical areas induces such hallucinations (Penfield & Perot, 1963; Salanova, Andermann, Olivier, Rasmussen, & Quesney, 1992). The fact that focal cortical resections can result in complete remission of epileptic hallucinations supports the notion that these hallucinations cannot be attributed to a release phenomenon. Such hallucinations can also arise from damage to primary sensory cortices, such as through metabolic alterations causing irritation of neighboring tissue. According to our model, irritative processes would be confined to aberrant activation of the module sensory experience.

Attentional Spotlight

In an influential hypothesis, Crick (1984) proposed that the thalamic reticular nucleus (TRN) acts as a searchlight to guide attention to certain features of the environment and thereby intensifies processing of these features. The thalamus is acknowledged as one of three important nodes in a network underlying selective attention that comprises the prefrontal cortex, the parietal cortex, and the thalamus (Kastner & Ungerleider, 2000). Direct evidence for a role of the TRN in guiding attention and enhancing perception has been reported in macaque monkeys (McAlonan, Cavanaugh, & Wurtz, 2006). The TRN is thought to facilitate sensory processing by facilitating detection and discrimination through the initiation of *burst-firing* (when a population of neurons fires with a high-frequency burst in contrast to a continuous low-frequency baseline firing) in the lateral geniculate nucleus (LGN). Although the encoding of an externally presented stimulus becomes distorted during such burst-firing (Guido, Lu, Vaughan, Godwin, & Sherman, 1995), the background noise decreases significantly, thereby enhancing signal detectability. Sherman (2001) argued that such bursts act as a wake-up call signaling environmental change to the cortex.

We propose that activation of the TRN in the absence of sensory input could explain the involuntary character of hallucinations. Such activation is possible via connections from the prefrontal cortex to the TRN (Zikopoulos & Barbas, 2006), via feedback from sensory association cortex, and via neurotransmitters such as dopamine and acetylcholine (Behrendt & Young, 2004). Our hypothesis is simple: Strong activation of the attentional spotlight yields a sensory experience. Normally, this is triggered by sensory input (the TRN is strongly connected to sensory cortex), resulting in a real percept that is correctly attributed to an external source. In some cases, however, the attentional spotlight can be strongly activated in the absence of sensory input, which will result in hallucinations. Thus, spontaneous overactivation of this area could lead to the emergence of hallucinations (Behrendt & Young, 2004; Manford & Andermann, 1998). This could occur as a consequence of neurotransmitter abnormalities (acetylcholine and dopamine modulate this system), impairment of sensory afferents, or aberrant input from frontal areas. Involvement of the reticular thalamic system is also of relevance to hypnagogic and hypnopompic hallucinations and may explain why complex visual hallucinations occur more frequently in drowsy states (Manford & Andermann, 1998). Paradoxical sleep states have been associated with increased subcortical release of dopamine, presynaptic inhibition of thalamic relay nuclei, and serotonergic disinhibition (Gottesman, 2004).

Cognitive Route

The present model assumes that hallucinations may arise from a fourth, more cognitive route, in which emotion, top-down perceptual mechanisms, and metacognitive functions (e.g., source/self-monitoring) all play a decisive role. This route is especially relevant for hallucinations in normal people and for psychotic hallucinations (e.g., in patients with schizophrenia and psychotic depression). The idea here is that an affective state (more specifically, stress and anxiety) negatively influences (i.e., perturbs) monitoring systems, resulting in external misattributions of internally generated events, but can also influence top-down factors such as perceptual expectations. This is indicated in Figure 7.1 by arrows from "Emotion and Motivation" toward "Monitoring" and toward "Top-Down Factors." As discussed in chapter 2, this volume, there is evidence that emotional factors can modulate verbal self-monitoring (Johns et al., 2001; Seal, Crowe, & Cheung, 1997) and source monitoring (Baker & Morrison, 1998; Larøi, Marczewski, & Van der Linden, 2004). Evidence that the affective state can influence perception and imagery comes from neuroimaging studies showing that amygdala activation in response to emotional stimuli can boost activation of perceptual areas (Dolan, 2002). Thus, an affective state can modulate and prime perception through top-down factors. Furthermore, a functional magnetic resonance imaging (fMRI) study has reported hyperactivation of the amygdala in (nonclinical) psychosis-prone individuals, which included hallucinatory experiences (Mohanty et al., 2005). This is consistent with Aleman and Kahn's (2005) proposal that increased amygdala activation may be associated with the positive symptoms of schizophrenia (i.e., hallucinations and delusions), whereas amygdala impairment may contribute to negative symptoms (e.g., affective flattening).

The top-down factors' subsystem in the model refers to the influence of prior knowledge, perceptual expectations, and attention on perception (as discussed in chap. 4, this volume). In Figure 7.1, excessive activation of such top-down factors can "push" images to the right within the Sensory Experience box. As a result, images will acquire stronger sensory and reality characteristics due to excessive top-down modulation and will therefore be more easily confused with bottom-up percepts. Evidence that top-down attention can activate primary cortical areas is provided in several fMRI studies of visual and auditory perception (Chawla, Rees, & Friston, 1999; Woldorff et al., 1993). Activation of the thalamus in top-down attention has also been reported in neuroimaging studies. Connections from the lateral prefrontal

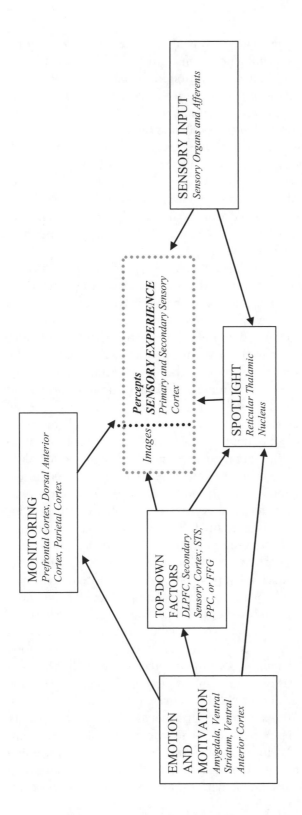

Figure 7.1. The role of emotion and motivation in cognitive processes. DLPFC = dorsolateral prefrontal cortex; STS = superior temporal sulcus; PPC = posterior parietal cortex; FFG = fusiform gyrus.

cortex to the thalamus may mediate top-down influences in normal circumstances, in which bottom-up influences constrain the LGN activation by inputs to the reticular nucleus. Hyperactivation in the lateral prefrontal cortex (which could be due to disinhibition by defective connections) or from emotion regulation areas in the orbitofrontal cortex to the reticular nucleus could lead to diminished control of the LGN and hence result in spontaneous burst activity affecting projections to the sensory association cortex. Such projections have been described by Zikopoulos and Barbas (2006), who suggested that these frontal regions target sensory tiers of the TRN to select relevant and motivationally significant signals. Alternatively, increased input into perceptual areas (e.g., Wernicke's area) from frontal areas (e.g., Broca's area) may affect the reticular nucleus via corticothalamic projections originating in the sensory association cortex.

As the reader may have noted, this mechanism of top-down influences largely overlaps with the mechanism of the attentional spotlight described above. In fact, it concerns a final common pathway (involving the TRN and the sensory association cortex) with different causative agents: top-down factors such as expectations generated in prefrontal regions versus direct influences (e.g., through acetylcholine) in the third route (i.e., activation of the attentional spotlight) described above. It is also possible that top-down influences act without any intervention from the thalamus. Future studies should examine this in more detail. Consistent with the top-down approach, neural network simulations have also shown that a mechanism of exuberant top-down processing can lead to the spontaneous activation of perceptual representations in the absence of sensory input (Hoffman & McGlashan, 2006).

The monitoring subsystem in the model refers to the metacognitive processes discussed in chapter 5 in which the cognitive system makes a decision regarding the source of perceptual events, that is, whether they are internally generated or externally presented. These two types of perceptual representation (images vs. bottom-up percepts) are shown in the Sensory Experience box in Figure 7.1. The vertical line between images and percepts denotes the criterion for classifying a perceptual event as internally generated imagery versus externally presented sensory information. The gradient by which some experience is likely to be classified as an image or as a bottom-up percept is strongly affected by two factors: vividness and sense of reality (Aggernæs, 1994; M. K. Johnson & Raye, 1981). *Vividness* refers to sensory, semantic, and contextual details: A bottom-up percept is generally clear and rich in such details, whereas images are much fainter (Kosslyn, 1994). The same holds for a sense of reality, which is of course influenced by vividness but can also be influenced by expectations and metacognitive factors. Faulty monitoring of one's mental processes could shift the criterion line to the left, thereby resulting in a misclassification of certain imagery experiences as being percepts originating from the outside. It is doubtful whether monitoring errors on their own can cause hallucinations, as it is unclear how thought, inner speech, or retrieved memories can be transformed into experiences with perceptual qualities just by virtue of their misattribution to an external origin (Behrendt & Young, 2004). However, when they interact with overactive top-down systems, such biases could contribute to erroneous perceptual decision making. Indeed, hallucinations in schizophrenia have been shown to be associated with self-monitoring errors, although these have not been consistently and exclusively linked to hallucinations (Ford & Mathalon, 2005). With regard to the neural basis of monitoring, the anterior cingulate cortex has been appointed a pivotal role (Frith, 1992), which has been confirmed by neuroimaging studies (Allen et al., 2005, 2007). The premotor cortex and superior temporal gyrus (in the case of verbal material) have also been implied in self-monitoring (McGuire et al., 1996).

Summary

In terms of the components delineated in the model (see Figure 7.1), our aim is to understand the occurrence of sensory experience in the absence of a corresponding sensory input. Normally, this is only possible via imagery, which by definition is the mental re-creation of a sensory experience. However, imagery has a willful component to it, and the perceptual characteristics of mental images are distinct from bottom-up percepts in that they are less clear and less vivid, contain fewer contextual details, and do not feel real (i.e., do not exist independent of one's own mental activity). Thus, the sensory experience that is activated by mental imagery is rather faint and could better be termed as being a pseudosensory experience. We have therefore located these types of images to the left side of the dotted line in the Sensory Experience box (see Figure 7.1), which depicts both a gradient in perceptual clarity and a gradient in terms of a sense of reality. In normal circumstances, only actual sensory input or the process of imagery can access and activate perceptual codes in the brain.

Monitoring centers "know" whether a sensory experience is externally presented or internally generated, because the former depends on activation of the bottom-up route and the latter depends on the top-down route. Only when an anomaly occurs can other types of internally generated perceptions emerge. Specifically, this can occur via three routes. First, imagery can be bypassed by aberrant hyperexcitation of attentional processes. These normally have limited access to perceptual codes, but activation of the sensory thalamic reticular system can fully activate such codes. Bottom-up information (i.e., input from sensory organs) is normally crucial for such activation to occur, but under certain circumstances these can be activated in the absence of such sensory input. This may involve neurotransmitter abnormalities (acetylcholine and dopamine modulate this system), impairment of sensory afferents, or aberrant input from frontal areas. This route is consistent with the irritation model. The second route consists of disinhibition of perceptual areas via impairment of connections or as a consequence of damage to neighboring tissue. This route is consistent with the perceptual release model. Both could be termed low-level routes and are characteristic of most neurological and pharmacological hallucinations. In terms of the model, this consists of hyperactivation of the perceptual attention component or impairment of the sensory input component. The third and final route is of a higher order, cognitive route that does not bypass imagery but that manipulates imagery processes. Affective states (particularly hyperarousal due to stress) can trigger internally oriented mental processes, such as absorption and imagery. This calls on attentional resources that can hence not be allocated to context and reality discrimination processing. Together with an external attribution bias or self-monitoring error (which may be motivationally enhanced by the ego-hostile content of the subjects' thoughts), this can lead to the shift from pseudoperception (or imagery) to perception. Thus, this route involves the emotion and motivation, top-down factors, and monitoring components. We would furthermore suggest that the exuberance of top-down factors plays a decisive role in this route.

In terms of neurological and pharmacological hallucinations, processes depicted in the right side of Figure 7.1 will be mainly implicated, whereas in psychotic hallucinations, processes depicted in the left side of the figure will be more strongly implicated. For all types of hallucinations, however, factors in the middle of the figure are most probably involved: attentional spotlight, top-down factors, and monitoring errors (e.g., external attribution). In neurological and pharmacological hallucinations, the latter might primarily be the consequence of the experience of hallucinations (i.e., these factors may be altered as a result of repeated experiences of hallucinations), whereas in psychiatric hallucinations, top-down and monitoring factors may play an important role in the emergence of the hallucinations (i.e., they may already be present before the generation of hallucinations).

PREDICTIONS

The present model elicits several hypotheses. First, it predicts differential roles of brain areas: the lateral prefrontal cortex for top-down factors, the anterior cingulate and premotor cortex for monitoring processes, the thalamus for the attentional spotlight, and the sensory association cortex for imagery. Research into the time course of regional activation during hallucinations would test hypotheses regarding the various brain networks involved in different types of hallucinations. For example, in drug-induced hallucinations, activation of the thalamus would be expected before activation of the sensory association cortex or more frontal areas, whereas in schizophrenic hallucinations, prefrontal activation might precede activation of thalamic and perceptual areas. Furthermore, the model predicts stronger effects of expectations in shaping perception in hallucinators compared with nonhallucinators. Cognitive tasks of perception in which expectations are manipulated could be devised to test this prediction in hallucination-prone compared with non-hallucination-prone individuals. It would also be of interest to study people in different affective states (which could be experimentally induced) to see whether this affects top-down processing and reports of detecting stimuli that were not actually presented. The prediction that neurotransmitters such as dopamine and acetylcholine will primarily affect the attentional spotlight can also be tested using pharmacological agents affecting dopaminergic or cholinergic systems in an fMRI study that modulates top-down perceptual attention.

One important challenge for future studies will be to delineate more precisely the mechanisms through which stored perceptual representations activate vivid sensory qualities into conscious awareness, in the absence of corresponding sensory input, and which factors are necessary and sufficient for hallucinations to occur. Another significant challenge is related to explaining why hallucinations in different modalities and with different contents arise in different clinical disorders and in different contexts. Why do auditory hallucinations and personally salient and emotionally charged hallucinations dominate in psychotic patients, whereas visual hallucinations and less personally salient and less emotionally charged hallucinations seem to dominate in neurological disorders? Why are other modalities (olfactory, tactile, somatic, etc.) less represented in the majority of clinical disorders? In terms of contexts, why were visual hallucinations and hallucinations with religious content more common in medieval Europe, whereas present-day European patients seem to have more auditory hallucinations and with less religious content? Why do Western (e.g., U.K.) patients commonly report, for example, auditory hallucinations that include running commentaries and instructions, whereas this is not the case for some non-Western patients (e.g., Saudi Arabia) whose auditory hallucinations often include superstitious and religious themes? There are no simple answers to these questions, and there has not been enough research to help us even begin to answer them. Nonetheless, these questions merit serious consideration.

Two conclusions can be drawn from some of the research presented in this book looking at variations (in terms of hallucination content and hallucination modalities) across clinical disorders and along historical and cultural lines. First, hallucinations seem to be shaped by the immediate environment and by the cultural values of those experiencing them. Second, hallucinations may be viewed as a form of personal expression, that is, as the expression of the person's concerns, feelings, past experiences, thoughts, and so on. Thus, the psychotic patient may have a greater need to express a range of thoughts, feelings, and concerns, and (auditory) hallucination is the more apt manner of expressing them. In contrast, in the neurological patient the need to express these personal concerns is not as marked, or it may be that the patient is able to express these personal concerns through other means and not necessarily via (visual) hallucinations.

That psychotic patients tend to express auditory hallucinations might be related to the fact that these personal concerns are more readily expressed in this modality; at the same time, we must not forget that visual hallucinations are also present and that these types of hallucinations are therefore also able to express these concerns. This would also help explain why olfactory, tactile, and somatic modalities are less represented in clinical disorders in general, and specifically in psychotic patients—that is, that the range and (emotional) depth of personal concerns are less readily expressed via these modalities. However, it might also be possible that the preponderance of auditory–verbal hallucinations in schizophrenia and related psychotic disorders is mainly due to neurobiological factors, such as a combination of certain genetic polymorphisms that disorganizes the attentional and language systems, and input to these systems from emotional systems.

The dominance of visual hallucinations in neurological patients may be a more direct reflection of the clinical disorder itself, especially relating to underlying neurophysiological mechanisms such as release phenomena due to lesions in sensory pathways or the arousal system and/or irritative processes acting on cortical centers. These ideas are clearly speculative and therefore need to be examined and eventually challenged by future research.

CONCLUSION

In sum, the hallucination riddle is far from being fully solved. There is still some ways to go before we are able to better understand this phenomenon. However, significant progress has been made in pinpointing the cognitive processes and brain systems involved in hallucinations. We are confident that a model incorporating multiple factors, including perceptual, cognitive, emotional, and metacognitive processes, acknowledges the complexity of hallucinations but at the same time can account for a wide range of published research findings. Indeed, such a model will provide a valuable heuristic for further research and ultimately provide important information to develop more effective treatment schemes for hallucinations. The next chapter examines treatment strategies.

CHAPTER HIGHLIGHTS

Four different routes (or a combination of these) are proposed that may result in a hallucination:

- release phenomena due to lesions in sensory pathways or the arousal system (brain stem, thalamus);

- irritative processes acting on cortical centers that integrate perceptual information;
- unconstrained activation of attentional processing that drives perceptual areas; and
- a cognitive route with key roles for affective state, top-down factors, and source/self-monitoring.

8

TREATMENT OF HALLUCINATIONS

A number of strategies can be used in the treatment of hallucinations. Important to underline here is that improvement mainly refers to a reduction in the distress a hallucination causes and the frequency of its occurrence, not simply its absence or disappearance. Therefore, when assessing treatment efficacy, it is important to use assessment strategies that address these aspects. For more information concerning the principal assessment strategies available for hallucinations, see the Appendix. It is also important to note that the treatment strategies presented in this chapter (with only a few exceptions) relate to the management of auditory hallucinations; in other words, few strategies have been developed for nonauditory hallucinations.

In this chapter, pharmacological treatments are briefly presented, followed by more detailed presentations of repeated transcranial magnetic stimulation, coping strategies, appraisals, metacognitive beliefs, psychoeducation (and in particular, normalization), cognitive behavior therapy (CBT; individual treatment and in groups), hallucinations-focused integrative treatment, and self-help. We end the chapter by addressing specific issues, including the importance of treating co-occurring psychopathological conditions and associated problems, trauma, the role of imagery, command hallucinations, the role of individuals' personal history, and positive or adaptive hallucinations.

Note that many of the distinctions used in the chapter are made for practical reasons, so there might be considerable overlap between sections and treatment strategies. For instance, interventions focusing on metacognitive beliefs or appraisals often also use strategies from CBT and/or psychoeducation. Also, for example, hallucinations-focused integrative treatment contains CBT, psychoeducation, coping training, and antipsychotic medication. An exhaustive review of the numerous intervention strategies that are available for treating hallucinations is beyond the scope of this chapter. As a result, some strategies may have been left out. Similarly, owing to lack of space, practical aspects of the treatment schemes have not been detailed. For more practical information, the reader is asked to consult the cited references.

MEDICATION

Although pharmacotherapy is largely effective in treating acute psychosis and in preventing the frequency of relapse, a significant proportion of patients continue to experience symptoms. For instance, between 10% and 60% of patients who adhere to drug treatment continue to experience psychotic symptoms (Curson, Patel, Liddle, & Barnes, 1988; Lindenmayer, 2000), and there is evidence that hallucinations can persist in 25% to 50% of patients even after adequate levels of medication have been prescribed (Pantelis & Barnes, 1996). Furthermore, medication noncompliance continues to present a particular problem. Cramer and Rosenheck (1998) found that, depending on the design adopted and the number of patients evaluated, nonadherence rates (to medication) in psychiatric patients ranged from 24% to 90%, with a mean nonadherence rate of around 60%. In one meta-analysis of studies examining the prevalence of medication nonadherence in patients with schizophrenia, Lacro, Dunn, Dolder, Leckband, and Jeste (2002) found a mean rate of nonadherence of 41% in studies with a strict set of study inclusion criteria and a 50% mean rate of nonadherence in studies with a stricter set of inclusion criteria. In another meta-analysis, the overall weighted mean rate of nonadherence (to both medication and scheduled appointments) was 26% (Nosé, Barbui, & Tansella, 2003). Also, although the arrival of atypical antipsychotic medication has been important in improving treatment for psychotic patients, compared with typical antipsychotic medication, they have been shown to be more efficient in the treatment of the negative symptoms of schizophrenia and seem to cause fewer unwanted extrapyramidal effects (Stip, 2000) and therefore do not necessarily show significantly greater efficacy for positive psychotic symptoms. Finally, antipsychotic drugs are effective for treating psychosis on the whole or for related conditions, but their specific effects for the treatment of hallucinations are poorly understood.

In addition to these general limitations of pharmacotherapy, attention is particularly warranted when considering treating hallucinations in nonadult populations (i.e., children and adolescents) and older (including dementia) populations. For instance, treating hallucinations in children and adolescents with pharmacotherapy should be questioned, especially because psychotic symptoms in many of these children discontinue without any medications (for a review, see Larøi, Van der Linden, & Goëb, 2006). Also, particular attention should be made when treating hallucinations in dementia patients. This issue is discussed in more detail at the end of the chapter, where particular populations are presented (i.e., dementia and neurological populations).

TRANSCRANIAL MAGNETIC STIMULATION

Transcranial magnetic stimulation (TMS), in particular repetitive TMS (rTMS), has been proposed as a treatment for hallucinations in schizophrenia. In TMS, a time-varying magnetic field is generated by a current pulse through a stimulator coil placed over a certain scalp position. The rapid rise and fall of the magnetic field induces a flow of current in the underlying brain tissue (diameter of approximately 2 to 3 centimeters), resulting in membrane depolarization and neural activation (Barker, 1991; Hallett, 2000). In particular, 1-Hz (or slow) rTMS is usually used in the context of hallucination treatment because it reduces brain excitability (for a review, see Hoffman & Cavus, 2002), in contrast to fast rTMS (>5 Hz; e.g., used in depression treatment), which enhances brain excitability. The idea here is that where rTMS coils are placed, these brain areas (e.g., speech perception areas) will be deactivated.

Aleman, Sommer, and Kahn (2007) recently performed a meta-analysis of studies using rTMS as a treatment for auditory hallucinations. A total of 15 studies were identified that reported empirical data regarding rTMS treatment of auditory hallucinations. Of these, 10 studies fulfilled inclusion criteria and were included in the treatment effect analysis. The total sample size for the 10 studies was 216. Most studies used highly similar techniques and treatment settings. That is, active rTMS was placed over the left temporoparietal cortex (the left temporoparietal cortex is generally identified as the position halfway between the T3 and P3 electrode positions of the International 10–20 System of Electrode Placement, following Hoffman et al., 2003), between 80% and 100% motor threshold is commonly used, and all studies used a frequency of 1 Hz.[1] All studies included a sham rTMS control condition or control group. In sham rTMS, the coil is rotated by 90 degrees, so the magnetic field does not enter the brain. Length of stimulation varied

---

[1]*Motor threshold* refers to the strength of the stimulus provided, which is the percentage of the total machine output that is required to produce movement of thumb or fingers.

between studies but was mainly between 15 and 20 minutes. Finally, the length of treatment varied from 4 days to 10 days. Results revealed a mean standardized gain effect size of .76, providing support for the efficacy of this treatment in reducing the severity of auditory hallucinations in schizophrenia. In contrast to the effects obtained on hallucinations, rTMS did not improve positive symptoms in general. Thus, the observed effect was specific to auditory hallucinations. With regard to the duration of the treatment, Aleman et al. (2007) did not observe larger effect sizes in studies that included more treatment sessions.

However, a number of issues remain. First, although the effect sizes in Aleman et al. (2007) went in a positive direction, some studies did not clearly support the therapeutic efficacy of rTMS on hallucinations (e.g., Fitzgerald et al., 2005; Lee et al., 2005; McIntosh et al., 2004; G. Saba et al., 2006). Future studies should investigate why certain patients respond to rTMS treatment, whereas others do not seem to improve. Indeed, there is evidence of individual differences regarding treatment effects. For instance, d'Alfonso et al. (2002) observed individual differences in the onset of the improvement. Duration of treatment effects may vary widely. Hoffman et al. (2003) reported that 52% of patients maintained improvement for at least 15 weeks.

The diverging findings might be related to individual variations in terms of the anatomical–functional locus of hallucination activity and/or speech processing areas. All studies stimulate left temporoparietal areas in rTMS, but hallucinations involve a much larger network (for a detailed discussion, see chap. 6, this volume). For instance, although studies have suggested the involvement of the left temporal cortex (e.g., Dierks et al., 1999), other studies have implicated the right temporal/temporoparietal cortex (e.g., Shergill, Brammer, Williams, Murray, & McGuire, 2000; Lennox, Park, Jones, & Morris, 1999) as well as other brain regions (e.g., Shergill, Brammer, et al., 2000; Silbersweig et al., 1995). In these patients, rTMS directed at the left (or contralateral) hemisphere may be less effective. Thus, to enhance efficacy, brain imaging methods might be applied to determine the functional locus of hallucination activity individually and to target these regions of interest with rTMS using a neuronavigator. A study by Langgut, Zowe, Spiessl, and Hajak (2006) used imaging-guided rTMS in a patient with medication-resistant auditory hallucinations to target exactly the area of excessive neuronal activity within the temporoparietal cortex. The authors reported that the intrusiveness, intensity, and frequency of the patient's hallucinations improved during the first 2 weeks of rTMS treatment. However, follow-up investigations after 2 and 5 weeks revealed an attenuation of this initially increased activity.

Three other studies have used functional magnetic resonance imaging (fMRI) to localize brain activity during hallucinations and target the active areas using rTMS. Jadri et al. (2007) reported the case of an 11-year-old boy with treatment-resistant childhood onset schizophrenia and auditory verbal hallucinations. When fMRI-guided rTMS over the left temporoparietal cortex was used, there was an improvement of 47% on the Auditory Hallucinations Rating Scale (Hoffman et al., 2003), and this improvement was also observed clinically—the boy was even able to attend school again. Hoffman et al. (2007) used fMRI-guided rTMS in 16 schizophrenia patients with resistant hallucinations and reported that delivering rTMS to left temporoparietal sites in Wernicke's area and the adjacent supramarginal gyrus was accompanied by a greater rate of auditory–verbal hallucination improvement compared with sham stimulation and rTMS delivered to anterior temporal sites. Finally, Sommer et al. (2007) compared the efficacy of fMRI-guided rTMS to conventional positioning of the coil using the International 10–20 system. Both groups improved to an equal extent. Additional research is needed to establish whether fMRI guidance yields better results. A limitation of fMRI guidance is that, to obtain reliable activation patterns, patients need to hallucinate with several intervals in the scanner; that is, activation during hallucinations and during epochs without hallucinations should be compared. The problem here is that most patients do not hallucinate with such intervals of several minutes altered by nonhallucination periods.

Also, little is known as to which cognitive mechanisms are being altered in effective rTMS treatment. In the only study to date to have examined this issue, Brunelin, Poulet, et al. (2006) examined cognitive mechanisms and found that effective rTMS treatment coincided with improvements in source monitoring functioning, which has been argued to be an important mechanism in hallucinations (see chap. 5, this volume). However, no other studies have examined other cognitive mechanisms underlying effective rTMS treatment in (auditory) hallucinations.

In a number of studies, assessment of hallucinations involves a combination of many hallucination characteristics (using a so-called composite score) so that when improvement is observed, this improvement may be related to several characteristics (e.g., frequency, loudness, content, number of voices, emotional distress, intensity) or to a combination of these. For instance, one widely used scale in rTMS studies is the Auditory Hallucinations Rating Scale (Hoffman et al., 2003), which is a seven-item scale measuring frequency, reality, loudness, number of voices, length, attentional salience, and distress level. Most studies report composite scores to measure improvement, making it difficult to say exactly which aspects of hallucinations are improved after rTMS treatment. However, in the few studies that do attempt to identify which hallucination characteristics are modified after rTMS treatment, improvement is usually attributed to reductions in hallucination frequency (Hoffman et al., 2005).

Interactions may occur between type of medication and effectiveness of rTMS. d'Alfonso et al. (2002) suggested that antipsychotic medication could influence rTMS efficacy. In particular, they found that although all 7 patients on clozapine showed improvement, the single patient on olanzapine showed worsening. In Hoffman et al. (2000), not all patients showed robust improvements after active rTMS, and one factor contributing to this variable response was suggested to be concurrent anticonvulsant drug treatment, which seemed to reduce rTMS effects. Also, symptoms prompting administration of anticonvulsant drugs (e.g., mood liability) were suggested to be negative predictors of rTMS response. Studies examining the effects of rTMS have also exclusively focused on auditory hallucinations and have not looked at the effects of rTMS in hallucinations from other modalities. One would presume that there is no change in these (i.e., nonauditory) hallucinations because the brain area stimulated in typical rTMS studies is less pertinent.

Another issue that needs further investigation is possible side effects related to rTMS treatment. A magnetic resonance imaging study indicated no structural brain changes in humans after high-dose rTMS (Niehaus, Hoffman, Grosse, Roricht, & Meyer, 2000), and Hoffman et al. (2003) did not find any indication of negative effects of active rTMS on cognition. However, more studies are needed that examine possible side effects in the context of rTMS treatment. It is important to note that the majority of rTMS studies include treatment-resistant patients. Therefore, this type of intervention must be viewed as a last-resort treatment—that is, in cases in which more conventional treatment schemes (e.g., antipsychotic medication, psychological interventions, psychosocial interventions, electroconvulsive therapy) have not been found to be effective in patients.

One study (Schreiber et al., 2002), not included in Aleman et al.'s (2007) meta-analysis because it is a case study, deserves mention because it is the only study to examine the efficacy of rTMS for command hallucinations. A schizophrenic patient with a 20-year history of auditory command hallucinations, responding poorly to conventional and novel neuroleptics, was treated with fast (10 Hz) rTMS administered to the right dorsolateral prefrontal cortex.[2] After 20 rTMS treatments, results showed that both the Brief Psychiatric Rating Scale and the Positive and Negative Syndrome Scale (PANSS; described in the Appendix) scores improved, but changes in other ratings scales (assessing depression, general mental state, sleep) were minor and nonsignificant. Important to note is that there were no changes in the content, intensity, and frequency of hallucinations as a result of rTMS treatment. At follow-up 6 weeks after the rTMS treatment ended, all scores (apart from PANSS) returned to pre-rTMS treatment baseline.

COPING STRATEGIES

Studies have shown that patients with schizophrenia make effortful attempts to overcome or cope with persistent positive symptoms such as hallu-

---

[2]This area was stimulated following documentation of right hypofrontality in pretreatment single photon emission computed tomography.

cinations. For instance, 60% to 90% of hallucinating schizophrenia patients use specific coping strategies (Carter, Mackinnon, & Copolov, 1996; Farhall & Gehrbe, 1997; Nayani & David, 1996; O'Sullivan, 1994). *Coping* has been defined as "constantly changing cognitive and behavioral efforts to manage particular external and/or internal demands that are appraised as taxing or exceeding the resources of the person" (Lazarus & Folkman, 1984, p. 141). Self-initiated self-coping is common in psychosis, indicating that individuals who feel overwhelmed by their psychotic experiences mobilize coping defenses. It has been shown that the degree of coping mobilized by the person is associated with severity of the psychotic experience and the level of distress and is aimed at improving subjective control over the experience. The presence of coping, therefore, may be conceived as an indicator of the response by a person who feels overwhelmed by the experience of psychosis. For a recent review of studies examining coping strategies for hallucinations in schizophrenia patients, please consult Farhall, Greenwood, and Jackson (2007).

Fallon and Talbot (1981) reported on 40 patients with schizophrenia who experienced auditory hallucinations every day. They found that the most commonly used strategies were modification of behavior, modification of sensory input, and cognitive techniques. The most common behavioral techniques consisted usually of increases in behavior such as lying down or walking, attending to hobbies or reading, listening to music or watching television, having interpersonal contact, and taking medication. Sensory modification mostly involved relaxation techniques such as relaxing or sleeping and doing physical exercise. The cognitive strategies mostly involved ignoring the auditory hallucinations, blocking thoughts by emptying the mind, or using competing distracting thoughts. The strategies did not vary with the age at onset or duration of the illness. The authors then distinguished between those with good or fair adaptation to the presence of persistent hallucinations and those who adapted poorly to their presence. However, analysis of the results did not reveal any clear group differences in terms of the types of coping strategies used. Fallon and Talbot concluded that successful coping appeared to result from the systematic application of widely used coping strategies, and there were individual differences in both the number and type of strategies used and whether these were successful.

Romme, Honig, Noorthoorn, and Escher (1992)[3] sent a questionnaire to 450 people responding to a television program about hearing voices. The vast majority (93%) reported that the voices were socially interfering, and 67% reported not being able to cope with them. The main coping strategies used were distraction (e.g., running, meditating), ignoring the voices, selective attention (e.g., concentrating on the pleasant voices), and setting limits

---

[3]The sample included in this study was unique in that it consisted of individuals who varied in their contact with psychiatric care.

(e.g., giving voices a set time during the day). They also compared people who reported coping with the voices with noncopers and found that distraction was the only strategy used significantly more often by the noncopers, whereas ignoring, selective listening, and setting limits were used more often by the copers.

O'Sullivan (1994) interviewed 40 patients (the majority with schizophrenia or schizoaffective disorder) attending a depot medication clinic who had experienced auditory hallucinations either in the past or at the time of the study. They found that participants used significantly more coping strategies with voices experienced as unpleasant than with voices experienced as pleasant. Strategies used to cope with the (unpleasant) auditory hallucinations fell into four main categories (on the basis of factor analysis): (a) active manipulation of attention (seeking the company of others, watching television, going somewhere quiet, trying to rest or relax, talking inwardly to oneself); (b) passive withdrawal (lying down, thinking of death or dying, bottling up one's feelings, trying to rest or relax); (c) cognitive changes (listening to or reasoning with the auditory hallucinations, trying to go to sleep); and (d) other types of strategies (reading the Bible, telling the auditory hallucinations to go away). Finally, almost four fifths of the strategies described by participants as "most useful" were reported to have been self-devised. Most of the others had been suggested to them by the doctor, and in all cases one strategy suggested was to take medication.

Carter et al. (1996) administered the coping strategies section of the Mental Health Research Institute Unusual Perception Schedule (MUP; see the Appendix for more information concerning this scale) to a group of 100 psychotic patients and confirmed the frequent use of self-developed methods of coping with auditory hallucinations. However, there was a lack of correspondence between use and efficacy of these techniques. That is, the most frequently tried strategies were not reported as being effective, and the most effective strategies had been tried by only a small proportion of patients. Efficacy was shown to be unrelated to demographic or illness characteristics of the patients. There was little evidence of learning or effects of experience. The number of strategies tried did not increase with age, and lower efficacy was reported among those who had experienced hallucinations over long periods. A significant proportion of the patients had tried only methods that offered partial or no effectiveness. Findings of the prevalent use of ineffective methods implies that patients do not develop useful techniques as part of the ongoing course of their illness. This might be related to the fact that some of the methods require specific skills or interests. They also found relationships between efficacy and the specific use of some strategies. Humming as well as using earplugs or headphones were highly efficacious strategies although few people had tried them.

Nayani and David (1996) asked a group of 100 psychotic patients (all of whom had experienced auditory hallucinations in the past 3 months) a series of questions concerning their hallucinations, including questions about coping strategies adopted to relieve their hallucinations. Results revealed that 76% of the patients were able to identify at least one activity that helped them deal with auditory hallucinations. Talking to somebody (63%), going to sleep (43%), thinking of something else (39%), listening to music (30%), and shouting at the voices to go away (28%) were among those most frequently reported by subjects. Participants were also asked whether any activities made things worse. Watching television (55%) and listening to the radio (28%) were often cited. In particular, with regard to watching television, patients remarked that the voices would often comment to them about certain programs or the television presenter's voice would transform into the hallucinated voice and address the patient directly.

Participants who regularly used several coping mechanisms tended to experience less distress, and insight was positively associated with the number of coping mechanisms used (i.e., the higher the insight, the greater the chance they attempt coping strategies). Also, coping seemed to be associated with the presence of pleasant or questioning voices. Nayani and David interpreted this as suggesting that some forms of psychotic experience may originate as coping strategies against the primary (unpleasant) experience (Dittmann & Schüttler, 1990; Romme & Escher, 1989).

Bak et al. (2001) found that coping strategies involving active problem solving (e.g., distraction, problem solving, help seeking, shifted attention, socialization, task performance, indulgence) in a group of patients with schizophrenia was associated with more experience of control over the psychotic experience than other coping styles, especially compared with symptomatic coping (e.g., following or obeying the symptoms, locking oneself in, compulsive behavior, self-mutilating behavior). Bak et al. (2003) reported similar findings in a general population study, in which need for care was associated with severity of psychotic experiences rather than with distress, mean level of control, or average number of coping strategies used. There were, however, qualitative differences concerning the type of coping strategy used in that those who resorted to the strategy of symptomatic coping experienced less control over their symptoms, and this strategy was used more frequently in the need-for-care group. Active coping, in contrast, was positively associated with control.

Studies suggest that teaching more effective coping strategies to children and adolescents with hallucinations is important. For instance, Escher, Delespaul, Romme, Buiks, and van Os (2003) found that baseline level of self-initiated coping was strongly associated with baseline severity of positive symptoms of psychosis, suggesting that coping is indeed a valid measure for the degree to which individuals attempt to "defend" themselves against the experience of being overwhelmed by their psychotic experiences. Also, it was found that higher levels of coping defenses at baseline were strongly predictive of depression at follow-up. The fact that active problem solving was the only coping style that was negatively associated with depression, whereas passive and avoidant styles had the strongest effect sizes (i.e., were most likely to be associated with depression), is in line with the idea that a tendency to feel overwhelmed by the voices (e.g., high power and omnipotence; see studies by Chadwick and Birchwood and collaborators below) fuels feelings of distress. Escher et al. also found that an active problem-solving coping style was the most effective in providing more experience of control over the psychotic experience.

Similarly, findings from Escher et al. (2004) suggest that improving children's and adolescents' ability to cope with emotions may be highly appropriate in some cases. There was evidence of a hierarchy: In a group of children for whom the onset of the voice hearing was associated with grief, almost all of the children stopped hearing voices and developed positively, whereas in a group of children for whom the onset of voices was related to divorce, physical illness, or sexual abuse, fewer children stopped hearing voices and more children showed negative development. Results revealed that receiving no care at all was the most successful and professional care was the least successful and was not significantly associated with the continuation or discontinuation of the voices. Escher et al. attributed this finding to at least two factors. First, in the group that received professional care, there were children who suffered multiple disorders such as learning disabilities and attention-deficit/hyperactivity disorder. Second, illness-oriented care (especially a medication-only treatment style) in this group was less effective in promoting development.

The second most effective form of care was the combination of professional and supplementary care. Escher et al. (2004) suggested that this was probably related to a more individual and creative approach to treatment and to the fact that professionals in this group had more knowledge about teaching children to cope with their emotions. The kinds of care that were experienced as helpful were mostly oriented to providing social support, promoting development, and helping to work through social problems. Mental health care seemed more promising when it was oriented toward helping the person feel safe (e.g., by reducing anxiety levels, normalizing the experience, providing information to the family), being supportive, and helping the person learn to cope with the voices. An important element seemed to be working through the problems (e.g., bereavement, problems in the home or at school, abuse, long-term physical illness) and working through the emotions involved. In general, treatment was successful when it was aimed at both positive development and discontinuation of the voices, not by suppressing them but rather by coping with them, giving them all due attention to the emotions involved.

Finally, Wahass and Kent (1997b) reported that cultural background has an effect on some aspects of coping but not others. Saudi Arabian and British patients both reported a widespread use of self-generated coping strategies. Furthermore, cessation methods, alterations in social activities, and individual engagement methods were used in similar proportions in the two groups. However, the majority of Saudi Arabian patients used strategies associated with their religion, whereas British patients were more likely to use distraction or physiologically based approaches.

These findings reveal that the type of coping strategy plays an important role. Therefore, exploration of coping strategies is a vital part of assessment. A number of assessment strategies to assess coping with psychotic symptoms are available, such as the Maastricht Assessment of Coping Strategies (Bak et al., 2001), and coping strategies are included in the Maastricht Voices Interview for Children (Escher, Romme, Buiks, Delespaul, & van Os, 2002b; see the Appendix for more information concerning these scales). Furthermore, findings suggest that more active strategies (e.g., ignoring, selective listening, setting limits, humming, using earplugs or headphones, distraction, problem solving, help seeking, shifted attention, socialization, task performance, indulgence, active problem solving) are more adaptive (e.g., are related to higher levels of control, are more effective, and are negatively associated with depression). In contrast, more passive strategies (e.g., watching television, symptomatic coping) seem more maladaptive for psychotic experiences such as hallucinations. In addition, the use of effective coping strategies may allow the patient a certain degree of autonomy (Dittmann & Schüttler, 1990). Studies also show that the majority of the coping strategies used by patients are those that they had devised themselves (O'Sullivan, 1994). Also, Carter et al. (1996) found that a significant proportion of patients had tried only methods that offered partial or no effectiveness. It is therefore important to consider such strategies and to take into account whether they help or hinder recovery. If there is evidence that the patient's coping strategies hamper development, it is up to the clinician to rectify this. Indeed, the clinician can assist the patient to reinforce certain strategies and point out other strategies that enhance some form of better self-control and a higher degree of well-being (Dittmann & Schüttler, 1990). Tarrier (2002) provided detailed, practical accounts of how to incorporate a coping strategy approach for psychotic symptoms. Finally, some patients find it instructive to discuss coping strategies with other individuals with hallucinations to find more effective ways of managing hallucinations (see the Self-Help section, below).

APPRAISALS

Chadwick and Birchwood (1994) argued that a coping strategy approach (wrongly) assumes that behavioral and affective responses (or coping strategies) are randomly assigned to hallucinators. Chadwick and Birchwood and collaborators further argued that much emotional (e.g., distress, depression, anxiety) and voice-driven behavior (e.g., coping strategies) appears to be mediated by people's beliefs about the voice's identity (who is the voice?), purpose (why is the voice talking to me and not someone else?), omnipotence (how powerful is the voice?), and control (see Birchwood & Chadwick, 1997; Chadwick & Birchwood, 1994, 1995; van der Gaag, Hageman, & Birchwood, 2003). For instance, they have shown that voices believed to be malevolent provoke fear and anger and are resisted, benevolent voices are associated with positive effect and are engaged, and voices construed as benign are associated with a greater diversity of coping strategies (Birchwood & Chadwick, 1997). Therefore, within this perspective, simply advising patients to use a different coping strategy is unlikely to be helpful because it may conflict with central beliefs.

In this perspective, interventions may center on how the individual attributes the experiences based on underlying beliefs. Techniques involve undermining the patient's central beliefs about auditory hallucinations in a systematic manner. Indeed, weakening maladaptive (core) beliefs and strengthening more adaptive ones have been shown to have positive effects (e.g., reduced distress, improved coping) in patients (Chadwick & Birchwood, 1994). Disputing a belief's veracity may involve a number of widely used cognitive techniques, such as hypothetical contradiction (e.g., the patient is asked if a hypothetical but contradictory occurrence would alter a belief) and verbal challenge (e.g., the patient is asked to question the evidence for his or her beliefs and to generate other plausible explanations). Later, beliefs are questioned more directly by, for example, pointing out inconsistencies and irrationality, and are then tested empirically by the patient. This approach has also been shown to be effective in a group format in which a significant reduction in conviction in beliefs about omnipotence and control was found (Chadwick, Sambrooke, Rasch, & Davies, 2000). A questionnaire that assesses the cognitive, behavioral, and affective reactions to voices has been developed (the Beliefs About Voices Questionnaire, described in the Appendix).

METACOGNITIVE BELIEFS

As was presented in chapter 5, this volume, a number of studies have found evidence of an association between metacognitive beliefs and the presence of hallucinations. As a reminder, metacognitive beliefs are beliefs that are linked to the interpretation, selection, and execution of particular thought processes. This may include beliefs about thought processes (e.g., "I do not trust my memory"), the advantages and disadvantages of various types of thinking (e.g., "I need to worry in order to work well" and "I could make myself sick with worrying"), and beliefs about the content of thoughts (e.g., "It is bad to think certain thoughts"). According to Morrison, Haddock, and Tarrier (1995), metacognitive beliefs that are inconsistent with intrusive thoughts (e.g., "Not being able to control my thoughts is a sign of weakness" and "I cannot ignore my worrying thoughts") lead to their external attribution as hallucinations and other psychotic symptoms such as delusions. Furthermore, it is argued that such a misattribution is maintained because it reduces cognitive dissonance. When the occurrence of intrusive thoughts does not comply with the person's metacognitive beliefs, an aversive state of arousal results (cognitive dissonance), which the person tries to escape by externalizing the intrusive thoughts (resulting in hallucinatory and delusional experiences) and thus maintaining consistency in his or her belief system. For instance, based on Morrison et al.'s (1995) view, a person who believes that one should control all thoughts yet at the same time frequently experiences uncontrollable thoughts would tend to attribute these thoughts as stemming from something other than him- or herself.

There are clinical implications of these studies that show that metacognitive beliefs may have a causal role in auditory hallucinations via the misattribution of intrusive thoughts. For instance, these studies reveal the need to perform a detailed assessment of patients' experiences of intrusive thoughts and metacognitive beliefs (with, e.g., the Meta-Cognitions Questionnaire;[4] Cartwright-Hatton & Wells, 1997). Treatment of hallucinations may involve challenging some of these metacognitive beliefs by using verbal or behavioral methods of reattribution and provide normalizing information regarding intrusive thoughts. Metacognitive-focused treatment strategies (Wells, 2000) that modify metacognitive beliefs and improve executive control over attention could also be highly useful. Another possible intervention could involve proposing alternatives to the beliefs that seem to maintain the hallucinations. In contrast, active suppression-based management strategies for auditory hallucinations are unlikely to be effective and may actually be involved in maintaining the hallucinations. Thus, behavioral experiments such as those suggested by Salkovskis and Kirk (1989) for use with obsessional patients may be used to demonstrate the paradoxical effects of suppression. Similarly, in those with negative metacognitive beliefs concerning voices (e.g., will make them go mad), a natural (spontaneous) reaction (or safety behavior) would be to suppress such intrusive experiences, which will most likely result in an increase of their frequency and intensity. Finally, if beliefs about the controllability of mental events are important, then these beliefs should be amenable to similar cognitive interventions, in particular, challenging cognitive distortions such as "should" statements and black-and-white thinking.

French, Morrison, Walford, Knight, and Bentall (2003) used a CBT approach with a group of high-risk cases to prevent the onset of psychosis. The approach directed treatment toward metacognitive beliefs, selective at-

---

[4]Note that a short form of this questionnaire also exists (Wells & Cartwright-Hatton, 2004) in addition to a version developed for adolescents (Cartwright-Hatton et al., 2004).

tention strategies, and the manipulation of safety behaviors. In particular, they found that engaging these individuals is feasible when a problem-oriented approach is adopted. Finally, patients included in this study clearly preferred a psychological approach to their problems over a medical one that requires pharmacological treatment.

García-Montes, Pérez-Álvarez, Balbuena, Garcelàn, and Cangas (2006) presented data showing that patients with auditory hallucinations and obsessive–compulsive disorder present similar forms of interpreting their thoughts. In particular, both groups see their thoughts as uncontrollable and dangerous and consider that these thoughts may come to have a direct effect on the world. These types of beliefs are related to what has been known as thought–action fusion (TAF; Shafran & Rachman, 2004). In general, TAF can be considered as a specific type of magical thinking or superstitious belief that involves faulty causal relationships between one's own thoughts and external reality. One intervention would be to point out that TAF is a normal phenomenon, that is, that many people are superstitious. Also based on this, it would seem reasonable to propose treatments that allow the patient with auditory hallucinations to reduce the importance of the power and danger that thoughts may have.

PSYCHOEDUCATION

For both patients and caregivers, psychoeducation is a valuable tool for knowing what is wrong with the patients and how the condition may have developed. This is especially true for a stigmatizing illness such as schizophrenia and for stigmatized experiences such as hallucinations. Indeed, a majority of people perceive those who "hear voices" as being violent and unstable, and believe they should be locked away (Cockshutt, 2004). However, history shows (fortunately) that attitudes toward and explanations for voice hearing vary over time (Leudar & Thomas, 2000; Watkins, 1998), therefore suggesting that they may be modified.

As we have seen several times, the distress related to hallucinations is crucial and causes a number of problems that need to be dealt with. On an individual level, distress associated with hallucinations may be alleviated (e.g., via the numerous techniques described in this book and elsewhere). However, distress associated with hallucinations may also be decreased on a societal level. That is, if attitudes in the general population concerning hallucinations were less negative and damaging, then this would make it much easier for those suffering from hallucinations to properly manage their experiences.

One frequently used psychoeducation technique is normalization. Normalization refers to the process by which thoughts, behaviors, moods, and experiences are compared and understood in terms of similar thoughts, behaviors, moods, and experiences attributed to other individuals who are not diagnosed as ill (Kingdon & Turkington, 2005). Studies have shown that normalization interventions in adult populations are successful in alleviating the distress associated with the presence of hallucinations and delusions (Kingdon & Turkington, 1994, 1996). It is important to communicate to those who hear voices that healthy individuals from the general population also have had hallucinatory experiences at one time or another and that hallucinations are not necessarily a sign of psychosis (see chap. 3, this volume). Such information can be liberating for people who believe that they are the only ones with such experiences or who think that such experiences automatically mean that they are mad.

Normalizing techniques may include presenting normal circumstances in which hallucinations can occur, such as deprivation states (sleep deprivation, sensory deprivation); posttraumatic stress disorder (PTSD; e.g., similarities between flashbacks and hallucinations) and other traumas (sexual and physical abuse); and organic (e.g., drug-induced, fever, drug or alcohol withdrawal states, brain stimulation), fear (e.g., hostage situations), bereavement, and trance states (e.g., those experienced in religious ceremonies). (Note that many of these factors are reviewed in chap. 3, this volume, in the section "Hallucinations in Nonclinical Groups.") Relating psychotic symptoms to beliefs in various nonscientific phenomena (e.g., belief in God, ghosts, superstitions, reincarnation, the Devil, thought transference, predicting future events, and horoscopes) that are common in the general population may also be recommended. These normalization factors may provide patients with alternative explanations to hallucinatory experiences and facilitate reattribution of hallucinations. Thought experiments may also be proposed, such as those describing transient disruptions of ordinary mental life (e.g., wondering whether the phone is actually ringing or whether it is one's imagination) that parallel the cognitive processes underlying psychotic experiences such as hallucinations (Garrett, Stone, & Turkington, 2006). Other aims of normalization include promoting an understanding of psychological phenomena that also resemble symptoms of schizophrenia; reducing "fear of going mad," isolation and feelings of isolation, and stigma (by others and self); and improving self-esteem (Kingdon & Turkington, 1994, 2005). However, when using normalization techniques, one should keep in mind that there also may be a risk of minimizing problems or failing to deal with the consequences or development of having the hallucinatory experiences (Kingdon & Turkington, 2005), which should be avoided. Finally, although normalization techniques are mainly used in adult populations, findings from studies suggest that such techniques may also be fruitful in children and adolescents with hallucinations. Indeed, a number of studies have shown that very few children and adolescents reveal their hallucinations to their associates (i.e., parents, siblings, friends, etc.; for a review of these studies, see Larøi et al., 2006).

However, treatment should include providing information not only to those individuals experiencing the hallucinations but also to their associates. Indeed, this latter group appears to appreciate and benefit from the reassurance that hearing voices does not necessarily mean that their family member or friend is crazy or that she or he has schizophrenia or another psychotic condition. Similarly, education campaigns concerning psychotic experiences geared toward the general public, schools, and primary health services also appear to be an important intervention strategy. Studies show that even brief educational courses on mental illness reduce stigmatizing attitudes among a wide variety of participants (Pinfold et al., 2003; Rüsch, Angermeyer, & Corrigan, 2005; Schulze, Richter-Werling, Matschinger, & Angermeyer, 2003).

COGNITIVE BEHAVIOR THERAPY

A number of studies have shown that cognitive behavior therapy (CBT) is effective in alleviating positive psychotic symptoms. For more information concerning the efficacy of CBT for psychotic symptoms, the reader may refer to the numerous excellent reviews and meta-analyses that have examined this issue (Dickerson, 2000; Garety, Fowler, & Kuipers, 2000; Gaudiano, 2005; R. A. Gould, Mueser, Bolton, Mays, & Goff, 2001; Haddock et al., 1998; Pilling et al., 2002; Rector & Beck, 2001; Shergill, Murray, & McGuire, 1998; Tarrier & Wykes, 2004; Wykes, 2004; Zimmerman, Favrod, Trieu, & Pomini, 2005).

What follows is a brief, nonexhaustive overview of some of the CBT studies that have provided results concerning hallucinations in particular. Both individual and group CBT are presented. We also present special populations and techniques briefly, such as mindfulness/acceptance-based CBT, functional CBT, CBT for psychotic patients with intellectual disabilities, CBT for older patients with visual hallucinations, and CBT for individuals in early phases of psychosis. For practical reasons, the term *cognitive behavior therapy* is used here, although some authors also use the term *cognitive therapy* (or CT).

Garety et al. (2000) noted that the general aims of CBT for psychotic patients are to reduce the distress and disability caused by psychotic symptoms, to reduce emotional disturbance, and to help the person to arrive at an understanding of psychosis to promote the active participation of the individual in the regulation of risk of relapse and social disability. Furthermore, Garety et al. conceptualized therapy as a series of six stages: (a) building and maintaining a therapeutic relationship; (b) using cognitive–behavioral coping strategies; (c) developing a new understanding of the experience of psychosis; (d) addressing delusions and hallucinations; (e) addressing negative self-evaluations, anxiety, and depression; and (f) managing risk of relapse and social disability.

Individual Cognitive Behavior Therapy

A number of studies have examined the effects of individual CBT on psychotic symptoms (which include hallucinations). On the whole, CBT seems effective in alleviating psychotic symptoms. For instance, in a meta-analysis of controlled studies examining the effectiveness of CBT on the positive symptom of schizophrenia,[5] Zimmerman et al. (2005) reported a mean weighted effect size of .37, representing a small to moderate effect size. Overall, this implies that a typical patient in the CBT group improved more than 64% of the control patients and that CBT increases the success rate of reducing positive symptoms from 41% to 59%.

In a randomized controlled trial, Valmaggia, van der Gaag, Tarrier, Pijnenborg, and Sloof (2005) compared CBT with supportive counseling in a group of patients with chronic schizophrenia. At posttreatment, there was a small, nonsignificant effect for CBT compared with supportive counseling for positive symptoms. Supplementary analyses showed that CBT was significantly more effective for alleviating physical characteristics and cognitive interpretations of auditory hallucinations but not for the emotional characteristics. However, these benefits were not sustained at follow-up (after 6 months).

Morrison (2002) described a case study in which CBT was used in the context of auditory hallucinations. The patient was 29 years old, with a diagnosis of bipolar disorder, although this changed to schizophrenia at the time of the intervention. His concerns were hearing voices, believing that there was a conspiracy against him, depression, unsatisfactory social life, and sleeping too much. These goals were then prioritized, and realistic goals were set in relation to each problem. For the hallucinations, the initial goals were set in relation to small changes that were meaningful to him and to measure changes (with the help of percentage ratings) in terms of control over voices and the distress caused by voices. Initially, intervention focused on the persecutory beliefs using mainly a series of event–thought–feeling–behavior cycles. When there was a clear decrease in belief ratings and distress ratings for persecutory beliefs, intervention strategies then focused on the auditory hallucinations. Because the event–thought–feeling–behavior framework was found to be useful for the patient, this was also used for the voices.

An examination of several weeks' worth of diaries revealed a number of common themes in the internal and external events that preceded voice activity, such as social situations (particularly small enclosed spaces with lots of people present), use of cannabis, use of alcohol, anxiety, and paranoid thoughts. Factors that appeared to make the voices worse included the above-mentioned triggers, as well as paying attention to the voices, resisting what they suggested doing, and driving a car. Factors that appeared to make the

---

[5]A total of 14 studies conducted between 1990 and 2004 were included in the meta-analysis.

voices easier to deal with included going to bed, sometimes having an alcoholic drink, and obeying the voices. Three major explanations were then identified: (a) the voices were from a higher power (this was the interpretation that the patient started with), (b) the voices were a form of mental illness, or (c) the voices were an unusual thought process (this interpretation was arrived at later on in the intervention). Concerning the first interpretation, evidence for (e.g., the voice can predict unlikely things happening, it feels physically very convincing) and against (e.g., it could be coincidence, a lot of what the voices predict does not occur) was documented throughout the intervention period and was discussed. The second interpretation (the voices being a form of mental illness) had been repeatedly presented to the patient by his psychiatrists. Evidence for this included, for example, the fact that he had been admitted several times to psychiatric hospitals, he had been given a diagnosis of bipolar disorder, and he was taking several medications. Evidence against this interpretation included the fact that hearing voices did not seem to happen at work and that medication was not always effective for the voices. Finally, concerning the last interpretation (voices being an unusual thought process), evidence for this included the fact that the voices could be a stress response or could be triggered by cannabis, and analysis of the content of the voices revealed that the voices often spoke about things that were of high personal salience to him. The patient was also given information concerning the prevalence of hearing voices in the general population (i.e., normalization), and discussions also concerned the nature and mechanisms of unwanted intrusive thoughts and their possible relation to hallucinations (e.g., thought–action fusion). Taken together, this information helped him conclude that there might be some link between his thoughts and his voices. For a more detailed account of this case, consult Morrison (2002). Kingdon and Turkington (2005) also provided practical information on how to work within a CBT approach with hallucinations.

Group Cognitive Behavior Therapy

Group CBT for psychotic symptoms, including hallucinations, has also been proposed. Treating groups would first have the obvious advantage of being able to treat more people compared with individual treatment. Also, people experiencing hallucinations often report the loneliness that the voices produce, and groups may be able to reduce these effects and combat the feelings of isolation that voice hearers report by sharing their experiences with others, identifying common factors that increase or decrease their experiences, and sharing natural coping strategies to increase the coping repertoire (Wykes, 2004). Important to note is that group CBT for voices may not be suitable for everyone, for instance, in an individual whose beliefs are disturbing to discuss in a group context. Also, group CBT may be used in conjunction with individual CBT. Previous studies of group treatment for voices have shown beneficial, albeit uncontrolled, effects (Chadwick et al., 2000; Gledhill, Lobban, & Sellwood, 1998; Pearlman & Hubbard, 2000; Trygstad et al., 2002; Wykes, Parr, & Landau, 1999). The only controlled, randomized study of group CBT to date (Wykes et al., 2005) showed that group CBT improved social functioning 6 months following therapy. However, there was no general effect of group CBT on the severity of hallucinations. Nonetheless, the results suggested that improvement on hallucinations could be observed where treatment started early and where very experienced therapists were involved.

Particular Cognitive Behavior Therapy Techniques and Populations

Newer approaches to CBT have explored the utility of adding mindfulness or acceptance-based techniques to treat psychotic symptoms (Bach & Hayes, 2002; Gaudiano & Herbert, 2006). For example, Gaudiano and Herbert examined the efficacy of mindfulness or acceptance-based CBT (or acceptance and commitment therapy; ACT) in a group of psychotic patients. In brief, ACT encourages individuals to accept and experience internal events nonjudgmentally (i.e., mindfully) while simultaneously working toward the pursuit of personally defined goals (Hayes, Strosahl, & Wilson, 1999). Psychotic inpatients were randomly assigned to either a control group (who received typical treatment) or a group receiving typical treatment in addition to individual sessions of ACT. Results at discharge from the hospital suggested short-term advantages in the ACT group in affective symptoms, overall improvement, social impairment, and distress associated with hallucinations. A follow-up assessment 4 months later revealed decreases in the believability of hallucinations for those in the ACT group. Furthermore, change in believability was strongly associated with change in distress.

Another recent development is functional CBT (fCBT). In general, one may view fCBT as a form of CBT whose particular aim is improving social, personal, and occupational functioning. In particular, Cather et al. (2005) argued that fCBT was developed to target (a) only symptoms that interfere with progress toward functional goals and (b) improved functioning as an explicit outcome of treatment. Although Cather et al. did not find that fCBT was significantly more efficient than psychoeducation in terms of symptom reduction, within-group effect sizes suggested an advantage for fCBT relative to psychoeducation for reducing positive symptoms, particularly auditory hallucinations.

CBT may also be used in relatively special populations. For instance, a series of studies have shown that CBT may be used for psychotic patients with intellectual or learning disabilities (Haddock, Lobban, Hatton, & Carson, 2004; Kirkland, 2005; Legget, Hurn, & Goodman, 1997; Oathamshaw & Haddock, 2006). Collerton and Dudley (2004) maintained that CBT may be used successfully for older people with visual hallucinations. Finally, CBT may also be used as an intervention in early stages of psychosis (e.g., Bechdolf et al., 2005).

Summary

Studies seem to suggest that CBT is a modestly effective treatment scheme for positive psychotic symptoms. Few studies have directly and specifically examined the positive effects of CBT on hallucinations, although one study (Valmaggia et al., 2005) did suggest that it may alleviate at least some features of hallucinations. One general limit of CBT is that it does not deal with the experiences (i.e., hallucinations) themselves but rather deals exclusively with reactions (e.g., distress) to the experiences. Furthermore, there is little evidence that CBT improves patients' depression, negative symptoms, or social functioning, and although studies indicate that CBT is more effective than routine care, the superiority of CBT is less evident when it is compared with other therapies that use equivalent amounts of one-to-one therapist attention (Dickerson, 2000). In addition, as pointed out by McKenna (2003), many of the CBT clinical trials have been lacking in methodological rigor (e.g., absence of a control and/or blind condition), and a number of studies have not shown a significant advantage (e.g., in terms of reducing global symptomatology, positive symptoms, or negative symptoms) for CBT compared with the control intervention (which usually consists of supportive counseling). Finally, Birchwood and Trower (2006) correctly argued that future CBT studies should be more theory driven to begin to clarify possible variables and mechanisms underlying effective treatment.

More studies examining the efficacy of CBT for hallucinations are clearly needed. The use of elaborate and well-designed case studies might be fitting in this context because CBT probably should be individualized, at least in part (like any other type of treatment). The reported modest effect sizes (Zimmerman et al., 2005) might be a reflection of this. Shergill et al. (1998) pointed out that the inclusion of case reports might inevitably result in a tendency toward the reporting of positive rather than negative findings. This is true, unless of course scientific journals begin to appreciate the clinical and theoretical import some negative findings may have. Also, if cases are sufficiently elaborate and detailed, this may result in the reporting of less successful features of the CBT, in addition to aspects that seemed to be alleviated by the treatment. Both positive and negative effects of CBT for hallucinations are valuable for clinicians and researchers. For a discussion of the advantages of the case study methodology, see Dattilio (2006).

HALLUCINATIONS-FOCUSED INTEGRATIVE TREATMENT

Hallucinations-focused integrative treatment (HIT) uses multiple modalities to maximize control of persistent auditory hallucinations. This approach integrates a number of different types of treatment strategies (e.g., CBT, supportive counseling, psychoeducation, coping training, mobile crisis intervention, and antipsychotic medication), and the intervention uses 20 one-hour sessions over 9 to 12 months (Jenner, 2002). HIT is different from most CBT programs in that both patient and relatives receive cognitive interventions and coping training.

In HIT there are a number of different modules: motivation, coping training, CBT, family treatment, psychoeducation, and medication. The motivation module involves moving away from a disease/medical model toward a focus based on consumer needs and demands. For instance, medication noncompliance is viewed as a request for medication adjustment, resistance is regarded as consumer complaints, and symptoms and behaviors are labeled positively. Furthermore, the patient selects the timing and order of therapeutic interventions, and interventions are accommodated to the patient's degree of awareness of the illness. The coping module involves teaching patients and relatives a repertoire of skills for anxiety management, for distracting patients' attention from the voices, and for focusing attention on the voices when necessary. Daily monitoring of the characteristics of the voices, contextual aspects, and coping and its effect is seen as crucial to developing appropriate coping strategies. The CBT module focuses on precipitating events; on emotional, cognitive, and behavioral actions or reactions; and on the reactions of others. Psychoeducation focuses on symptoms and on problem solving. In the family treatment module, joint sessions with the patient and relatives are favored. Relatives monitor their feelings, cognitions, and behavior toward the patient, and patients in turn monitor their relatives' reactions. Relatives are trained in positive labeling and in selectively reinforcing the patient's coping behavior, self-care, and daily activities. Finally, medication is provided according to typical guidelines resembling those of the American Psychiatric Association.

Studies suggest that HIT is effective for chronic schizophrenic patients (Jenner, Nienhuis, van de Willige, & Wiersma, 2006; Jenner, Nienhuis, Wiersma, & van de Willige, 2004; Jenner, van de Willige, & Wiersma, 1998, 2006; Wiersma, Jenner, Nienhuis, & van de Willige, 2004; Wiersma, Jenner, van de Willige, Spakman, & Nienhuis, 2001) and for psychotic adolescents (Jenner & van de Willige, 2001) with auditory hallucinations. Also, these positive effects have been shown to last as long as 9 or 18 months after treatment (Jenner et al., 2004; Jenner, Nienhuis, et al., 2006; Wiersma et al., 2004).

In a randomized controlled trial, Jenner et al. (2004) compared patients in routine care with those with HIT. Results revealed significant group differences at a 9-month follow-up for distress and amount of interference with daily functioning and total burden of voices but not for frequency of voices, duration of voices, and control over voices. Similar results were reported in a randomized controlled trial comparing HIT and treatment as usual (Jenner, Nienhuis, et al., 2006), where HIT demonstrated significant posttreatment (at 18-month follow-up) improvements for the following hallucination characteristics: amount and threat of negative content, distress and amount of interference with daily functioning, and the total burden of the voices. There were no significant differences between the two groups at the 18-month follow-up for frequency and duration and the level of control over voices. In a naturalistic prospective design, Jenner and van de Willige (2001) examined the effectiveness of HIT in a group of 14 first-episode adolescents with both acute and chronic auditory hallucinations. Results showed that 9 patients were free of voices for at least 2 consecutive months after treatment. Furthermore, satisfaction with the program was high, and findings suggested that the interventions were helpful in motivating formerly drug-refusing (noncompliant) adolescents to accept drugs in later instances.

Stant et al. (2003) examined the cost-effectiveness of HIT in patients with schizophrenia with a history of persistent auditory hallucinations. In this study, costs (in and outside the health care sector) and outcomes were registered prospectively during a period of 18 months for patients who received the HIT program and for patients in a care-as-usual condition. Mean costs for the whole study period per patient in the HIT group ($18,237) were lower than the mean costs per patient in the care-as-usual group ($21,436), although this difference did not reach statistical significance. Supplementary analyses (which took into account skewed distributions of cost variables) indicated that future cost differences will, in most cases, be in favor of the HIT program. In terms of symptomatology (measured with the PANSS; see the Appendix), results were in favor of the HIT group, although differences did not reach a statistically significant level.

SELF-HELP

Many patients find that discussing their symptoms with others experiencing the same symptoms is beneficial. It may help them realize that they are not alone in having these experiences. Also, such discussions may bring to light effective coping strategies of which they were not previously aware. Romme and Escher (2000) provided some guidelines for self-help interventions. They distinguished between two types of self-help groups. One is from a clinical perspective, in which a clinician is present to facilitate discussions and provide information based on medical practice and research. Another involves organizing self-help groups of voice hearers without the presence of mental health professionals, thus enabling access to information from a variety of sources and not just from a medical source. The two types of self-help are not necessarily mutually exclusive, and the appropriateness of the type of self-help will probably vary between individuals and may change over time. For more details concerning ways of working within a self-help perspective, consult Romme and Escher (2000).[6] Also important to add is that a number of self-help organizations for voice hearers exist in a number of countries, such as the Hearing Voices Network in the United Kingdom, the National Empowerment Center in the United States, and the Stichting Weerklank in the Netherlands. (Information concerning many of these organizations are included in Romme & Escher, 2000.) Reading relevant (self-help) literature might also be helpful to some. A number of information handouts for hallucinations are available to the public, such as the one included in Kingdon and Turkington (2005). Also, the National Health Service in the United Kingdom has published a self-help guide for hallucinations ("Understanding Voices and Disturbing Beliefs"). Finally, self-help workbooks exist, such as "Working With Voices" (Coleman & Smith, 1997). As Romme and Escher (2000) pointed out, it is important for clinicians to have some knowledge of these self-help organizations, and where such groups are not readily available to voice hearers, to help organize such groups themselves.

IMPORTANCE OF TREATING CO-OCCURRING PSYCHOPATHOLOGICAL CONDITIONS AND ASSOCIATED PROBLEMS

It is well known that a number of psychiatric conditions frequently co-occur with psychotic disorders. For instance, Kessler et al. (1994) reported that 79% of patients with schizophrenia had at least one comorbid psychiatric disorder, and 59% had more than three comorbid psychiatric disorders. In a group of 96 psychotic patients, it was found that the total lifetime prevalence of psychiatric comorbidity was 57.3% (Cassano, Pini, Saettoni, Rucci, & Del'Osso, 1998). Studies have found obsessive–compulsive disorder to be comorbid in 24% to 45% of schizophrenic patients (Berman et al., 1998; Lysaker et al., 2000; Nechmad et al., 2003; Poyurovsky et al., 2001), 17% of patients with schizophrenia also have social anxiety (Cosoff & Hafner, 1990), 20% suffer from panic disorder (Turnbull & Bebbington, 2001), and as many as 60% of patients with schizophrenia also suffer from substance abuse (Fowler, Carr, Carter, & Lewin, 1998). Thus, comorbidity, at least in the context of schizophrenia, seems to be the rule rather than the exception.

Studies with nonclinical adult participants have also revealed relations between self-reported hallucinations and depression and anxiety (Allen et al., 2005; Lewandowski et al., 2006; Paulik, Badcock, & Maybery, 2006; Verdoux et al., 1998; for more detailed information concerning some of these studies, see chap. 3, this volume, and in particular the section "Hallucinations in Nonclinical Groups"). Hallucinations in children and adolescents

---

[6]Note that this book has been translated from Dutch into a number of languages, including English, French, Spanish, Swedish, Danish, and German.

also have been associated with various psychopathological disorders and conditions (e.g., mood disorders, substance abuse, PTSD, anxiety disorders, dissociative experiences, migraine, Tourette's syndrome). Furthermore, characteristics of hallucinations and delusions may modulate the degree of comorbidity (Dhossche, Ferdinand, Van der Ende, Hofstra, & Verhulst, 2002; Yoshizumi, Murase, Honjo, Kaneko, & Murakami, 2004), and high levels of anxiety and depression are important hallucination continuation factors (Escher et al., 2004; for a review of this literature, see Larøi, Van der Linden, & Goëb, 2006). Studies also have reported that the presence of hallucinations in patients with dementia related to Alzheimer's disease and Parkinson's disease is associated with coexisting psychopathological conditions such as anxiety and depression (Aarsland, Larsen, Cummings, & Lake, 1999; Cohen-Mansfield, 2003; Cooper, Mungas, Verma, & Weiler, 1991; Fénelon, Mahieux, Huon, & Ziégler, 2000; Inzelberg, Kipervasser, & Korczyn, 1998; Sanchez-Ramos, Ortoll, & Paulson, 1996; Teri et al., 1999). Although few studies have examined the issue of the co-occurrence of psychopathological conditions in hallucinations in normal, old-age populations, one study that did examine this issue reported that hallucinations were related to higher levels of depression (Turvey et al., 2001).

Stress vulnerability models (e.g., Zubin & Spring, 1977; Zuckerman, 1999) suggest a link between neurotic (or emotional) disorders and psychotic disorders. In such models, for instance, the emotional stress created by a comorbid anxiety disorder could push a person over his or her threshold. In a review of the literature, Freeman and Garety (2003) provided convincing evidence of the link between neurosis and psychosis and, in particular, between hallucinations and neurosis, for both the development and the maintenance of these experiences.

Therefore, proposing intervention strategies for these coexisting conditions seems crucial. Also, because hallucinations' content is many times mood congruent, this work will most probably also involve working with aspects that are indirectly related to hallucinations, such as improving self-esteem and levels of depression. Indeed, studies reveal that the effective treatment of coexisting psychopathological disorders has positive effects on hallucinations. For instance, Morrison (2002) described a case study in which CBT was used in the context of hallucinations and where aspects of the content of voices (e.g., the voice telling the patient that he would never get a girlfriend, the voice calling him names) were discussed as perhaps reflecting low self-esteem. As a consequence, work aimed at improving sense of self-worth was agreed on between the patient and the clinician. Results revealed a reduction of hallucination scores at postintervention compared with preintervention.

Good (2002) used CBT to treat a comorbid social phobia in a schizophrenia patient with hallucinations and found that his intervention resulted in significant drops in the patient's scores for hallucinations, delusions, social phobia, agoraphobia, anxiety, and depression. However, treatment interventions in this study were not directly addressed for hallucinations. Dudley, Dixon, and Turkington (2005) reported the case of a patient with schizophrenia suffering from a specific phobia (fear of dogs), agoraphobia, auditory hallucinations (of sounds and derogatory comments), and delusional beliefs. Because the patient placed his fear of dogs at the top of the list, treatment focused on this, in addition to focusing on the patient's avoidance of public places (agoraphobia), both with the help of a standard habituation program. Some treatment interventions were directly addressed for hallucinations, although this mostly involved normalization. Results revealed a significant reduction of psychotic symptoms, including hallucinations.

In a study including children and adolescents hearing voices, Escher et al. (2004) found that in a high percentage of cases, hearing voices was associated with serious problems in daily life, within the family, at school, and so forth. In many cases, the voices disappeared when these problems were solved and the children's development took a positive turn.

TRAUMA

Traumatic experiences in the past or present seem to play an important role as either hallucination triggers or important hallucination development factors. An extensive and relatively recent body of evidence reveals that a high prevalence of (childhood) sexual and physical abuse is related to hallucinations. (For more detail concerning this issue, see chap. 4, this volume; see also W. Larkin & Morrison, 2006; Morrison, Frame, & Larkin, 2003; Read, Perry, Moskowitz, & Connolly, 2001; Read, van Os, Morrison, & Ross, 2005.) For instance, one study (Hardy et al., 2005) found that of 75 individuals with nonaffective psychosis and who experienced current hallucinations, approximately half (55%) of the sample experienced a subjectively significant trauma (a trauma experienced in the past that still affected them). The traumas that were most often associated with hallucinations were sexual abuse and bullying. Furthermore, a subgroup of patients had at least one type of phenomenological association between their traumas and their hallucinations (e.g., intrusive hallucinations were more likely in individuals who had also experienced an intrusive trauma). On the basis of this large body of research, authors have proposed a number of probable relationships between the experiences of trauma and psychosis; that is, some psychotic patients may develop PTSD in response to their psychosis, some may develop psychosis as a result of traumatic experiences, some may develop both, and some may develop a vicious circle between their PTSD symptoms and their psychosis (Morrison et al., 2003).

It has been argued that psychotic experiences such as hallucinations may emerge as a coping strategy for trauma, especially in those individuals with positive (metacognitive) beliefs about unusual experiences (Morrison et al., 2003). Studies suggest that people who have been abused as children are more likely to be abused as adults. However, sexual and physical abuse cases remain unidentified by mental health staff (especially those with a predominantly biological-genetic approach to mental disorders), and patients diagnosed as psychotic or schizophrenic are asked about abuse even less often than other patients. Information about the links between life events (childhood trauma, bereavement, drug abuse, urban living) and hallucinations can be helpful in reducing distress and may provide an alternative explanation for hallucinations. Also, the continual presence of traumatic life events may later develop into a comorbid PTSD in some patients, which may actually be perceived as more distressing than the hallucinations themselves. Certain studies also show that the relationship between (sexual or physical) abuse and hallucinations is demonstrated by the dose effect, with the more severe forms of abuse being related to particularly high rates of hallucinations. Finally, several studies have found that the content of hallucinations experienced by, for example, abuse survivors is frequently related to the abuse, such as consisting of flashback elements, concrete details of episodes of traumatic victimization, increased reference to evil or to the devil, or a tendency to view auditory hallucinations as malevolent (for a review, see Read et al., 2005).

This research revealing relations between traumatic life events and hallucinations has important clinical implications. For instance, including questions about trauma and life events both in the past and present during assessment is vital.[7] Indeed, it is unlikely that patients will spontaneously disclose abuse, and few professionals ask their patients about this. Mueser et al. (1998) found that although 48% of patients with severe mental illness qualified for a diagnosis of PTSD, only 2% had actually received such a diagnosis in their records. Morrison et al. (2003) proposed that, in light of the high prevalence rates of traumatic life events in patients with psychosis and other mental disorders, services that receive such patients should be designed with the minimization of trauma in mind (e.g., alternative to hospital admission, provide normalization information concerning the prevalence of psychotic symptoms in the general population and provide education concerning symptoms of trauma and the prevalence of PTSD in response to psychosis). Another obvious consequence of this research is that we are now beginning to clarify what interventions may be particularly helpful for people who experience psychosis and have suffered traumatic life events. For instance, psychological treatment utilized for PTSD patients (e.g., imaginal exposure, re-

---

[7]A number of assessment strategies exist for (traumatic) life events and vary from respondent-based or checklist methods (e.g., the Life Event Record [Coddington, 1972]; the Life Events Checklist [Gray, Litz, Hsu, & Lombardo, 2004; J. H. Johnson & McCutcheon, 1980]; the Traumatic Life Events Questionnaire [Kubany et al., 2000]); relatively complete, interview-based schedules (e.g., the Stressful Life Events Schedule [Williamson et al., 2003]); and extensive semistructured interview methods (e.g., the Life Events and Difficulties Schedule [G. W. Brown, Bifulco, & Harris, 1987]).

appraising the meaning of the traumatic event) may also prove appropriate for psychotic patients with evidence of past traumatic experiences. Finally, there are also implications for prevention. For example, providing appropriate help for child abuse survivors in the mental health system might reduce or prevent a great number of individuals developing problems with their hallucinations (e.g., prevent them from becoming clinical cases).

THE ROLE OF IMAGERY

Recurrent images are often associated with hallucinations. For example, people who hear voices will frequently have an image of the perceived source of the voice (e.g., God, the devil, their next-door neighbor) or an image that is associated with the content of the voice. There is a large body of work showing that imagery occurs in patients with anxiety disorders, obsessive–compulsive disorder, and social phobia (see Morrison, Beck, et al., 2002). Studies have also shown this to be the case in patients with psychotic symptoms, in particular those with hallucinations. For instance, Morrison, Beck, et al. (2002) found that in a group of 35 patients who were experiencing hallucinations and/or delusions, the majority of patients (74.3%) reported images, and most were recurrent and associated with affect, beliefs, and memories. Common themes included, for example, images about traumatic memories and images about the perceived source or content of voices. Furthermore, images about traumatic memories appear similar to the vivid images or flashbacks present in patients with PTSD, and the former may well lead patients to develop PTSD-like phenomena in relation to their hallucinations. Also, in auditory hallucinations, images were mainly related to the perceived source of the voice (e.g., spirits of friends, an alien sphere, and a neighbor shouting through a bullhorn) or the content of the voices (e.g., abusing young girls or stabbing someone). The results suggest that mental imagery is implicated in the maintenance of hallucinations and support the view that similar processes are involved in the maintenance of both anxiety and psychosis (Morrison, 2001).

The clinical implications of this are that images can be a useful way of accessing personal meaning and core beliefs and that these images can be modified to become less distressing or powerful. Furthermore, some patients may use the images as evidence in support of their beliefs about voices. It is thus important to reduce the frequency of such images or alter the content or meaning of such images. Hackmann (1997) reported that effective modification of persistent images can require specific imagery-related interventions such as modifying the ending of an image, introducing humor to the image, or having an adult establish control in the image. Another intervention may include helping patients realize that just because they can image something does not mean it is true (similar to thought–action fusion). There are no intervention studies for hallucinations, although Morrison (2004) successfully used imagery-based treatment strategies in the case of a patient suffering from delusions.

COMMAND HALLUCINATIONS

As mentioned in chapter 2, command hallucinations may be considered as a particular subtype of auditory hallucinations in that the voice is experienced as commanding rather than commenting. Relations between command hallucinations and action (i.e., compliance) and between command hallucinations and dangerousness are complex (for a review, see Braham, Trower, & Birchwood, 2004). Nonetheless, one study (Erkwoh, Willmes, Eming-Erdmann, & Kunert, 2002) found that there is a significantly higher risk of complying to command hallucinations in patients for whom the voices are familiar or are accepted as real (i.e., are uncritical) and where there are posthallucinatory affective reactions (i.e., nonindifference). Beck-Sander, Birchwood, and Chadwick (1997) explored factors influencing command hallucinations during auditory hallucinations and found that the beliefs patients hold about their voices were important in determining whether patients complied with commands and the affect generated.

Finally, Mackinnon, Copolov, and Trauer (2004) also examined factors associated with compliance and resistance to command hallucinations. They found that patients with command hallucinations reported the voices more negatively than those who did not hear commands, were more likely to describe the voices as being like relays or stuck (i.e., resembling obsessive-compulsive thoughts), used a greater number of specific coping methods, and were more likely to have negative symptoms and a wider range of delusional content. Mackinnon et al. concluded that these (and other) findings suggest that command hallucinations may warrant special therapeutic attention.

One CBT intervention program has been specifically developed for command hallucinations that does not depend on reducing the experience of voices but on reducing the perceived power of voices to harm the individual (or others). Trower et al. (2004) conducted a randomized controlled trial comparing this form of CBT with treatment as usual for command hallucinations. They found that CBT was effective for command hallucinations. In particular, there were large and significant reductions in compliance behavior, and this intervention (compared with treatment as usual) improved degree of conviction in the power and superiority of the voices and need to comply, as well as in levels of distress and depression. Finally, these differences were maintained at 12 months' follow-up. For more detailed information concerning the theoretical and practical aspects of this form of CBT for command hallucinations, consult Byrne, Birchwood, Trower, and Meaden (2006).

ROLE OF INDIVIDUALS' PERSONAL HISTORY

Romme and Escher (2000) described a unique approach that is based on analyzing the relationship between the patient's personal history and hearing voices (done with the help of the Maastricht Voices Interview for Children, described in the Appendix). This approach is particularly based on research showing relations between hallucinations and (traumatic) life events. In a collaboration between the voice hearer and the therapist, a report of the voices ensues, and this enables the development of a hypothesis that not only helps make sense of the voices for the interviewer but also, and more importantly, gives voice hearers meaning to the voices.

Romme and Escher (2000) identified three distinct phases in the process of learning to cope with voices: the startling phase (dominated by the feeling of being overwhelmed by the strange, new experiences and the inability to talk about the experiences); the organization phase (when the voice hearer has grown more used to the voices and is actively seeking coping strategies); and the stabilization phase (characterized by a growing feeling of control and identity with the voices). Techniques may involve short-, medium, and long-term techniques that are particularly (but not exclusively) relevant to one of the three phases. For example, short-term techniques are related to extending control over the voices; in particular, treatment involves anxiety management, trying out medication, providing information and health education, and offering support to both the patient and the family. Medium-term techniques tackle specific interactions between the hearer and the voices and may involve individual treatment (e.g., normalizing, coping strategies, and influencing beliefs) and getting involved in self-help groups. Finally, the long-term techniques aim at dealing with voices in everyday living to reintegrate into society. These final techniques can be particularly challenging to put into action because much of the distress and lack of control of voices are related to attitudes in the voice hearers' immediate surroundings and in society in general.

POSITIVE OR ADAPTIVE HALLUCINATIONS

As mentioned in chapter 2, a number of studies have revealed that some individuals perceive their hallucinations as positive or adaptive. This might have therapeutic implications. For example, patients may have come to rely on their pleasurable hallucinations and may be less motivated to change. Treatment would be fundamentally different for patients with primarily disturbing hallucinations than for patients with pleasurable hallucinations. In the latter case, the patients might not be very motivated to change because they do not perceive the hallucinations to be negative or problematic. Also, in such patients, noncompliance with treatment might be related to this. For example, Miller, O'Connor, and DePasquale (1993; described in more detail in chap. 2, this volume) found that a sizable minority of patients did not want their voices to disappear as a consequence of treatment. Indeed, seen in this light, removing hallucinations may actually be counterindicated in some patients. Perhaps the most effective strategy would be to attempt to help the patient view his or her voice as an important and cherished companion, while at the same time trying to avert the patient from viewing the voices as coming from a dreaded and unfriendly opponent. Therefore, intervention in these cases might focus on other issues such as adjustment to daily life and even how these positive experiences might actually interfere with social functioning. For instance, findings from Favrod, Grasset, Spreng, Grossenbacher, and Hodé (2004) suggest that patients who interpret their voices as being positive or benevolent may be considered, erroneously, as requiring less therapy than patients with malevolent voices. Indeed, results from this study showed that benevolent voices may affect social functioning in a negative manner; in particular, they were associated with poor communication.

PARTICULAR POPULATIONS

With few exceptions, many of the treatment strategies mentioned so far in this chapter have been developed with psychotic patients with hallucinations in mind. However, as mentioned several times in this volume, other categories of patient may also suffer from hallucinations (nonpsychotic, neurological, etc.). Consequently, because all these different clinical populations with hallucinations vary in terms of their clinical makeup and etiology, this must also be taken into account when considering treatment strategies for these patients. In this section, some examples of such particular populations are presented (those with dementia, Parkinson's disease, and Charles Bonnet syndrome). Although in certain cases it may be appropriate to apply intervention strategies (i.e., described in this volume) developed for psychotic patients in these and other nonpsychotic patients, a number of considerations must be made for these patients, and specific intervention strategies for these populations must also be developed and implemented. Because the treatment literature for hallucinations is clearly dominated by strategies for psychotic patients, there is therefore a paucity of strategies for nonpsychotic patients. Future researchers and clinicians are therefore urged to address this paucity.

Dementia

Particular attention and prudence is warranted when considering whether (and eventually, how) to treat hallucinations observed in patients with dementia. For a detailed presentation of pharmacological treatment strategies for psychotic symptoms in dementia patients, see Ballard, O'Brian, James, and Swann (2001). Documentation of the effectiveness of these agents in patients with dementia is largely lacking (Hoeh, Gyulai, Weintraub, & Streim, 2003). Studies fail to demonstrate significant advantage over placebo (L. S. Schneider, Pollock, & Lyness, 1990), long-term efficacy has not been addressed sufficiently, and there is a paucity of well-controlled studies (e.g., placebo-controlled, double-blind trials). Those studies that do find therapeutic effects of these agents on psychotic symptoms in dementia only show moderate improvement, provide nonspecific effects, may result in considerable side effects such as confusion that may greatly worsen the situation, and may result in the development of tolerance, dependence, or accelerated cognitive decline, even in atypical antipsychotics (Jeste & Lacro, 2000).

Furthermore, poor compliance with medication and interactions with other drugs are additional complications associated with pharmacological treatments in this population (Rao & Lyketsos, 1998). Older adults are also more likely to take multiple medications, thus increasing the likelihood of potential drug interactions (Douglass & Levine, 2000). Also, antipsychotic agents were constructed for psychiatric patients who differ significantly from patients with dementia in terms of phenomenology of symptoms, neurobiological substrates of symptoms, and clinical makeup. For instance, there is limited evidence to support any involvement of dopaminergic systems in the psychotic phenomena of dementia. Recent studies have suggested that cholinesterase inhibitors are effective in alleviating visual hallucinations in Lewy Body Dementia (McKeith et al., 2005; Mori, Ikeda, Fukuhara, Nestor, & Tanabe, 2006). Furthermore, this improvement may be due, at least in part, to improved attentional function or an increased level of alertness.

There are a number of important questions to ask before implementation of pharmacological treatments in older patients. In general, one is recommended to first seek out possible nonpharmacological interventions for the patient (Tariot, 1996). The presence of hallucinations in older patients is often related to sensory deprivation and/or vision loss (some of this research is described in chap. 3, this volume). Hallucinations have been consistently related to vision loss, and people with poor vision may be more likely to misidentify objects. Another possible explanation of the presence of hallucinations is related to the sensory deprivation notion, whereby people experience hallucinations in the absence of the stimulation of sensory areas by external objects. Interventions in these cases may simply involve providing visual or auditory aids (eyeglasses, enhanced-contrast materials, improved lighting, and hearing aids) or providing sensory input through auditory or tactile channels. Also, inappropriate sensory stimulation may play a role in the development and maintenance of hallucination in older populations. Various stimuli have been clinically reported to cause hallucinations. For instance, a reflection in a bathroom mirror or in a window at night may lead an older person with dementia to believe that someone is in the same room or on the other side of a door. Here, intervention may simply involve removing a mirror, placing a curtain over a window, or shutting off an intercom system, television, or bright light.

Another early (nonpharmacological) intervention is to assess and eventually modify environmental factors that aggravate the symptom(s). Education for the patient and caregiver in terms of the disorder and the problem behavior (and how to manage it and possibly alleviate it or reduce its impact) is another possible strategy. Early in the process, clinicians must also ask themselves if the symptoms are actually bothersome or harmful to the patient (or whether they are harmless and acceptable) and whether it is actually the patient's entourage who finds the behavior harmful, bizarre, dangerous, and so on. Also, in the light of a psychotic episode in patients with dementia, one must ask oneself if there is need for (pharmacological) treatment at all, as certain episodes may simply be a one-time episode. Also, one must consider the optimal treatment duration. Here, studies reveal that although short-term treatment may be needed, rarely will there be need for long-term, chronic antipsychotic treatment. Finally, there is the question of treatment modification: Are the symptoms stable or not? Certain conditions will not require much treatment modification because symptoms are usually relatively stable.

According to Ballard et al. (2001), the decision as to whether to treat patients with dementia for psychotic symptoms depends on a number of factors: the distress experienced by the patient, the distress experienced by their caregivers, practical management problems specifically relating to the symptom (do the psychotic symptoms result in any major practical management problems that are difficult to overcome with treatment of the symptoms?), the frequency with which the symptom occurs, and the natural course of the symptom. Few patients with dementia are greatly distressed by their psychotic symptoms (Ballard, Saad, et al., 1995; Gilley, Whalen, Wilson, & Bennett, 1991). Indeed, some hallucinations provide comfort to the person and do not need to be addressed. For instance, some find talking to deceased loved ones a pleasant and comforting experience. Hallucinations that do not have a negative impact usually do not require treatment. Therefore, treatment should only be considered if there is a substantial level of distress either to the person with dementia or to the caregiver. Studies show that many people experience these symptoms on only a few occasions per week, with less than a quarter experiencing them more than once a day (Ballard, Saad, et al., 1995). Even if distressing, if the symptom occurs on a very infrequent basis, there might not be a basis for treatment, and a strategy based on providing practical support at the times when the symptoms tend to occur may be more profitable.

Another consideration is related to the natural course of psychotic symptoms. Follow-up studies suggest, for example, that almost 50% of these symptoms resolve spontaneously within 3 months (Ballard et al., 1997). The symptoms most likely to persist are those that have already been present for 3 months at the time of assessment. Hence, if one is presented with a newly occurring psychotic symptom of only a few weeks' duration, unless the symptom is especially distressing or problematic, the most pertinent course may be to monitor carefully for a few weeks or months, during which time it may well resolve spontaneously. This is especially important when taking into consideration that the optimal time for response for pharmacological interventions may be 6 weeks or longer. If, however, after having considered all these issues, it is deemed that pharmacological treatment is the only realistic option, a cautious, closely monitored trial (with low doses) is indicated. For more detailed information concerning nonpharmacological treatment schemes for dementia patients, see Ballard et al. (2001); Cohen-Mansfield (2003); and Carlson, Fleming, Smith, and Evans (1995).

Parkinson's Disease

Because visual hallucinations in Parkinson's disease are commonly considered to be a side effect of dopaminergic therapy (primarily levodopa), researchers have suggested that reducing or withdrawing medication may reduce hallucinations. However, this usually increases motor disability in patients. Henderson and Mellers (2000) pointed out that when worsening motor symptoms exclude any further reduction in medication while at the same time increasing medication will cause a worsening of psychosis, then treatment with an atypical antipsychotic agent should be considered. In this context, recent studies have suggested that one potentially effective pharmacologic treatment (which in addition avoids the adverse side effects associated with dopaminergic therapy) for hallucinations in Parkinson's disease is cholinesterase inhibitors (Wolters, 2006).

It is important to underline that much evidence suggests that hallucinations in Parkinson's disease are not a simple dopaminergic adverse event (for more detailed information concerning this issue, see chaps. 3 and 7, this volume; also refer to Fénelon et al., 2000). One study reported that the occurrence of vivid dreams (and not the occurrence of hallucinations or delusions) was most strongly related to levels of levodopa doses. Furthermore, studies have shown that a number of cognitive, affective, pharmacological, and environmental factors play important roles in the genesis of visual hallucinations in Parkinson's disease. For instance, Sanchez-Ramos et al. (1996) found that sleep disturbance, levodopa, psychosis, depression, and dementia were associated with hallucinations. Fénelon et al. (2000) reported that when hallucinators and nonhallucinators were compared, significant differences were found in terms of (higher in hallucinators) age, duration of disease, severity of motor state, level of depressive symptoms, level of cognitive impairment, daytime somnolence, and a history of ocular pathology, but levodopa-equivalent dose did not differ significantly between the two groups. Therefore, treatment should also take into account these (and other) factors when attempting to alleviate hallucinations in Parkinson's disease.

Unfortunately, however, little work has been done in the area of developing nonpharmacological treatment interventions for hallucinations in Parkinson's patients. Nevertheless, Sanchez-Ramos et al. (1996) provided the following recommendations: modify the environment to protect the patient, enhance orientation by light personal contact and stimulation, make an effort to avoid the effect of sensory and motor deprivation (which is particularly evident in advanced Parkinson's disease), and help the patient and patient's entourage accept the hallucinations (especially when they are non-threatening).

Charles Bonnet Syndrome

Eperjesi and Akbarali (2004) reviewed three types of interventional strategies for Charles Bonnet syndrome (CBS): visual management, pharmacological management, and social management. (Note, however, that many of the studies examining the efficacy of these strategies included small samples in uncontrolled trials.) In terms of visual management, studies have shown that hallucinations attributed to CBS may disappear after treatment of the underlying cause of visual impairment or blindness, such as cataract extraction, treatment of subretinal hemorrhage, and implementation of optical devices. Important to note is that hallucinations may decrease in severity and eventually cease as the eye disease grows worse. The efficacy of pharmacological interventions for CBS hallucinations is less clear, with some authors claiming that they may have an effect (Batra, Bartels, & Wormstall, 1997) and others maintaining that they have no effect on hallucinations (Hosty, 1990; Teunisse, Zitman, & Raes, 1994; Tuelth, Cheong, & Samander, 1995). According to Eperjesi and Akbarali, probably the best form of intervention for CBS consists of social management. This may include providing contact with a sympathetic professional, giving reassurance of the benign nature of the hallucinations, counseling, psychoeducation (e.g., giving an explanation of the syndrome's cause using the phantom limb analogy, explaining that CBS is not related to mental illness), and limiting social isolation (ideally having patients join psychoeducation groups). Other important intervention strategies may include psychotherapy and treatment of possible complications such as depression (Fernandez, Lichtshein, & Vieweg, 1997).

SUMMARY

This chapter has described several intervention strategies for hallucinations. It is difficult to claim that one strategy or a group of strategies is more efficient than others, because studies have not directly compared the efficacy of these strategies in patients with hallucinations. Clinicians should, however, be familiar with the majority of these intervention strategies (and also be aware of their respective advantages and disadvantages) so that the most appropriate and individualized treatment may be provided for their patients. Furthermore, many of the intervention strategies described in this chapter may be used jointly in the same patient. For example, van der Gaag (2006) provided theoretical arguments for combining cognitive (in particular CBT, which provides psychological remission) and biological (in particular pharmacotherapy, which provides biological remission) interventions to maximize the chance for full recovery and remission of delusions and auditory hallucinations. The HIT program is also a good example of this, whereby several types of interventions may be proposed more or less simultaneously in the same patient (e.g., antipsychotic medication, coping training, psychoeducation, CBT, family treatment). Also, clinicians will probably need to adjust treatment programs over time. For instance, although psychoeducation may be seen as an important intervention early on, other strategies (e.g., CBT) may be integrated in later sessions. Similarly, in patients who show good improvement with individual CBT, the clinician may then propose group CBT.

CHAPTER HIGHLIGHTS

- A number of intervention strategies are available that may alleviate or eliminate hallucinations.
- No single strategy clearly arises from the scientific literature as being the most effective for hallucinations, and more research is needed to prove the specific efficacy of some of these strategies in the context of hallucinations.
- This suggests that treatment should be individualistic and that several intervention strategies should be used simultaneously.

APPENDIX:
ASSESSMENT INSTRUMENTS
FOR HALLUCINATIONS

The various available instruments for hallucinations are briefly described in this Appendix. Important to note is that although we attempted to have as exhaustive a review as possible of assessment strategies, some may not be mentioned. For lack of space, only the most widely used assessment strategies are included. There are four different sections, covering assessment strategies for adult populations, children and adolescents, older (nonclinical) individuals, and patients with dementia. This Appendix will end with a discussion of some of the clinical implications related to a comprehensive assessment of hallucinations. Finally, it is important to note that not only should assessment include a detailed evaluation of the hallucinations themselves, as well as the contexts in which they appear, but the assessment of medical and psychiatric problems and the presence of adverse life events is also essential.[1] Here is a list of the assessment instruments that are described in this Appendix:

- *Scales for adult populations*: Positive and Negative Syndrome Scale, Mental Health Research Institute Unusual Perception Schedule, Psychotic Symptom Rating Scales, Beliefs About Voices Questionnaire, Launay–Slade Hallucination Scale, Verbal Hallucinations Questionnaire, command hallucinations scales (Voice Compliance Scale, Voice Power Differential Scale), Institute of Psychiatry Visual Hallucinations Interview, Auditory Hallucinations Rating Scale, Topography of Voices Rating Scale, Positive Symptoms for Cocaine-Induced Psychosis.
- *Assessment strategies for children and adolescents*: Youth Self Report, Diagnostic Interview Schedule for Children, Kiddie—Schedule for Affective Disorders and Schizophrenia for School-Age Children, Maastricht Voices Interview for Children.
- *Assessment strategies for patients with dementia*: CERAD Behavior Rating Scale for Dementia, Behavioral Pathology in Alzheimer's Disease Rating Scale, Columbia University Scale for Psychopathology in Alzheimer's Disease, Neuropsychiatric Inventory, Visual Changes in Parkinson's Disease.
- *Another relevant scale*: Maastricht Assessment of Coping Strategies.

---

[1]References concerning assessment strategies for traumatic life events are included in chapter 8, this volume, in the section titled "Trauma."

It is worth examining how hallucinations are assessed in two of the most widely used assessment strategies for schizophrenic and psychotic patients: the Positive and Negative Syndrome Scale (PANSS; Kay, Fiszbein, & Opler, 1987) and the Scale for the Assessment of Positive Symptoms (SAPS; Andreasen, 1984). In the PANSS, there is only one hallucinations dimension, in which hallucinations are assessed along a 7-point severity scale (*absent, minimal, slight, average, moderately severe, severe, extreme*). However, different hallucination modalities are not assessed, and hallucination characteristics (e.g., frequency, control, triggers, emotional aspects, localization, physical qualities) are not included. In the SAPS, auditory (general, voices commenting, voices conversing), somatic or tactile, olfactory, and visual hallucinations are assessed individually along a 6-point severity scale (*none, questionable, mild, moderate, marked, severe*); however, hallucination characteristics (e.g., frequency, control, triggers, emotional aspects, localization, physical qualities) are not assessed.

Mental Health Research Institute Unusual Perception Schedule

The Mental Health Research Institute Unusual Perception Schedule (MUPS; Carter, Mackinnon, Howard, Zeegers, & Copolov, 1995) is a semistructured assessment tool for auditory hallucinations. It consists of items assessing various aspects of hallucinations, such as physical characteristics (e.g., frequency, when during the day, localization, volume, clarity), personal characteristics (e.g., sex of the voice; number of voices; known voice or not; whether in first, second, or third person), relations and emotion (e.g., relation with the voice, emotional state during the experience, associated emotions), form and contents (e.g., linguistic complexity, repeated contents, commands), cognitive processes (e.g., delusional activity, language or accent), perception of the experience (e.g., imaginary vs. real, hallucinations in other modalities), and psychosocial aspects (e.g., triggers, strategies used, role of medication). Subjects are asked to refer to the most recent hallucinatory episode to answer the questions. Although the MUPS is a highly extensive and detailed scale (with 365 items in total), clinicians are not obliged to use the whole scale but rather may use just certain modules.

Psychotic Symptom Rating Scales

The Psychotic Symptom Rating Scales (PSYRATS; Haddock, McCarron, Tarrier, & Faragher, 1999) is a self-report instrument consisting of two parts, one designed to rate auditory hallucinations and the other to measure delusions. In particular, the auditory hallucination section consists of 11 items assessing dimensions (based on a 5-point scale) of frequency, duration, location, loudness, beliefs concerning the origin of voices (varying from the belief that they are solely internally generated to solely from external causes), amount of negative content of voices, degree of negative content, amount of distress, intensity of distress, disruption of life caused by voices, and controllability of voices. Finally, the number of voices (over the past week) and the form of the voices (first person, second person, third person; single words or phrases without pronouns) are assessed. The scales have been found to have excellent interrater reliability (Haddock et al., 1999).

Beliefs About Voices Questionnaire

The Beliefs About Voices Questionnaire (BAVQ; Chadwick & Birchwood, 1995) is a 30-item self-report instrument that measures how people perceive and respond to their verbal auditory hallucinations. It includes five subscales: (a) Malevolence (e.g., "My voice is evil"), (b) Benevolence (e.g., "My voice wants to help me"), (c) Omnipotence (e.g., "My voice is very powerful"), (d) Resistance (e.g., "When I hear my voice, I usually think of preventing it from talking"), and (e) Engagement (e.g., "When I hear my voice, I usually seek its advice"). Among these five subscales, three relate to beliefs about voices (Malevolence, Benevolence, and Omnipotence), and two measure emotional and behavioral reactions to the voices (Resistance and Engagement). All responses are rated by checking "yes" or "no." Individuals who hear more than one voice are asked to complete the questionnaire for their predominant voice. The BAVQ shows acceptable levels of reliability, validity, and stability on test–retest over 1 week (Chadwick & Birchwood, 1995).

A revised version of the BAVQ has also been developed (the Revised Beliefs About Voices Questionnaire; BAVQ–R; Chadwick, Lees, & Birchwood, 2000) to address two weaknesses in the original BAVQ: Participants answered "yes" or "no" to each of the items, and there was only 1 item concerning omnipotence. Thus, the revised version contains a total of 35 items (including 5 new items pertaining to omnipotence), and responses are rated on a 4-point scale (*disagree, unsure, agree slightly,* and *agree strongly*). Results from Chadwick et al. (2000) revealed that the BAVQ–R was more reliable and sensitive to individual differences than the BAVQ and that the BAVQ–R reliably measures omnipotence.

Launay–Slade Hallucination Scale

The Launay–Slade Hallucination Scale (LSHS; Launay & Slade, 1981) is a questionnaire for measuring hallucinatory experiences in both the clinical (Kot & Serper, 2002; Levitan, Ward, Catts, & Hemsley, 1996; Serper, Dill, Chang, Kot, & Elliot, 2005; Young, Bentall, Slade, & Dewey, 1987) and nonclinical populations (Aleman, Nieuwenstein, Böcker, & de Haan, 2001; Bentall & Slade, 1985b; Larøi, Marczewski, & Van der Linden, 2004;

Larøi & Van der Linden, 2005b; Morrison, Wells, & Nothard, 2000, 2002; Paulik, Badcock, & Maybery, 2006; Waters, Badcock, & Maybery, 2003). The original scale was designed to assess hallucinatory experiences in the carceral population and consisted of 12 items. However, a number of changes have since been made to the LSHS, including changing the negative response items to positive ones and substituting the true-and-false format with a 5-point scale (Bentall & Slade, 1985b); incorporating additional items measuring predisposition to visual hallucinations, predisposition to auditory hallucinations, vividness of imagery, and daydreaming (Morrison et al., 2002); and adding items assessing other subtypes of hallucinations, including visual, olfactory, haptic, gustatory, hypnagogic, and hypnopompic hallucinations (Larøi, Marczewski, & Van der Linden, 2004; Larøi & Van der Linden, 2005b).

The internal structure of the LSHS has been examined on numerous occasions (Aleman, Nieuwenstein, et al., 2001; Larøi, Marczewski, & Van der Linden, 2004; Larøi & Van der Linden, 2005b; Levitan et al., 1996; Morrison et al., 2000; Paulik et al., 2006; Serper et al., 2005; Waters, Badcock, & Maybery, 2003). Larøi and Van der Linden (2005b) performed principal-components analysis on a revised version of the LSHS and found evidence of five factors that were characterized as representing items related to (a) sleep-related hallucinatory items, (b) vivid daydreams, (c) intrusive or vivid thoughts, (d) auditory hallucinations, and (e) visual hallucinations.

Verbal Hallucinations Questionnaire

The Verbal Hallucinations Questionnaire (Barrett & Etheridge, 1992) consists of 13 descriptions of verbal hallucination experiences (e.g., "Sometimes I have thought I heard people say my name . . . like in a store when you walk past some people you don't know . . . but I know they didn't really say my name so I just go on" and "I sometimes hear my thoughts aloud. I actually hear them spoken outside my head when no one really said anything"). This questionnaire was primarily based on Posey and Losch's (1983) hallucinations questionnaire. However, this scale has a certain number of limitations. The psychometric properties of the Verbal Hallucinations Questionnaire have never been examined, little or no information is available concerning the scale, such as how items were selected, and few studies have used this instrument. Another limitation is that the Verbal Hallucinations Questionnaire only assesses hallucinations in the verbal modality. Finally, subjects are asked to respond to certain items that are very precise or that relate to idiosyncratic hallucinatory experiences. For example, subjects are asked to describe the frequency of verbal hallucinations that occur in a car.[2] Certain aspects inher-

---

[2] "Sometimes when I am driving in my car, I hear my own voice from the backseat. It sounds like it is little short statements . . . usually soothing . . . like 'It'll be all right' or 'Now, just calm down' "; "I drive a lot at night. Sometimes I hear sounds in the backseat like people talking . . . just a word here and there, but no one is there" (Barrett & Caylor, 1998, p. 211).

ent in these items are highly pertinent to the onset of hallucinations in such items (e.g., occurring at night, presence of fatigue), but not all subjects experience this type of verbal hallucination in the given context (i.e., in a car), or they may take place in other contexts (e.g., in one's own house, at work, while using public transport). In a similar vein, two items describe overly specific contexts (i.e., in the house) that tap into highly similar experiences (i.e., hearing one's name).[3]

Command Hallucinations Scales

Some assessment tools have been developed for use (but not exclusively) in the context of command hallucinations. The Voice Compliance Scale (Beck-Sander, Birchwood, & Chadwick, 1997) is an observer-rated scale to measure the frequency of command hallucinations and the level of compliance or resistance with each identified command. The Voice Power Differential Scale (Birchwood, Meaden, Trower, Gilbert, & Plaistow, 2000) measures the perceived relative power differential between voice and voice hearer with regard to the components of power, including strength, confidence, respect, ability to inflict harm, superiority, and knowledge. There are seven items, and each is rated on a 5-point scale and yields a total power score.

Institute of Psychiatry Visual Hallucinations Interview

The Institute of Psychiatry Visual Hallucinations Interview (Santhouse, Howard, & ffytche, 2000) was developed[4] from a previous unstructured survey (ffytche & Howard, 1999). Participants are questioned about various phenomenological categories of pathological visual experience, such as temporal aspects (e.g., duration of individual hallucinations, length of time subjects have been hallucinating, frequency), emotional content (pleasant, unpleasant, neutral), localization (e.g., in front of the subject, out of the corner of the eye, in their blind area), detail and physical characteristics (e.g., more detail than real objects, whole scenes or individual objects or figures, can you see through them, flashes, lines, colors, zigzags, regular or irregular patterns, face without a body, words, letters, musical notes, numbers), and triggers (e.g., if they appear when the participant's eyes are closed, if they disappear when the participant blinks or moves his or her head). In addition, there are exclusion questions (e.g., visions associated with sound or talking, dizziness,

---

[3]"Last summer I was in the backyard. Suddenly I heard my husband call my name from inside the house. He sounded like something was wrong and his voice was loud and clear. I ran in but nobody was in the house. He was out in the garage and hadn't called at all"; "Sometimes when I'm in the house all alone, I hear a voice call my name . . . it's just once . . . like 'Sally' " (Barrett & Caylor, 1998, p. 211)
[4]This instrument was originally developed for assessing hallucinations in eye disease but has also been used in other populations, such as patients with dementia (see Mosimann et al., 2006).

or strange smells; occurrence only in bed or on waking from sleep; history of psychiatric and/or neurological disorders; frightening visions of small animals, snakes, maggots).

Auditory Hallucinations Rating Scale

The Auditory Hallucinations Rating Scale (Hoffman et al., 2003) contains seven items measuring frequency (0 = *stopped*; 9 = *relatively uninterrupted*), reality (0 = *indistinguishable from own thoughts*; 5 = *very real*), loudness (0 = *too faint to be heard properly*; 5 = *yelling or screaming*), number of voices, length (0 = *no words heard*; 4 = *multiple sentences*), attentional salience (1 = *doesn't affect me at all*; 7 = *the only thing that is important and I pay attention to is my voices*), and distress level (1 = *not distressing at all*; 5 = *often produces significant fear or anxiety*).

Topography of Voices Rating Scale

The Topography of Voices Rating Scale (Hustig & Hafner, 1990) is a self-report questionnaire that includes items measuring the loudness, clarity, level of distress, and intrusiveness of auditory–verbal hallucinations. Each item is rated on a 5-point scale.

Positive Symptoms for Cocaine-Induced Psychosis

The Positive Symptoms for Cocaine-Induced Psychosis (SAPS–CIP; Cubells et al., 2005) is based on the SAPS described previously (Andreasen, 1984). As in the SAPS, the SAPS–CIP assigns numerical severity scores to symptoms. Symptoms in the following domains are evaluated: delusions, hallucinations, and cocaine-related behaviors (e.g., compulsive foraging for cocaine), and these are further divided into categories according to phenomenology: type of delusions, sensory modality of hallucinations, and type of cocaine-related behavior. Regarding hallucinations, the division of scoring along sensory modalities (visual, auditory, somatic/tactile, and olfactory) was retained. However, on the basis of pilot work, the original SAPS differentiation of Schneiderian first-rank hallucinations (i.e., voices commenting on the subject and voices conversing with each other) was collapsed into the auditory hallucinations section.

Summary

The above-mentioned scales have various advantages in relation to each other. Compared with the other scales, the MUPS is probably the most complete scale in terms of its ability to take into account the greatest number of phenomenological characteristics. Although the LSHS may be used in a clinical context, its particular strength is its usefulness in research contexts, especially in studies including both clinical and nonclinical subjects. Furthermore, not only are different types and hallucination modalities (e.g., auditory, visual, olfactory, tactile hallucinations, and hypnagogic and hypnopompic hallucinations) assessed in more recent versions of this scale (e.g., Larøi, Marczewski, & Van der Linden, 2004; Larøi & Van der Linden, 2005b), the presence of phenomena such as vivid imagery, daydreams, or intrusive thoughts is also evaluated. Although the BAVQ does not elicit detailed and wide-ranging information concerning phenomenological characteristics of hallucinations to the same degree as, for example, the MUPS, it does provide the clinician and researcher with related and crucial information concerning how subjects react in the face of hallucinatory experiences.

ASSESSMENT STRATEGIES FOR CHILDREN AND ADOLESCENTS

Youth Self Report

The Youth Self Report (YSR; Achenbach, 1991) is a questionnaire for children and adolescents ages 11 to 18 consisting of 17 competence items and 103 problem items covering emotional and behavioral problems during the previous 6 months. Items can be scored 0 (*not true*), 1 (*somewhat or sometimes true*), or 2 (*very true or often true*). Hallucination items of the YSR include Item 40 ("I hear sounds or voices that other people think aren't there") and Item 70 ("I see things that other people think aren't there"). A drawback of the YSR is that it can only be used for older children (not younger than 11 years). In addition, only 2 hallucination items are included. Finally, hallucinations characteristics (e.g., frequency, severity, degree of control, emotional content and emotional reactions, triggers) are not evaluated.

Diagnostic Interview Schedule for Children

The schizophrenia section of the Diagnostic Interview Schedule for Children (DISC–C; A. Costello, Edelbrock, Kalas, Kessler, & Klaric, 1982) asks five questions: (a) "Some people believe in mind reading or being psychic. Have other people read your mind?"; (b) "Have you ever had messages sent just to you through television or radio?"; (c) "Have you ever thought that people are following you or spying on you?"; (d) "Have you heard voices other people can't hear?"; and (e) "Has something ever gotten inside your body or has your body changed in some strange way?" The questions are scored with a 3-point response scale (1 = *no*; 2 = *yes, likely*; 3 = *yes, definitely*). Downsides of the DISC–C include the fact that there is only one item concerning hallucinations. Furthermore, all items are endorsed on a present or absent basis; that is, no Likert scales are utilized. Finally, dimensions concerning various characteristics (e.g., frequency, severity, degree of control, emotional content and emotional reactions, triggers) of hallucinations are not incorporated.

Kiddie—Schedule for Affective Disorders and Schizophrenia for School-Age Children

The Kiddie—Schedule for Affective Disorders and Schizophrenia for School-Age Children (K–SADS) is a semistructured symptom-oriented diagnostic interview protocol derived from the adult SADS (Endicott & Spitzer, 1978). It is designed for children ages 6 to 18 years. Hallucinations (that are not related to sleep) are divided into three broad categories: (a) nondiagnostic auditory hallucinations (e.g., hearing nonverbal noises such as footsteps or knocking, hearing one's name being called without any other verbal hallucinations), (b) diagnostic hallucinations (e.g., hearing one or more voices saying at least one word other than one's own name), and (c) nonauditory hallucinations (visual, tactile, or somatic and olfactory hallucinations). Hallucinatory phenomena are then rated according to six different characteristics: experienced location of the origin of the hallucinations, whether other family members shared or fostered the experience, frequency, severity, and the degree to which the hallucinations were thematically and temporally consistent with depressed mood. Shortcomings of the K–SADS include the fact that certain hallucination characteristics are absent, in particular, the emotional content and emotional reactions related to the experiences. Also, triggers are not included for hallucinations, and neither are aspects such as coping techniques and beliefs.

Maastricht Voices Interview for Children

The Maastricht Voices Interview for Children (MIK; Escher, Romme, Buiks, Delespaul, & van Os, 2002b) was derived from the Maastricht Voices Interview for Adults (Romme & Escher, 2000). It contains several items related to the experience of hearing voices. This includes number of voices, frequency, emotional tone, and triggers of the voice. In addition, the degree of coping mobilized by the voices, attributions of voices (i.e., the presence of secondary explanations), and the presence of life events (based on a list of 22 common childhood events) are assessed. Finally, the child is specifically asked whether the voice was related to some past stressful life event or trauma. Limitations of the MIK include the fact that only (verbal) auditory hallucinations are assessed and that although a number of hallucination characteristics are assessed, they are mostly evaluated on a yes/no basis or are asked as open-ended questions, making it difficult to quantify responses.

Summary

These scales were not specifically designed to assess hallucinations. As a consequence, they contain far too few items relating to such experiences, and the few items that are included are not detailed enough in terms of their various characteristics (e.g., severity, frequency, control, triggers, emotional aspects, control). The only exception is the MIK, although this scale only assesses auditory hallucinations, and answers are not readily quantifiable.

ASSESSMENT STRATEGIES FOR OLDER, NONCLINICAL POPULATIONS

No assessment strategies have been developed with the older (nonclinical) population in mind. As a consequence, what follows is a presentation of studies examining hallucinations in older, nonclinical populations and brief descriptions of the assessment strategies used in each study. (These studies are described in more detail in chap. 3, this volume).

In Turvey et al. (2001), the question concerning hallucinations that proxy interviewees were asked consisted of the following question: "Does (name of participant in the study) ever see or hear things that are not really there—yes or no?" Thus, in this study, hallucinations were simply recorded as present or absent, and no further questions were asked to expand on the phenomenology of these symptoms. Livingston, Kitchen, Manela, Katona, and Copeland (2001) used the persecution, perceptual distortion, and affective response to delusions and hallucinations subsections of the Geriatric Mental State Schedule (Copeland et al., 1976) to identify people who had these symptoms in the month prior to the study. The hallucinations section rates clearly abnormal or puzzling experiences in all sensory modalities. Whether they occur when the respondent is awake and whether the respondent judges the experience to be real are also evaluated. Note that in this study, the prevalence of perceptual distortion (and not necessarily hallucinations) was the experience of interest. Furthermore, data were not presented concerning how subjects responded to "follow-up" definitions of the perceptual disturbances (i.e., whether they occurred in an awake state and subjects' realness judgments), making unclear the extent to which the perceptual disturbances could be considered hallucinations. For example, subjects who responded affirmatively to the perceptual disturbance question but who were not in an awake state and who were highly uncertain as to the "realness" of the experience cannot be considered to have had hallucinations. In Lyketsos et al. (2000), the Neuropsychiatric Inventory was used, which is described below.[5] Finally, participants in Cole, Dowson, Dendukuri, and Belzile (2002)

---

[5]As a reminder, both individuals with and without dementia were included in this study.

were asked if they had heard any sounds, noises, music, or voices where there did not seem to be a source for the sound. Those who reported auditory hallucinations (i.e., those who responded either "possibly" or "probably" to the first item) were asked to describe the sounds and to indicate whether the sounds were heard in the left, right, or both ears; whether it originated inside or outside the head; and whether they believed that other people could hear the sound. A hallucination score was computed by summing up the scores of responses to the four questions about hallucinations (heard sound, location of sound, source of sound, others can hear sound).

It is clear that hallucinations have not been assessed appropriately in studies including older, nonclinical individuals because they have mostly consisted of self-constructed scales. However, there is no reason why already established scales for the nonclinical population (e.g., LSHS) should not be used. For instance, in a revised version of the LSHS (Larøi, Marczewski, & Van der Linden, 2004; Larøi & Van der Linden, 2005b), one item ("On certain occasions I have felt the presence of someone close who had passed away") was included with the older adult population in mind (although nonelderly individuals respond affirmatively to this item) and has been administered to older populations (Larøi, DeFruyt, van Os, Aleman, & Van der Linden, 2005).

ASSESSMENT STRATEGIES FOR PATIENTS WITH DEMENTIA

CERAD Behavior Rating Scale for Dementia

The CERAD Behavior Rating Scale for Dementia (BRSD; Tariot et al., 1995) came out of the Consortium to Establish a Registry for Alzheimer's Disease (CERAD) initiative and was designed to assess behavioral symptoms in patients with dementia. Items cover a wide range of behaviors, including anxiety and fearfulness, depressive behaviors, restlessness, memory-related problems, socially inappropriate behavior, hallucinations, and delusions. It consists of 51 items rated according to frequency of occurrence on a scale of 1 (*occurred on only 1 or 2 days during the past month*) to 4 (*occurred on 16 or more days in the past month*). It takes approximately 45 minutes to administer. There are 2 items that are directly related to hallucinations: "Has the subject heard voices or sounds when there was no sound?" and "Has the subject seen things or people that were not there?" If there is an affirmative answer to an item, the respondent is asked to describe the experience. Also, the degree of clarity of the experiences is rated (i.e., vague or clear). The CERAD is mainly pertinent for Alzheimer's patients. Advantages of this scale include the fact that it is part of a nationally administered battery (CERAD). However, because the maximum frequency is "16 or more days in the past month," it does not distinguish between behaviors that occur frequently (e.g., once every 1 or 2 days) or very frequently (e.g., several times a day). Thus, the CERAD may be less pertinent for very frequent behavior (e.g., hallucinations in Lewy body dementia) and may have limited usefulness in detecting subtle changes or treatment effects. Also, severity of symptoms is not assessed.

Behavioral Pathology in Alzheimer's Disease Rating Scale

The Behavioral Pathology in Alzheimer's Disease Rating Scale (BE-HAVE–AD; Reisberg et al., 1987) was designed to assess the characteristic behavioral and cognitive symptomatology that commonly occurs in patients with Alzheimer's disease, behaviors that are frequently disturbing to the caregivers of Alzheimer's patients, and potentially remediable behaviors in Alzheimer's disease (mostly through pharmacological interventions). The BEHAVE–AD is a 25-item scale that rates symptoms on a scale from 0 to 3 (0 = *not present*; 1 = *vague: not clearly defined*; 2 = *clearly defined*; 3 = *verbal or physical actions or emotional responses to the hallucinations*). Time taken to complete the BEHAVE–AD is approximately 20 minutes. Subscales include hallucinations, paranoid and delusional ideation, activity disturbances, aggressiveness, diurnal rhythm disturbances, affective disturbance, anxieties and phobias, and a global rating of the impact of all behavior problems combined on the caregiver and patient. Each symptom is rated on a 4-point severity scale. For hallucinations, each modality is assessed (visual, auditory, olfactory, haptic, others), followed by its severity (not present, vague or not clearly defined, clearly defined hallucination of objects or persons, verbal or physical actions or emotional responses to the hallucinations). Monteiro et al. (2001) developed a version of the BEHAVE–AD that includes a frequency component for each of the 25 items (the Behavioral Pathology in Alzheimer's Disease—Frequency-Weighted Severity Scale; BEHAVE–AD–FW). Advantages of the BEHAVE–AD include the fact that it is useful with outpatients and nursing home patients and it has been shown to be useful for both patients with moderate dementia and patients with severe dementia (Reisberg, Franssen, Sclan, Kluger, & Ferris, 1989). Shortcomings include the fact that it is only pertinent for Alzheimer's patients and is mostly useful in prospective studies of pharmacologically remediated symptoms.

Columbia University Scale for Psychopathology in Alzheimer's Disease

The Columbia University Scale for Psychopathology in Alzheimer's Disease (CUSPAD; Devanand et al., 1992) is a short, semistructured instrument that can be administered by a trained lay interviewer for use in cross-sectional and long-term follow-up studies in a screening context. Particular emphasis was placed on the use of specific follow-up questions in this scale to help establish operational definitions for the presence of psychotic features in Alzheimer's disease. The scale takes between 10 and 25 minutes to administer and focuses on symptoms during the past month. There is a single explicit question for each item to facilitate its use by lay interviewers. In addition to hallucinations, delusions, wandering, verbal outbursts, violence, agitation, and sundowning constitute the items for behavioral disturbance. Also, items for depression are included. For each symptom, there is an initial question (present or absent), and in cases in which the symptom is present, follow-up questions are asked. For hallucinations, the follow-up questions first include rating if it is vague or clear, and then questions concerning the modality of the hallucinations are assessed (auditory, visual, olfactory, tactile, others). Advantages of the CUSPAD include the fact that it is easy to administer and contains questions pertaining to insight for items. Limitations include the fact that it was primarily constructed for use with patients with Alzheimer's disease. Being that it is a screening instrument, the CUSPAD assesses a relatively restricted range of behavior (mostly related to Alzheimer's disease) and lacks differential diagnostic capacity.

Neuropsychiatric Inventory

The Neuropsychiatric Inventory (NPI; Cummings et al., 1994) was developed to assess a wide range of behaviors encountered in dementia patients, to provide means of distinguishing between frequency and severity of behavioral changes, and to facilitate rapid (10 minutes) behavioral assessment through the use of screening questions. Questions were based on behavior observed in different dementias. In addition to questions about hallucinations, questions about delusions, agitation/aggression, dysphoria, anxiety, euphoria, apathy, disinhibition, irritability/lability, aberrant motor activity, nighttime disturbances, and appetite or eating change are included. These items were chosen because they also have the potential to distinguish between dementias that produce different types of behavioral disturbances. For hallucinations, after the screening question (presence or absence), questions concerning the modality are assessed (auditory, visual, olfactory, tactile, gustatory, others), and then the frequency (less than once per week, about once per week, several times a week but less than everyday, daily or essentially continuously present), severity (produce little distress in the patient, more disturbing to the patient but can be redirected by the caregiver, very disturbing to the patient and difficult to redirect), and the degree of caregiver distress are evaluated. Information is gathered from caregivers who are familiar with the patient's behavior who have at least daily contact with the patient. Advantages of the NPI include the fact that there are screening questions (minimizing administration time), both frequency and severity are scored, and a wide range of psychopathology is evaluated. It can also be used for several types of dementia patients. A version exists for use with nursing home residents (NPI–NH; Wood et al., 2000), and there is an adjunct scale for assessing caregiver distress (NPI–D; Kaufer et al., 1998).

Visual Changes in Parkinson's Disease Questionnaire

The Visual Changes in Parkinson's Disease Questionnaire (Barnes & David, 2001) comprises items covering the nature and properties of the patients' visual hallucinations, such as temporal factors (frequency, duration, onset), content (quantity, color, clarity, movement), subjective concomitants (affect, arousal level, perceived control), and external factors (triggers, eyes open or closed, lighting conditions).

Summary

In general, the above-mentioned measurement strategies for patients with dementia suffer from a number of common shortcomings. There are limitations in the instruments' accuracy (especially related to underestimation) as a result of items being based on informant ratings. Many of the instruments are too general; that is, they are relevant for dementia in general. At the same time, certain disorders are underrepresented, in particular Parkinson's disease (with the exception of the Visual Changes in Parkinson's Disease Questionnaire). In general, either severity or frequency is scored, even though both aspects provide highly informative data. Finally, many of the instruments lack differential diagnosis capacity.

ANOTHER RELEVANT SCALE:
THE MAASTRICHT ASSESSMENT OF COPING STRATEGIES

The Maastricht Assessment of Coping Strategies (MACS; Bak et al., 2001) is a semistructured interview that asks patients about the presence of a list of 24 symptoms related to psychosis. Both auditory hallucinations and nonverbal hallucinatory experiences (visual, olfactory, gustatory or tactile hallucinations) are included in this list. If a symptom is present, subjects are asked whether it has been present in the last week or month and to indicate (on a 7-point scale) the degree of distress associated with the symptom (varying from *no distress* to *very distressing*). In terms of coping strategies, patients are asked to name all the strategies used to alleviate the distress caused by the symptom. These coping strategies are categorized by the interviewer on the basis of a list of 14 different coping strategies. Factor analysis has identified five coping domains: active problem solving (distraction, problem solving, help seeking), passive illness behavior (prescribed medication, nonprescribed substances, physical change), active problem avoiding (shifted attention, socialization, task performance, indulgence), passive problem avoiding (isolation, nonspecific activities, suppression), and symptomatic behavior. Results from Bak et al. (2001) indicate that the MACS has good interrater and test–retest reliability.

CLINICAL IMPLICATIONS OF A COMPREHENSIVE ASSESSMENT OF HALLUCINATIONS

There are significant clinical implications of taking the multitude of hallucination characteristics into account, as can be done with some of the aforementioned assessment strategies (Larøi, 2006). For instance, it may provide patients with important information regarding their own experiences. Carter et al. (1995) reported that after patients were assessed with a comprehensive assessment instrument (the MUPS), many commented on how examining the different aspects of their auditory hallucinations provided them with new insight regarding their anxieties and fears, and perhaps even offered them new or different coping strategies for dealing with them. On the contrary, not taking these experiences into account might have disastrous effects. In many patients, for example, these experiences have been going on for a number of years and have become a part of their identity. Nayani and David (1996) suggested that a process of "accretion" occurs in schizophrenic patients with auditory hallucinations and that, over time, an individual suffering from hallucinations is apt to become more involved with the voices (e.g., have dialogues with them, describe them in more detail). Therefore, allowing the patient to talk about these experiences may have important positive clinical implications, whereas not being able to talk about them could have serious negative consequences.

Relations between patient and clinician may also be improved if one takes into account the phenomenological diversity of hallucinations. Chadwick and Birchwood (1995) mentioned that completing their hallucinations questionnaire (i.e., the BVAQ) seemed to ease communication with patients, perhaps because it conveyed some understanding of the hallucinatory experience. Similarly, Stephane, Thuras, Nasrallah, and Georgopoulos (2003) remarked that most patients in their study welcomed the opportunity of talking about their experiences and that this procedure seemed to enhance the therapeutic alliance. J. S. Strauss (1989) aptly noted,

> When closer attention is paid to patients' reports of their experiences, one key phenomenon suggested is the importance of the interaction between the person and the disorder. This interaction evolves over time and has implications for understanding, studying, and treating schizophrenia and related disorders. (p. 179)

One reason for this might be that routine and detailed inquiry into the wide variety of aspects of hallucinations may increase empathy with patients.

Taking into account the phenomenological diversity of hallucinations may help individualize treatment and management. For instance, treatment would be fundamentally different for a patient with primarily disturbing hallucinations versus patients with pleasurable hallucinations. In the latter case, the patient might not be very motivated to change because he or she does not perceive the hallucinations as negative or problematic. Also, in such patients, noncompliance with treatment might be related to this. For example, Miller, O'Connor, and DePasquale (1993) found that a sizable minority of patients did not want their voices to disappear as a consequence of treatment. Indeed, seen in this light, removing hallucinations may actually be counterindicated in some patients. Furthermore, because hallucinations' content is many times mood congruent, this work will most probably also involve working with aspects that are indirectly related to hallucinations, such as improving self-esteem and levels of depression.

Research has suggested that it is the phenomenological characteristics of hallucinations (and not simply, for instance, the presence of hallucinations) that are improved after effective treatment or that are associated with important risk factors. For instance, Fialko et al. (2006) found that suicidal ideation in a group of psychotic patients was clearly related to the emotional characteristics of auditory hallucinations (e.g., amount and degree of negative content, the amount of time the voices caused distress and the intensity of the distress) but not to other hallucination characteristics (e.g., frequency, duration, loudness, location). Miller (1996) observed that the (positive) antipsychotic effect on patients with schizophrenia was not an on-off switch phenomenon but in most cases was a qualitative change, with decreasing intensity, frequency, and emotional impact. As Miller (1996) herself commented, if a "presence versus absence of hallucinations" was used as an outcome criterion, the patients would have been classified as treatment nonresponders with respect to their hallucinations. A. R. Larkin (1979) found that hallucination control, intensity, and overt behavior changed significantly after inpatient treatment in his sample of patients. Therefore, therapeutic interventions should be directed at the phenomenological aspects of hallucinations, and furthermore, it is these aspects that merit detailed and systematic assessment when evaluating treatment efficacy.

Looking into more detail of the phenomenology of the hallucinations may open up new therapeutic avenues in certain patients. Hallucinations may implicate positive and/or adaptive emotional reactions (e.g., provide companionship, raise self-esteem, help sooth or relax the subject), yet studies have not examined how these reactions may influence hallucination formation and maintenance. A better understanding of the factors and mechanisms underlying adaptive emotional reactions in hallucinations may provide the clinician with ways of helping patients maintain these reactions. In addition, patients with predominantly negative emotional reactions to hallucinations may be instructed on how to reverse, as it were, this vicious circle of relating negative affect with the presence of hallucinations.

Furthermore, clinical work might involve helping the patient bring forth obscure positive descriptions of their hallucinations. For instance, Lowe (1973) found that the list of negative descriptions of hallucinations was much broader and much longer than was the list of positive adjectives describing hallucinations. The choice of negative, compared with positive, descriptions of the hallucinations was probably more accessible to these patients, creating a bias toward negative, compared with positive, hallucinations in patients. Similarly, Morrison (2002) presented a case study in which it became apparent that there were a number of positive beliefs about the voices that were preventing intervention from being maximally effective and may have contributed to their maintenance. This may be related to such a bias toward negative aspects associated with hallucinations. Romme and Escher (1989) found that the most fruitful strategies were to select the positive voices, listen and talk only to them, and try to understand them. For example, in one patient, such a positive voice asked such insightful and helpful questions as "How do you hear us, and in what way do we talk to you?"

Taking into account the phenomenological diversity of hallucinations may also help provide important information concerning changes in the patient's condition. Research shows that localizations of hallucinations may change over time. For example, voices that were initially heard as coming from outside via the ears may eventually be perceived as being located within the hearer's own head or body (Romme, Honig, Noorthoorn, & Escher, 1992). Furthermore, these changes may occur according to the hearer's mental and emotional state (e.g., when a person is stressed or upset, their voices may be loud and they may experience them as coming from outside).

Wykes (2004) noted this evidence in variation in the phenomenology of hallucinations. For instance, sometimes voices appear to be actual people in the same room or a different place but occurring outside the head. Sometimes they are inside the head and possibly being transmitted there by an unseen force. On yet other occasions, the person is unclear whether the voices are indeed his or her own thoughts or might switch between these explanations. Similarly, the content of the voices might also change over time, with some people feeling that the voice is positive and helpful, or there may be changes in the content over very brief periods of time or between different voices at the same time. Many of these variations occur in the absence of evidence for changes in medication, either in prescription or in adherence. The fact that there is evidence of changes in voices' phenomenological characteristics even when they are described as treatment resistant shows that they are still malleable and that there is room for optimism in their treatment. Similarly, A. R. Larkin (1979) reported that hallucinatory content in a group of schizophrenia patients was threatening and isolating in the acute phase but more socially focused during remission. Also, patients sometimes observe that the voices are at one time "telling jokes," whereas at another point in time they "become mean." It is therefore plausible that these variations in the phenomenology reflect important changes in the patient's emotional state.

REFERENCES

Aarsland, D., Larsen, J. P., Cummings, J. L., & Lake, K. (1999). Prevalence and clinical correlates of psychotic symptoms in Parkinson disease: A community-based study. *Archives of Neurology, 56,* 595–601.

Achenbach, T. (1991). *Manual for the Youth Self-Report and 1991 profile.* Burlington: University of Vermont, Department of Psychiatry.

Aggernæs, A. (1994). Reality testing in schizophrenics. *Nordic Journal of Psychiatry, 48,* 47–54.

Aleman, A. (2001). Hallucinations and the cerebral hemispheres. *Journal of Psychiatry and Neuroscience, 26,* 64.

Aleman, A., Böcker, K. B. E., & de Haan, E. H. F. (1999). Disposition towards hallucination and subjective versus objective vividness of imagery in normal subjects. *Personality and Individual Differences, 27,* 707–714.

Aleman, A., Böcker, K. B. E., & de Haan, E. H. F. (2001). Hallucinatory predisposition and vividness of auditory imagery: Self-report and behavioral indices. *Perceptual and Motor Skills, 93,* 268–274.

Aleman, A., Böcker, K. B. E., Hijman, R., de Haan, E. H. F., & Kahn, R. S. (2002). Hallucinations in schizophrenia: Imbalance between imagery and perception? *Schizophrenia Research, 57,* 315–316.

Aleman, A., Böcker, K. B. E., Hijman, R., de Haan, E. H. F., & Kahn, R. S. (2003). Cognitive basis of hallucinations in schizophrenia: Top-down mechanisms. *Schizophrenia Research, 64,* 175–185.

Aleman, A., & de Haan, E. H. F. (1998). On redefining hallucination. *American Journal of Orthopsychiatry, 68,* 656–658.

Aleman, A., Formisano, E., Koppenhagen, H., Hagoort, P., de Haan, E. H. F., & Kahn, R. S. (2005). The functional neuroanatomy of metrical stress evaluation of perceived and imagined spoken words. *Cerebral Cortex, 15,* 221–228.

Aleman, A., & Kahn, R. S. (2005). Strange feelings: Do amygdala abnormalities dysregulate the emotional brain in schizophrenia? *Progress in Neurobiology, 77,* 283–298.

Aleman, A., Nieuwenstein, M., Böcker, K. B. E., & de Haan, E. H. F. (2000). Mental imagery and perception in hallucination-prone individuals. *Journal of Nervous and Mental Disease, 188,* 830–836.

Aleman, A., Nieuwenstein, M., Böcker, K. B. E., & de Haan, E. H. F. (2001). Multidimensionality of hallucinatory predisposition: Factor structure of the Launay–Slade Hallucination Scale in a normal sample. *Personality and Individual Differences, 30,* 287–292.

Aleman, A., Sommer, I. E., & Kahn, R. S. (2007). Efficacy of slow transcranial magnetic stimulation in the treatment of resistant auditory hallucinations in schizophrenia: A meta-analysis. *Journal of Clinical Psychiatry, 68,* 416–421.

Ali, J. A. (2002). Musical hallucinations and deafness: A case report and review of the literature. *Neuropsychiatry, Neuropsychology and Behavioral Neurology, 15,* 66–70.

Al-Issa, I. (1977). Social and cultural aspects of hallucinations. *Psychological Bulletin, 84,* 570–587.

Al-Issa, I. (1978). Sociocultural factors in hallucinations. *International Journal of Social Psychiatry, 24,* 167–176.

Al-Issa, I. (1995). The illusion of reality or the reality of an illusion? Hallucinations and culture. *British Journal of Psychiatry, 166,* 368–373.

Allen, P., Amaro, E., Fu, C. H., Williams. S. C., Brammer, M. J., Johns, L. C., & McGuire, P. K. (2007). Neural correlates of the misattribution of speech in schizophrenia. *British Journal of Psychiatry, 190,* 162–169.

Allen, P., Freeman, D., Johns, L., & McGuire, P. (2006). Misattribution of self-generated speech in relation to hallucinatory proneness and delusional ideation in healthy volunteers. *Schizophrenia Research, 84,* 281–288.

Allen, P., Freeman, D., McGuire, P., Garety, P., Kuipers, E., Fowler, D., et al. (2005). The prediction of hallucinatory predisposition in non-clinical individuals: Examining the contribution of emotion and reasoning. *British Journal of Clinical Psychology, 44,* 127–132.

Allen, P., Johns, L. C., Fu, C. H. Y., Broome, M. R., Vythelingum, G. N., & McGuire, P. K. (2004). Misattribution of external speech in patients with hallucinations and delusions. *Schizophrenia Research, 69,* 277–287.

Altman, H., Collins, M., & Mundy, P. (1997). Subclinical hallucinations and delusions in nonpsychotic adolescents. *Journal of Child Psychology and Psychiatry, 38,* 413–420.

Amador, X. F., & David, A. S. (2004). *Insight and psychosis* (2nd ed.). Oxford, England: Oxford University Press.

American Psychiatric Association. (1987). *Diagnostic and statistical manual of mental disorders* (3rd ed., rev.). Washington, DC: Author.

American Psychiatric Association. (1994). *Diagnostic and statistical manual of mental disorders* (4th ed.). Washington, DC: Author.

Andreasen, N. C. (1984). *The Scale for the Assessment of Positive Symptoms (SAPS).* Iowa City: University of Iowa Press.

Andreasen, N. C., & Flaum, M. (1991). Schizophrenia: The characteristic symptoms. *Schizophrenia Bulletin, 17,* 27–49.

Arnold, T. (1806). *Observations on the nature, causes and preventions of insanity* (2nd ed.). London: Philips.

Asaad, G., & Shapiro, B. (1986). Hallucinations: Theoretical and clinical overview. *American Journal of Psychiatry, 143,* 1088–1097.

Asaad, G., & Shapiro, B. (1987). Reply: What about the bicameral mind? *American Journal of Psychiatry, 144,* 5.

Atkinson, J. R. (2006). The perceptual characteristics of voice-hallucinations in deaf people: Insights into the nature of subvocal thought and sensory feedback loops. *Schizophrenia Bulletin, 32,* 701–708.

Atkinson, J. R., Gleeson, K., Cromwell, J., & O'Rourke, S. (2007). Exploring the perceptual characteristics of voice hallucinations in deaf people. *Cognitive Neuropsychiatry, 12,* 339–361.

Baba, A., & Hamada, H. (1999). Musical hallucinations in schizophrenia. *Psychopathology, 32,* 242–251.

Bach, P., & Hayes, S. C. (2002). The use of acceptance and commitment therapy to prevent the rehospitalization of psychotic patients: A randomized controlled trial. *Journal of Consulting and Clinical Psychology, 70,* 1129–1139.

Badcock, J. C., Waters, F. A. V., Maybery, M. T., & Michie, P. T. (2005). Auditory hallucinations: Failure to inhibit irrelevant memories. *Cognitive Neuropsychiatry, 10,* 125–136.

Baillarger, J. (1886). Physiologie des hallucinations. Les deux théories [Psychology of hallucinations. The two theories]. *Annales médico–psychologiques. Journal de l'aliénation mentale et de la médecine légale des aliénés, 4,* 19–39.

Bak, M., Myin-Germeys, I., Hanssen, M., Bijl, R., Vollebergh, W., Delespaul, P., & van Os, J. (2003). When does experience of psychosis result in a need for care? A prospective general population study. *Schizophrenia Bulletin, 29,* 349–358.

Bak, M., van der Spil, F., Gunther, N., Radstake, S., Delespaul, P., & van Os, J. (2001). Maastricht Assessment of Coping Strategies (MACS–I): A brief instrument to assess coping with psychotic symptoms. *Acta Psychiatrica Scandinavica, 103,* 453–459.

Baker, C. A., & Morrison, A. P. (1998). Cognitive processes in auditory hallucinations: Attributional biases and metacognition. *Psychological Medicine, 28,* 1199–1208.

Ballard, C., Bannister, C., Graham, C., Oyebode, F., & Wilcock, G. (1995). Associations of psychotic symptoms in dementia sufferers. *British Journal of Psychiatry, 167,* 537–540.

Ballard, C., Harrison, R. W. S., Lowery, K., & McKeith, I. G. (1996). Noncognitive symptoms in Lewy body dementia. In R. H. Perry, I. G. McKeith, & E. K. Perry (Eds.), *Dementia with Lewy bodies* (pp. 67–84). Cambridge, England: Cambridge University Press.

Ballard, C., Holmes, C., McKeith, I., Neill, D., O'Brien, J., Cairns, N., et al. (1999). Psychiatric morbidity in dementia with Lewy bodies: A prospective clinical and neuropathological comparative study with Alzheimer's disease. *American Journal of Psychiatry, 156,* 1039–1045.

Ballard, C., O'Brian, J., Coope, B., Fairbairn, A., Abid, F., & Wilcock, G. (1997). A prospective study of psychotic symptoms in dementia sufferers: Psychosis in dementia. *International Psychogeriatrics, 9,* 57–64.

Ballard, C. G., O'Brian, J., James, I., & Swann, A. (2001). *Dementia: Management of behavioural and psychological symptoms.* Oxford, England: Oxford University Press.

Ballard, C. G., Saad, K., Patel, A., Gahir, M., Solis, M., Coope, B., & Wilcock, G. (1995). The prevalence and phenomenology of psychotic symptoms in dementia sufferers. *International Journal of Geriatric Psychiatry, 10,* 477–485.

Barber, T. X., & Calverley, D. S. (1964). An experimental study of "hypnotic" (auditory and visual) hallucinations. *Journal of Abnormal and Social Psychology, 63*, 13–20.

Barker, A. T. (1991). An introduction to the basic principles of magnetic nerve stimulation. *Journal of Neurophysiology, 8*, 26–37.

Barnes, J., & David, A. S. (2001). Visual hallucinations in Parkinson's disease: A review and phenomenological survey. *Journal of Neurology, Neurosurgery, and Psychiatry, 70*, 727–733.

Barrett, T. R., & Caylor, M. R. (1998). Verbal hallucinations in normals: V. Perceived reality characteristics. *Personality and Individual Differences, 25*, 209–221.

Barrett, T. R., & Etheridge, J. B. (1992). Verbal hallucinations in normals: I. People who hear "voices." *Applied Cognitive Psychology, 6*, 379–387.

Barrett, T. R., & Etheridge, J. B. (1994). Verbal hallucinations in normals: III. Dysfunctional personality correlates. *Personality and Individual Differences, 16*, 57–62.

Barta, P. E., Pearlson, G. D., Powers, R. E., Richards, S. S., & Tune, L. E. (1990). Auditory hallucinations and smaller superior temporal gyral volume in schizophrenia. *American Journal of Psychiatry, 147*, 1457–1462.

Batra, A., Bartels, M., & Wormstall, H. (1997). Therapeutic options in Charles Bonnet syndrome. *Acta Psychiatrica Scandinavica, 96*, 129–133.

Bebbington, P. E., Bhugra, D., Brugha, T., Singleton, N., Farrell, M., Jenkins, R., et al. (2004). Psychosis, victimization, and childhood disadvantage: Evidence from the second British National Survey of Psychiatric Morbidity. *British Journal of Psychiatry, 185*, 220–226.

Bebbington, P. E., & Nayani, T. (1995). The psychosis screening questionnaire. *International Journal of Methods in Psychiatric Research, 5*, 11–19.

Bechdolf, A., Veith, V., Schwarzer, D., Schormann, M., Stamm, E., Janssen, B., et al. (2005). Cognitive–behavioral therapy in the pre-psychotic phase: An exploratory study. *Psychiatry Research, 136*, 251–255.

Beck, A. T., & Rector, N. A. (2003). A cognitive model of hallucinations. *Cognitive Therapy and Research, 27*, 19–52.

Beck-Sander, A., Birchwood, M., & Chadwick, P. (1997). Acting on command hallucinations: A cognitive approach. *British Journal of Clinical Psychology, 36*, 139–148.

Behrendt, R.-P. (1998). Underconstrained perception: A theoretical approach to the nature and function of verbal hallucinations. *Comprehensive Psychiatry, 39*, 236–248.

Behrendt, R.-P., & Young, C. (2004). Hallucinations in schizophrenia, sensory impairment and brain disease: A unifying model. *Behavioral and Brain Sciences, 27*, 771–787.

Belenky, G. L. (1979). Unusual visual experiences reported by subjects in the British Army study of sustained operations, Exercise Early Call. *Military Medicine, 144*, 695–696.

Bentaleb, L. A., Beauregard, M., Liddle, P., & Stip, E. (2002). Cerebral activity associated with auditory verbal hallucinations: A functional magnetic resonance imaging case study. *Journal of Psychiatry and Neuroscience, 27,* 110–115.

Bentall, R. P. (1990). The illusion of reality: A review and integration of psychological research on hallucinations. *Psychological Bulletin, 107,* 82–95.

Bentall, R. P. (1995). Brains, biases, deficits and disorders. *British Journal of Psychiatry, 167,* 153–155.

Bentall, R. P. (1996). At the centre of a science of psychopathology? Characteristics and limitations of cognitive research. *Cognitive Neuropsychiatry, 1,* 265–273.

Bentall, R. P. (2000). Hallucinatory experiences. In E. Cardeña, S. J. Lynn, & S. Krippner (Eds.), *Varieties of anomalous experience: Examining the scientific evidence* (pp. 85–120). Washington, DC: American Psychological Association.

Bentall, R. P. (2003). *Madness explained: Psychosis and human nature.* London: Penguin Books.

Bentall, R. P., Baker, G. A., & Havers, S. (1991). Reality monitoring and psychotic hallucinations. *British Journal of Clinical Psychology, 30,* 213–222.

Bentall, R. P., & Slade, P. D. (1985a). Reality testing and auditory hallucinations: A signal detection analysis. *British Journal of Clinical Psychology, 24,* 159–169.

Bentall, R. P., & Slade, P. D. (1985b). Reliability of a scale measuring disposition towards hallucination: A brief report. *Personality and Individual Differences, 6,* 527–529.

Berman, I., Merson, A., Viegner, B., Losonczy, M. F., Pappas, D., & Green, A. I. (1998). Obsessions and compulsions as a distinct cluster of symptoms in schizophrenia: A neuropsychological study. *Journal of Nervous and Mental Disease, 186,* 150–156.

Berrios, G. E. (1985). Hallucinosis. In J. A. M. Fredericks (Ed.), *Neurobehavioral disorders* (pp. 561–572). Amsterdam: North Holland/Elsevier Science.

Berrios, G. E. (1990). Musical hallucinations: A historical and clinical study. *British Journal of Psychiatry, 156,* 188–194.

Berrios, G. E. (1996). *The history of mental symptoms: Descriptive psychopathology since the 19th century.* Cambridge, England: Cambridge University Press.

Berrios, G. E. (2005). On the fantastic apparitions of vision by Johannes Müller. *History of Psychiatry, 16,* 229–246.

Betts, G. H. (1909). *The distribution and functions of mental imagery.* New York: Columbia University.

Bick, P. A., & Kinsbourne, M. (1987). Auditory hallucinations and subvocal speech in schizophrenic patients. *American Journal of Psychiatry, 144,* 222–225.

Biederman, I. (1972, July 7). Perceiving real-world scenes. *Science, 177,* 77–80.

Bien, C. G., Benninger, F. O., Urbach, H., Schramm, J., Kurthen, M., & Elger, C. E. (2000). Localizing value of epileptic visual auras. *Brain, 123,* 244–253.

Bingley, T. (1958). Mental symptoms in temporal lobe epilepsy and temporal gliomas. *Acta Psychiatrica et Neurologica Scandinavica, 33*(Suppl. 120), 1–151.

Birchwood, M., & Chadwick, P. (1997). The omnipotence of voices: Testing the validity of a cognitive model. *Psychological Medicine, 27,* 1345–1353.

Birchwood, M., Meaden, A., Trower, P., Gilbert, P., & Plaistow, J. (2000). The power and omnipotence of voices: Subordination and entrapment by voices and significant others. *Psychological Medicine, 30,* 337–344.

Birchwood, M., & Trower, P. (2006). The future of cognitive–behavioural therapy for psychosis: Not a quasi-neuroleptic. *British Journal of Psychiatry, 188,* 107–108.

Black, D. W., & Nazrallah, A. (1989). Hallucinations and delusions in 1,715 patients with unipolar and bipolar affective disorders. *Psychopathology, 22,* 28–34.

Blakemore, S.-J., & Frith, C. (2003). Disorders of self-monitoring and the symptoms of schizophrenia. In T. Kircher & A. David (Eds.), *The self in neuroscience and psychiatry* (pp. 407–424). Cambridge, England: Cambridge University Press.

Blakemore, S.-J., Smith, J., Steel, R., Johnstone, E. C., & Frith, C. D. (2000). The perception of self-produced sensory stimuli in patients with auditory hallucinations and passivity experiences: Evidence for a breakdown in self-monitoring. *Psychological Medicine, 30,* 1131–1139.

Blakemore, S.-J., Wolpert, D. M., & Frith, C. D. (2002). Abnormalities in the awareness of action. *Trends in Cognitive Sciences, 6,* 237–242.

Bleuler, E. (1950). *Dementia praecox or the groups of schizophrenias.* New York: International Universities Press. (Original work published 1908)

Böcker, K. B. E., Hijman, R., Kahn, R. S., & de Haan, E. H. F. (2000). Perception, mental imagery and reality discrimination in hallucinating and non-hallucinating schizophrenic patients. *British Journal of Clinical Psychology, 39,* 397–406.

Boschi, S., Adams, R. E., Bromet, E. J., Lavelle, J. E., Everett, E., & Galambos, N. (2000). Coping with psychotic symptoms in the early phases of schizophrenia. *American Journal of Orthopsychiatry, 70,* 242–252.

Bourguignon, E. (1970). Hallucinations and trance: An anthropologist's perspective. In W. Keup (Ed.), *Origins and mechanisms of hallucinations* (pp. 83–90). New York: Plenum Press.

Bracha, H. S., Cabrera, F. J., Karson, C. N., & Bigelow, L. B. (1985). Lateralization of visual hallucinations in chronic schizophrenia. *Biological Psychiatry, 20,* 1132–1136.

Bracha, H. S., Wolkowitz, O. M., Lohr, J. B., Karson, C. N., & Bigelow, L. B. (1989). High prevalence of visual hallucinations in research participants with chronic schizophrenia. *American Journal of Psychiatry, 146,* 526–528.

Braham, L. G., Trower, P., & Birchwood, M. (2004). Acting on command hallucinations and dangerous behavior: A critique of the major findings in the last decade. *Clinical Psychology Review, 24,* 513–528.

Brasić, J. R. (1998). Hallucinations. *Perceptual and Motor Skills, 96,* 851–877.

Brébion, G., Amador, X., David, A., Malaspina, D., Sharif, Z., & Gorman, J. M. (2000). Positive symptomatology and source monitoring failure in schizophrenia: An analysis of symptom-specific effects. *Psychiatry Research, 95,* 119–131.

Brébion, G., Amador, X., Smith, M. J., Malaspina, D., Sharif, Z., & Gorman, J. M. (1999). Opposite links of positive and negative symptomatology with memory errors in schizophrenia. *Psychiatry Research, 88*, 15–24.

Brébion, G., David, A. S., Jones, H. M., Ohlsen, R., & Pilowsky, L. S. (2007). Temporal context discrimination in patients with schizophrenia: Associations with auditory hallucinations and negative symptoms. *Neuropsychologia, 45*, 817–823.

Brébion, G., Gorman, J. M., Amador, X., Malaspina, D., & Sharif, Z. (2002). Source monitoring impairments in schizophrenia: Characterization and associations with positive and negative symptomatology. *Psychiatry Research, 112*, 27–39.

Brett, E. A., & Starker, S. (1977). Auditory imagery and hallucinations. *Journal of Nervous and Mental Disease, 164*, 394–400.

Brewer, E. C. (2005). *Dictionary of phrase and fable* (J. Ayto, Ed.). New York: Collins. (Original work published 1898)

Broughton, R. (1982). Neurology and dreaming. *Psychiatric Journal of the University of Ottawa, 7*, 101–110.

Brown, G. W., Bifulco, A., & Harris, T. O. (1987). Life events, vulnerability and onset of depression: Some refinements. *British Journal of Psychiatry, 150*, 30–42.

Brown, J. W. (1985). Hallucinations: Imagery and the microstructure of perception. In P. J. Vinken, G. W. Bruyn, H. L. Klawans, & J. A. M. Fredericks (Eds.), *Handbook of clinical neurology* (pp. 351–372). Amsterdam: Elsevier Science.

Bruder, G., Rabinowicz, E., Towey, J., Brown, A., Kaufmann, C. A., Amador, X., et al. (1995). Smaller right ear (left hemisphere) advantage for dichotic fused words in patients with schizophrenia. *American Journal of Psychiatry, 152*, 932–935.

Brunelin, J., d'Amato, T., Brun, P., Bediou, B., Kallel, L., Senn, M., et al. (2007). Impaired verbal source monitoring in schizophrenia: An intermediate trait vulnerability marker? *Schizophrenia Research, 89*, 287–292.

Brunelin, J., Poulet, E., Bediou, B., Kallel, L., Dalery, J., d'Amato, T., & Saoud, M. (2006). Low frequency repetitive transcranial magnetic stimulation improves source monitoring deficit in hallucinating patients with schizophrenia. *Schizophrenia Research, 81*, 41–45.

Bryer, J., Nelson, B., Miller, J., & Krol, P. (1987). Childhood sexual and physical abuse as factors in adult psychiatric illness. *American Journal of Psychiatry, 144*, 1426–1430.

Bullen, J. G., Hemsley, D. R., & Dixon, N. F. (1987). Inhibition, unusual perceptual experiences and psychoticism. *Personality and Individual Differences, 8*, 687–691.

Burns, A., Jacoby, R., & Levy, R. (1990). Psychiatric phenomena in Alzheimer's disease: II. Disorders of perception. *British Journal of Psychiatry, 157*, 76–81.

Butler, R. W., Mueser, K. T., Sprock, J., & Braff, D. L. (1996). Positive symptoms of psychosis in posttraumatic stress disorder. *Biological Psychiatry, 39*, 839–844.

Byrne, S., Birchwood, M., Trower, P. E., & Meaden, A. (2006). *A casebook of cognitive behavior therapy for command hallucinations: A social rank theory approach.* East Sussex, England: Routledge.

Campbell, R. J. (2004). *Campbell's psychiatric dictionary* (8th ed.). Oxford, England: Oxford University Press.

Cangas, A. J., Errasti, J. M., García-Montes, J. M., Álvarez, R., & Ruiz, R. (2006). Metacognitive factors and alterations of attention related to predisposition to hallucinations. *Personality and Individual Differences, 40,* 487–496.

Cangas, A. J., García-Montes, J. M., de Lemus, M. L., & Olivencia, J. J. (2003). Social and personality variables related to the origin of auditory hallucinations. *International Journal of Psychology and Psychological Therapy, 3,* 195–208.

Carlson, D. L., Fleming, K. C., Smith, G. E., & Evans, J. M. (1995). Management of dementia-related behavioural disturbances: A nonpharmacologic approach. *Mayo Clinic Proceedings, 70,* 1108–1115.

Carter, D. M., Mackinnon, A., & Copolov, D. L. (1996). Patients' strategies for coping with auditory hallucinations. *Journal of Nervous and Mental Disease, 184,* 159–164.

Carter, D. M., Mackinnon, A., Howard, S., Zeegers, T., & Copolov, D. L. (1995). The development and reliability of the Mental Health Research Institute Perceptions Schedule (MUPS): An instrument to record auditory hallucinatory experience. *Schizophrenia Research, 16,* 157–165.

Cartwright-Hatton, S., Mather, A., Illingworth, V., Brocki, J., Harrington, R., & Wells, A. (2004). Development and preliminary validation of the Meta-Cognitions Questionnaire—Adolescent version. *Journal of Anxiety Disorders, 18,* 411–422.

Cartwright-Hatton, S., & Wells, A. (1997). Beliefs about worry and intrusions: The Meta-Cognitions Questionnaire and its correlates. *Journal of Anxiety Disorders, 11,* 279–296.

Cassano, G. B., Pini, S., Saettoni, M., Rucci, P., & Del'Osso, L. (1998). Occurrence and clinical correlates of psychiatric comorbidity in patients with psychotic disorders. *Journal of Clinical Psychiatry, 59,* 60–68.

Cather, C., Penn, D., Otto, M. W., Yovel, I., Mueser, K. T., & Goff, D. C. (2005). A pilot study of functional cognitive behavioral therapy (fCBT) for schizophrenia. *Schizophrenia Research, 74,* 201–209.

Catts, S. V., Armstrong, M. S., Norcross, K., & McConaghy, N. (1980). Auditory hallucinations and the verbal transformation effect. *Psychological Medicine, 10,* 139–144.

Chadwick, P., & Birchwood, M. (1994). The omnipotence of voices: A cognitive approach to auditory hallucinations. *British Journal of Psychiatry, 164,* 190–201.

Chadwick, P., & Birchwood, M. (1995). The omnipotence of voices: II. The Beliefs About Voices Questionnaire (BAVQ). *British Journal of Psychiatry, 166,* 773–776.

Chadwick, P., Lees, S., & Birchwood, M. (2000). The revised Beliefs About Voices Questionnaire (BAVQ-R). *British Journal of Psychiatry, 177,* 229–232.

Chadwick, P., Sambrooke, S., Rasch, S., & Davies, E. (2000). Challenging the omnipotence of voices: Group cognitive behaviour therapy for voices. *Behaviour Research and Therapy, 38,* 993–1003.

Chandiramani, K., & Varma, V. K. (1987). Imagery in schizophrenic patients compared to normal controls. *British Journal of Medical Psychology, 60,* 335–341.

Chang, J. B., Wang, P. N., Chen, W. T., Liu, C. Y., Hong, C. J., Lin, K. N., et al. (2004). ApoE epsilon4 allele is associated with incidental hallucinations and delusions in patients with AD. *Neurology, 63,* 1105–1107.

Chapman, F. M., Dickinson, J., McKeith, I., & Ballard, C. (1999). Association among visual hallucinations, visual acuity, and specific eye pathologies in Alzheimer's disease: Treatment implications. *American Journal of Psychiatry, 156,* 1983–1985.

Chawla, D., Rees, G., & Friston, K. J. (1999). The physiological basis of attentional modulation in extrastriate visual areas. *Nature Neuroscience, 2,* 671–676.

Chédru, F., Feldman, F., Améri, A., Salès, J., & Roth, M. (1996). Visual and auditory hallucinations in a psychologically normal woman. *Lancet, 348,* 896.

Cheyne, J. A., Newby-Clark, I. R., & Rueffer, S. D. (1999). Relations among hypnagogic and hypnopompic experiences with sleep paralysis. *Journal of Sleep Research, 8,* 313–317.

Cheyne, J. A., Rueffer, S. D., & Newby-Clark, I. R. (1999). Hypnagogic and hypnopompic hallucinations during sleep paralysis: Neurological and cultural construction of the night-mare. *Consciousness and Cognition, 8,* 319–337.

Choong, C., Hunter, M. D., & Woodruff, P. W. (2007). Auditory hallucinations in those populations that do not suffer from schizophrenia. *Current Psychiatry Reports, 9,* 206–212.

Close, H., & Garety, P. (1998). Cognitive assessment of voices: Further developments in understanding the emotional impact of voices. *British Journal of Clinical Psychology, 37,* 173–188.

Cockshutt, G. (2004). Choices for voices: A voice hearer's perspective on hearing voices. *Cognitive Neuropsychiatry, 9,* 9–11.

Coddington, R. D. (1972). The significance of life events as etiologic factors in diseases of children: I. A survey of professionals. *Journal of Psychosomatic Research, 16,* 205–213.

Cohen, L. H. (1938). Imagery and its relations to schizophrenic symptoms. *Journal of Mental Science, 84,* 284–346.

Cohen-Mansfield, J. (2003). Nonpharmacologic interventions for psychotic symptoms in dementia. *Journal of Geriatric Psychiatry and Neurology, 16,* 219–224.

Cole, M. G., Dowson, L., Dendukuri, N., & Belzile, E. (2002). The prevalence and phenomenology of auditory hallucinations among elderly subjects attending an audiology clinic. *International Journal of Geriatric Psychiatry, 17,* 444–452.

Coleman, R., & Smith, M. (1997). *Working with voices, victim to victor.* Gloucester, England: Handsell.

Collerton, D., & Dudley, R. (2004). A cognitive behavioural framework for the treatment of distressing visual hallucinations in older people. *Behavioural and Cognitive Psychotherapy, 32,* 1–13.

Collerton, D., Perry, E., & McKeith, I. (2005). Why people see things that are not there: A novel perception and attention deficit model for recurrent complex visual hallucinations. *Behavioral and Brain Sciences, 28,* 737–794.

Colloby, S. J., Pakrasi, S., Firbank, M. J., Perry, E. K., Piggott, M. A., Owens, J., et al. (2006). In vivo SPECT imaging of muscarinic acetylcholine receptors using (R,R) (123)I-QNB in dementia with Lewy bodies and Parkinson's disease dementia. *Neuroimage, 33*, 423–439.

Comer, N. L., Madow, L., & Dixon, J. J. (1967). Observations of sensory deprivation in a life-threatening situation. *American Journal of Psychiatry, 124*, 164–169.

Conn, R., & Posey, T. B. (2000). Dichotic listening in college students who report auditory hallucinations. *Journal of Abnormal Psychology, 109*, 546–549.

Cooper, J. K., Mungas, D., Verma, M., & Weiler, P. D. (1991). Psychotic symptoms in Alzheimer's disease. *International Journal of Geriatric Psychiatry, 6*, 721–726.

Copeland, J. R., Kelleher, M. J., Kellett, J. M., Gourlay, A. J., Gurland, B. J., Fleiss, J. L., & Sharpe, L. (1976). A semi-structured clinical interview for the assessment of diagnosis and mental state in the elderly: The Geriatric Mental State Schedule. 1. Development and reliability. *Psychological Medicine, 6*, 439–449.

Copolov, D. L., Mackinnon, A., & Trauer, T. (2004). Correlates of the affective impact of auditory hallucinations in psychotic disorders. *Schizophrenia Bulletin, 30*, 163–171.

Copolov, D. L., Seal, M. L., Maruff, P., Ulusoy, R., Wong, M. T. H., Tochon-Danguy, H. J., & Egan, G. F. (2003). Cortical activation associated with the experience of auditory hallucinations and perception of human speech in schizophrenia: A PET correlation study. *Psychiatry Research: Neuroimaging, 122*, 139–152.

Copolov, D. L., Trauer, T., & Mackinnon, A. (2004). On the non-significance of internal versus external auditory hallucinations. *Schizophrenia Research, 69*, 1–6.

Cosoff, S. J., & Hafner, J. (1990). The prevalence of comorbid anxiety in schizophrenia. *Australian and New Zealand Journal of Psychiatry, 33*, 67–72.

Costello, A., Edelbrock, C., Kalas, R., Kessler, M., & Klaric, S. (1982). *NIMH Diagnostic Interview for Children: Child version.* Rockville, MD: National Institute of Mental Health.

Costello, C. G. (1992). Research on symptoms versus research on syndromes: Arguments in favor of allocating more research time to the study of symptoms. *British Journal of Psychiatry, 160*, 304–308.

Cowell, P. E., Kostianovsky, D. J., Gur, R. C., Turetsky, B. I., & Gur, R. E. (1996). Sex differences in neuroanatomical and clinical correlations in schizophrenia. *American Journal of Psychiatry, 153*, 799–805.

Cramer, J. A., & Rosenheck, R. (1998). Compliance with medication regimens for mental and physical disorders. *Psychiatric Services, 49*, 196–201.

Crick, F. (1984). Function of the thalamic reticular complex: The searchlight hypothesis. *Proceedings of the National Academy of Sciences USA, 81*, 4586–4590.

Critchley, M. (1951). Types of visual perseveration: "Paliopsia" and "illusory visual spread." *Brain, 74*, 267–299.

Cubells, J. F., Feinn, R., Pearson, D., Burda, J., Tang, Y., Farrer, L. A., et al. (2005). Rating the severity and character of transient cocaine-induced delusions and hallucinations with a new instrument, the Scale for Assessment of Positive Symptoms for Cocaine-Induced Psychosis (SAPS–CIP). *Drug and Alcohol Dependence*, 80, 23–33.

Cullberg, J., & Nybäck, H. (1992). Persistent auditory hallucinations correlate with the size of the third ventricle in schizophrenic patients. *Acta Psychiatrica Scandinavica*, 86, 469–472.

Cummings, J. L., Mega, M., Gray, K., Rosenberg-Thompson, S., Carusi, D. A., & Gornbein, J. (1994). The Neuropsychiatric Inventory: Comprehensive assessment of psychopathology in dementia. *Neurology*, 44, 2308–2314.

Currie, S., Heathfield, K. W. G., Henson, R. A., & Scott, D. F. (1971). Clinical course and prognosis of temporal lobe epilepsy: A survey of 666 patients. *Brain*, 92, 173–190.

Curson, D. A., Patel, M., Liddle, P. F., & Barnes, T. R. E. (1988). Psychiatric morbidity of a long stay hospital population with chronic schizophrenia and implications for future community care. *British Medical Journal*, 297, 819–822.

d'Alfonso, A. A. L., Aleman, A., Kessels, R. P. C., Schouten, E. A., Postma, A., Van der Linden, J. A., et al. (2002). TMS of auditory cortex in schizophrenia: Effects on hallucinations and neurocognition. *Journal of Neuropsychiatry and Clinical Neurosciences*, 14, 77–79.

Dary, M., Eustache, F., Viader, F., & Lechevalier, B. (1994). Hallucinations (ou hallucinoses) auditives chez une patiente atteinte de maladie d'Alzheimer probable [Auditory hallucinations (or hallucinoses) in a patient with probable Alzheimer's disease]. *Revue de Neuropsychologie*, 4, 469–481.

Dattilio, F. N. (2006). Does the case study have a future in the psychiatric literature? *International Journal of Psychiatry in Clinical Practice*, 10, 195–203.

David, A. S. (1993). Cognitive neuropsychiatry? *Psychological Medicine*, 23, 1–5.

David, A. S. (1994). The neuropsychology of auditory–verbal hallucinations. In A. S. David & J. Cutting (Eds.), *The neuropsychology of schizophrenia* (pp. 269–312). Hove, England: Erlbaum.

David, A. S. (1999). Auditory hallucinations: Phenomenology, neuropsychology and neuroimaging update. *Acta Psychiatrica Scandinavica*, 99(Suppl. 395), 95–104.

David, A. S. (2004). The cognitive neuropsychiatry of auditory verbal hallucinations: An overview. *Cognitive Neuropsychiatry*, 9, 107–124.

David, A. S., & Lucas, P. (1993). Auditory–verbal hallucinations and the phonological loop: A cognitive neuropsychological study. *British Journal of Clinical Psychology*, 32, 431–441.

David, A. S., Malmberg, A., Lewis, G., Brandt, L., & Allbeck, P. (1995). Are there neurological and sensory risk factors for schizophrenia? *Schizophrenia Research*, 14, 247–251.

David, A. S., Woodruff, P. W. R., Howard, R., Mellers, J. D. C., Brammer, M., Bullmore, E., et al. (1996). Auditory hallucinations inhibit exogenous activation of auditory association cortex. *NeuroReport*, 7, 932–936.

Davies, M. F., Griffin, M., & Vice, S. (2001). Affective reactions to auditory hallucinations in psychotic, evangelical and control groups. *British Journal of Clinical Psychology, 40*, 361–370.

Delespaul, P., deVries, M., & van Os, J. (2002). Determinants of occurrence and recovery from hallucinations in daily life. *Social Psychiatry and Psychiatric Epidemiology, 37*, 97–104.

Della Sala, S., Francescani, A., Muggia, S., & Spinnler, H. (1998). Variables linked to psychotic symptoms in Alzheimer's disease. *European Journal of Neurology, 5*, 553–560.

Dennett, D. (1991). *Consciousness explained.* Boston: Little, Brown.

Devanand, D. P., Miller, L., Richard, M., Marder, K., Bell, K., Mayeux, R., & Stern, Y. (1992). The Columbia University Scale for Psychopathology in Alzheimer's Disease. *Archives of Neurology, 49*, 371–376.

Dhossche, D., Ferdinand, R., Van der Ende, J., Hofstra, M. B., & Verhulst, F. (2002). Diagnostic outcome of self-reported hallucinations in a community sample of adolescents. *Psychological Medicine, 32*, 619–627.

Dickerson, F. B. (2000). Cognitive behavioral psychotherapy for schizophrenia: A review of recent empirical studies. *Schizophrenia Research, 43*, 71–90.

Diederich, N. J., Goetz, C. G., & Stebbins, G. T. (2005). Repeated visual hallucinations in Parkinson's disease as disturbed external/internal perceptions: Focused review and a new integrative model. *Movement Disorders, 20*, 130–140.

Dierks, T., Linden, D. E., Jandl, M., Formisano, E., Goebel, R., Lanfermann, H., & Singer, W. (1999). Activation of Heschl's gyrus during auditory hallucinations. *Neuron, 22*, 615–621.

Ditman, T., & Kuperberg, G. R. (2005). A source-monitoring account of auditory verbal hallucinations in patients with schizophrenia. *Harvard Review of Psychiatry, 13*, 280–299.

Dittmann, J., & Schüttler, R. (1990). Disease consciousness and coping strategies of patients with schizophrenic psychosis. *Acta Psychiatrica Scandinavica, 82*, 318–322.

Dolan, R. J. (2002, November 8). Emotion, cognition, and behavior. *Science, 298*, 1191–1194.

Dolgov, I., & McBeath, M. K. (2005). A signal-detection-theory representation of normal and hallucinatory perception. *Behavioral and Brain Sciences, 28*, 761–762.

Douglass, M. A., & Levine, D. P. (2000). Hallucinations in an elderly patient taking recommended doses of cyclobenxaprine. *Archives of Internal Medicine, 160*, 1373.

Drevets, W. C., & Rubin, E. H. (1989). Psychotic symptoms and the longitudinal course of senile dementia of the Alzheimer's type. *Biological Psychiatry, 33*, 536–541.

Duda, J. E. (2004). Pathology and neurotransmitter abnormalities of dementia with Lewy bodies. *Dementia and Geriatric Cognitive Disorders, 17*(Suppl. 1), 3–14.

Dudley, R., Dixon, J., & Turkington, D. (2005). CBT for a person with schizophrenia: Systematic desensitization for phobias led to positive symptom improvement. *Behavioural and Cognitive Psychotherapy, 33*, 249–254.

du Feu, M., & McKenna, P. J. (1999). Prelingually profoundly deaf schizophrenic patients who hear voices: A phenomenological analysis. *Acta Psychiatrica Scandinavica, 99*, 453–459.

Eaton, W. E., Romanoski, A., Anthony, J. C., & Nestadt, G. (1991). Screening for psychosis in the general population with a self-report interview. *Journal of Nervous and Mental Disease, 179*, 689–693.

Ellason, J., & Ross, C. (1997). Childhood trauma and psychiatric symptoms. *Psychological Reports, 80*, 447–450.

Endicott. J., & Spitzer, R. L. (1978). A diagnostic interview: The Schedule for Affective Disorders and Schizophrenia. *Archives of General Psychiatry, 35*, 837–844.

Ensink, B. (1992). *Confusing realities: A study on child sexual abuse and psychiatric symptoms*. Amsterdam: Free University Press.

Ensum, I., & Morrison, A. P. (2003). The effects of focus of attention on attributional bias in patients experiencing auditory hallucinations. *Behaviour Research and Therapy, 41*, 895–907.

Eperjesi, F., & Akbarali, N. (2004). Rehabilitation in Charles Bonnet syndrome: A review of treatment options. *Clinical and Experimental Optometry, 87*, 149–152.

Erkwoh, R., Willmes, K., Eming-Erdmann, A., & Kunert, H. J. (2002). Command hallucinations: Who obeys and who resists when? *Psychopathology, 35*, 272–279.

Escher, A., Delespaul, P., Romme, M., Buiks, A., & van Os, J. (2003). Coping defence and depression in adolescents hearing voices. *Journal of Mental Health, 12*, 91–99.

Escher, A., Morris, M., Buiks, A., Delespaul, P., van Os, J., & Romme, M. (2004). Determinants of outcome in the pathways through care for children hearing voices. *International Journal of Social Welfare, 13*, 208–222.

Escher, S., Romme, M., Buiks, A., Delespaul, P., & van Os, J. (2002a). Formation of delusional ideation in adolescents hearing voices: A prospective study. *American Journal of Medical Genetics, 114*, 913–920.

Escher, S., Romme, M., Buiks, A., Delespaul, P., & van Os, J. (2002b). Independent course of childhood auditory hallucinations: A sequential 3-year follow-up study. *British Journal of Psychiatry, 181*(Suppl. 43), 10–18.

Esquirol, E. (1817). Hallucination. In Adelon et al. (Eds.), *Dictionnaire des sciences médicales par une société de médecines et de chirurgiens* [Dictionary of medical sciences by a society of doctors and surgeons] (Vol. 20, pp. 64–71). Paris: Panckoucke.

Esquirol, J. E. D. (1832). Sur les illusions des sens chez les aliénes [On the illusions of sense among the insane]. *Archives Générales de Médecine, 2*, 5–23.

Esquirol, J. E. D. (1965). *Mental maladies: A treatise on insanity*. New York: Hafner. (Original work published 1845)

Evans, C. L., McGuire, P. K., & David, A. S. (2000). Is auditory imagery defective in patients with auditory hallucinations? *Psychological Medicine, 30,* 137–148.

Evers, S., & Ellger, T. (2004). The clinical spectrum of musical hallucinations. *Journal of the Neurological Sciences, 227,* 55–65.

Ey, H. (1973). *Traité des hallucinations* [Treatise on hallucinations] (Vols. 1–2). Paris: Masson.

Fallon, I. R. H., & Talbot, R. E. (1981). Persistent auditory hallucinations: Coping mechanisms and implications for management. *Psychological Medicine, 11,* 329–339.

Farah, M. J., & Smith, A. F. (1983). Perceptual interference and facilitation with auditory imagery. *Perception and Psychophysics, 33,* 475–478.

Farhall, J., & Gehrbe, M. (1997). Coping with hallucinations. Exploring stress and coping framework. *British Journal of Clinical Psychology, 36,* 259–261.

Farhall, J., Greenwood, K. M., & Jackson, H. J. (2007). Coping with hallucinated voices in schizophrenia: A review of self-initiated strategies and therapeutic interventions. *Clinical Psychology Review, 27,* 476–493.

Farley, J., Woodruff, R., & Guze, S. (1968). The prevalence of hysteria and conversion symptoms. *British Journal of Psychiatry, 114,* 1121–1125.

Favrod, J., Grasset, F., Spreng, S., Grossenbacher, B., & Hodé, Y. (2004). Benevolent voices are not so kind: The functional significance of auditory hallucinations. *Psychopathology, 37,* 304–308.

Feinberg, I. (1978). Efference copy and corollary discharge: Implications for thinking and its disorders. *Schizophrenia Bulletin, 4,* 636–640.

Feinstein, A., & Ron, M. A. (1990). Psychosis associated with demonstrable brain disease. *Psychological Medicine, 20,* 793–803.

Fénelon, G., Mahieux, F., Huon, R., & Ziégler, M. (2000). Hallucinations in Parkinson's disease. *Brain, 123,* 733–745.

Fénelon, G., Marie, S., Ferroir, J. P., & Guillard, A. (1993). Hallucinose musicale: 7 cas [Musical hallucinosis: 7 cases]. *Revue Neurologique, 149,* 462–467.

Fénelon, G., Thobois, S., Bonnet, A.-M., Broussolle, E., & Tison, F. (2002). Tactile hallucinations in Parkinson's disease. *Journal of Neurology, 249,* 1699–1703.

Fenton, G. W., & McRae, D. (1989). Musical hallucinations in a deaf elderly woman. *British Journal of Psychiatry, 155,* 401–403.

Fernandez, A., Lichtshein, G., & Vieweg, W. V. R. (1997). The Charles Bonnet syndrome: A review. *Journal of Nervous and Mental Disease, 185,* 195–200.

Fernyhough, C. (2004). Alien voices and inner dialogue: Towards a developmental account of auditory verbal hallucinations. *New Ideas in Psychology, 22,* 49–68.

Festinger, L. (1957). *A theory of cognitive dissonance*. Stanford, CA: Stanford University Press.

ffytche, D. H., & Howard, R. J. (1999). The perceptual consequences of visual loss: "Positive" pathologies of vision. *Brain, 122,* 1247–1260.

ffytche, D. H., Howard, R. J., Brammer, M. J., David, A., Woodruff, P., & Williams, S. (1998). The anatomy of conscious vision: An fMRI study of visual hallucinations. *Nature Neuroscience, 1,* 738–742.

Fialko, L., Freeman, D., Bebbington, P. E., Kuipers, E., Garety, P. A., Dunn, G., & Fowler, D. (2006). Understanding suicidal ideation in psychosis: Findings from the Psychological Prevention of Relapse in Psychosis (PRP) trial. *Acta Psychiatrica Scandinavica, 114,* 177–186.

Finkel, S. I., Costa, S. E., Cohen, G., Miller, S., & Sartorius, N. (1996). Behavioral and psychological signs and symptoms of dementia: A consensus statement on current knowledge and implications for research and treatment. *International Psychogeriatrics, 8*(Suppl. 3), 497–500.

Fischer, C. E., Marchie, A., & Norris, M. (2004). Musical and auditory hallucinations: A spectrum. *Psychiatry and Clinical Neurosciences, 58,* 96–98.

Fitzgerald, P. B., Benitez, J., Daskalakis, J. Z., Brown, T. L., Marston, N. A., de Castella, A., & Kulkarni, J. (2005). A double-blind sham-controlled trial of repetitive transcranial magnetic stimulation in the treatment of refractory auditory hallucinations. *Journal of Clinical Psychopharmacology, 24,* 358–362.

Flaum, M., Andreasen, N. C., Swayze, V. W., II, O'Leary, D. S., & Alliger, R. J. (1994). IQ and brain size in schizophrenia. *Psychiatry Research, 53,* 243–257.

Flavell, J. H. (1979). Metacognition and cognitive monitoring: A new era of cognitive–developmental inquiry. *American Psychologist, 34,* 906–911.

Flavell, J. H., & Ross, L. (1981). *Social cognitive development: Frontiers and possible features.* New York: Cambridge University Press.

Ford, J. M., & Mathalon, D. H. (2005). Corollary discharge dysfunction in schizophrenia: Can it explain auditory hallucinations? *International Journal of Psychophysiology, 58,* 179–189.

Ford, J. M., Roach, B. J., Faustman, W. O., & Mathalon, D. H. (2007). Synch before you speak: Auditory hallucinations in schizophrenia. *American Journal of Psychiatry, 164,* 458–466.

Formisano, E., Kim, D. S., Di Salle, F., van de Moortele, P. F., Ugurbil, K., & Goebel, R. (2003). Mirror-symmetric tonotopic maps in human primary auditory cortex. *Neuron, 40,* 859–869.

Forstl, H., Besthorn, C., Geiger-Kabisch, C., Sattel, H., & Schreiter-Gasser, U. (1993). Psychotic features and the course of Alzheimer's disease: Relationship to cognitive, electroencephalographic and computerized tomography findings. *Acta Psychiatrica Scandinavica, 87,* 395–399.

Foss, J. (2004). Good science, bad philosophy. *Behavioral and Brain Sciences, 27,* 791–792.

Fowler, I. L., Carr, V. J., Carter, N. T., & Lewin, T. J. (1998). Patterns of current and lifetime substance use in schizophrenia. *Schizophrenia Bulletin, 24,* 443–455.

Freeman, D., & Garety, P. A. (2003). Connecting neurosis and psychosis: The direct influence of emotion on delusions and hallucinations. *Behaviour Research and Therapy, 41,* 923–947.

French, P., Morrison, A. P., Walford, L., Knight, A., & Bentall, R. P. (2003). Cognitive therapy for preventing transition to psychosis in high risk individuals: A case series. *Behavioural and Cognitive Psychotherapy, 31,* 53–67.

Freud, S. (1938). The interpretation of dreams. In A. A. Brill (Ed. & Trans.), *The basic writings of Sigmund Freud* (pp. ???). New York: Random House. (Original work published 1900)

Freud, S. (1966). *The psychopathology of everyday life* (J. Strachey, Trans.). London: Ernest Benn. (Original work published 1901)

Frith, C. D. (1987). The positive and negative symptoms of schizophrenia reflect impairments in the perception and initiation of action. *Psychological Medicine, 17,* 631–648.

Frith, C. D. (1992). *The cognitive neuropsychology of schizophrenia.* Hove, England: Erlbaum.

Frith, C. (1999). How hallucinations make themselves heard. *Neuron, 22,* 414–415.

Frith, C. D., & Dolan, R. J. (1997). Brain mechanisms associated with top-down processes in perception. *Philosophical Transactions of the Royal Society of London, Series B: Biological Sciences, 352,* 1221–1230.

Frith, C. D., & Done, D. J. (1989). Experiences of alien control in schizophrenia reflect a disorder in the central monitoring of action. *Psychological Medicine, 19,* 359–363.

Gallagher, A. G., Dinin, T. G., & Baker, L. V. J. (1994). The effects of varying auditory input on schizophrenic hallucinations: A replication. *British Journal of Medical Psychology, 67,* 67–76.

Galton, F. (1943). *Inquiries into human faculty and its development* (2nd ed.). London: Dent. (Original work published 1883)

García-Montes, J. M., Pérez-Álvarez, M., Balbuena, C. S., Garcelàn, S. P., & Cangas, A. J. (2006). Metacognitions in patients with hallucinations and obsessive–compulsive disorder: The superstition factor. *Behavior Research and Therapy, 44,* 1091–1104.

García-Montes, J. M., Pérez-Álvarez, M., & Fidalgo, A. M. (2003). Influence of the suppression of self-discrepant thoughts on the vividness of perception of auditory illusions. *Behavioural and Cognitive Psychotherapy, 31,* 33–44.

Garety, P. A., Bebbington, P., Fowler, D., Freeman, D., & Kuipers, E. (2007). Implications for neurobiological research of cognitive models of psychosis: A theoretical paper. *Psychological Medicine, 37,* 1377–1391.

Garety, P. A., Fowler, D., & Kuipers, E. (2000). Cognitive–behavioral therapy for medication-resistant symptoms. *Schizophrenia Bulletin, 26,* 73–86.

Garety, P. A., Kuipers, E., Fowler, D., Freeman, D., & Bebbington, P. E. (2001). A cognitive model of the positive symptoms of psychosis. *Psychological Medicine, 31,* 189–195.

Garralda, M. E. (1984). Hallucinations in children with conduct and emotional disorders: II. The follow-up study. *Psychological Medicine, 14,* 597–604.

Garrett, M., Stone, D., & Turkington, D. (2006). Normalizing psychotic symptoms. *Psychology and Psychotherapy: Theory, Research and Practice, 79,* 595–610.

Gaser, C., Nenadic, I., Volz, H. P., Buchel, C., & Sauer, H. (2004). Neuroanatomy of "hearing voices": A frontotemporal brain structural abnormality associated with auditory hallucinations in schizophrenia. *Cerebral Cortex, 14,* 91–96.

Gaudiano, B. A. (2005). Cognitive behavior therapies for psychotic disorders: Current empirical status and future directions. *Clinical Psychology: Science and Practice, 12,* 33–50.

Gaudiano, B. A., & Herbert, J. D. (2006). Acute treatment of inpatients with psychotic symptoms using acceptance and commitment therapy: Pilot results. *Behavior Research and Therapy, 44,* 415–437.

Gauntlett-Gilbert, J., & Kuipers, E. (2003). Phenomenology of visual hallucinations in psychiatric conditions. *Journal of Nervous and Mental Disease, 191,* 203–205.

Gazzaniga, M. S. (1995). Consciousness and the cerebral hemispheres. In M. S. Gazzaniga (Ed.), *The cognitive neurosciences* (pp. 1391–1400). Cambridge, MA: MIT Press.

Gazzaniga, M. S., Ivry, R. B., & Mangun, G. R. (2002). *Cognitive neuroscience.* New York: Norton.

Gilley, D. W., Whalen, M. E., Wilson, R. S., & Bennett, D. A. (1991). Hallucinations and associated factors in Alzheimer's disease. *Journal of Neuropsychiatry and Clinical Neurosciences, 3,* 371–376.

Gledhill, A., Lobban, F., & Sellwood, W. (1998). Group CBT for people with schizophrenia: A preliminary evaluation. *Behavioural and Cognitive Psychotherapy, 26,* 63–75.

Glicksohn, J., & Barrett, T. R. (2003). Absorption and hallucinatory experience. *Applied Cognitive Psychology, 17,* 833–849.

Glicksohn, J., Steinbach, I., & Elimalach-Malmilyan, S. (1999). Cognitive dedifferentiation in eidetics and synaesthesia: Hunting for the ghost once more. *Perception, 28,* 109–120.

Goetz, C.G., Pappert, E. J., Blasucci, L. M., Stebbins, G. T., Ling, Z. D., Nora, M. V., & Carvey, P. M. (1998). Intravenous levodopa in hallucinating Parkinson's patients: High dose challenge does not precipitate hallucinations. *Neurology, 50,* 515–517.

Good, J. (2002). The effect of treatment of a comorbid anxiety disorder on psychotic symptoms in a patient with a diagnosis of schizophrenia: A case study. *Behavioural Cognitive Psychotherapy, 30,* 347–350.

Goodwin, D. W., Alderton, P., & Rosenthal, R. (1971). Clinical significance of hallucinations in psychiatric disorders. *Archives of General Psychiatry, 24,* 76–80.

Goodwin, F. K., & Jamison, K. R. (1990). *Manic-depressive illness.* Oxford, England: Oxford University Press.

Gottesman, C. (2004). Paradoxical sleep and schizophrenia have the same neurobiological support. *Behavioral and Brain Sciences, 27,* 794–795.

Gould, L. N. (1948). Verbal hallucinations and activity of vocal musculature. *American Journal of Psychiatry, 105,* 367–372.

Gould, L. N. (1949). Auditory hallucinations and subvocal speech. *Journal of Nervous and Mental Disease, 109,* 418–427.

Gould, L. N. (1950). Verbal hallucinations and automatic speech. *American Journal of Psychiatry, 107,* 110–119.

Gould, R. A., Mueser, K. T., Bolton, E., Mays, V., & Goff, D. (2001). Cognitive therapy for psychosis in schizophrenia: An effect size analysis. *Schizophrenia Research, 48,* 335–342.

Gouzoulis-Mayfrank, E., Heekeren, K., Neukirch, A., Stoll, M., Stock, C., Daumann, J., et al. (2006). Inhibition of return in the human $5HT_{2A}$ agonist and NMDA antagonist model of psychosis. *Neuropsychopharmacology, 31,* 431–441.

Graham, J., Grunewald, R., & Sagar, H. (1997). Hallucinosis in idiopathic Parkinson's disease. *Journal of Neurology, Neurosurgery and Psychiatry, 63,* 434–440.

Gray, M. J., Litz, B. T., Hsu, J. L., & Lombardo, T. W. (2004). Psychometric properties of the Life Events Checklist. *Assessment, 11,* 330–341.

Green, M. F., Hugdahl, K., & Mitchell, S. (1994). Dichotic listening during auditory hallucinations in patients with schizophrenia. *American Journal of Psychiatry, 151,* 357–362.

Green, M. F., & Kinsbourne, M. (1989). Auditory hallucinations in schizophrenia: Does humming help? *Biological Psychiatry, 25,* 633–635.

Green, M. F., & Kinsbourne, M. (1990). Subvocal activity and auditory hallucinations: Clues for behavioural treatments. *Schizophrenia Bulletin, 16,* 617–625.

Green, P., & Preston, M. (1981). Reinforcement of vocal correlates of auditory hallucinations by auditory feedback: A case study. *British Journal of Psychiatry, 139,* 204–208.

Gregory, R. L. (1978). Illusions and hallucinations. In E. C. Carterette & M. P. Friedman (Eds.), *Handbook of perception: Vol. 9. Perceptual processing.* New York: Academic Press.

Griffiths, T. D. (2000). Musical hallucinosis in acquired deafness: Phenomenology and brain substrate. *Brain, 123,* 2065–2076.

Grimby, A. (1993). Bereavement among elderly people: Grief reactions, post-bereavement hallucinations and quality of life. *Acta Psychiatrica Scandinavica, 87,* 72–80.

Grimby, A. (1998). Hallucinations following the loss of a spouse: Common and normal events among the elderly. *Journal of Clinical Gerontology, 4,* 65–74.

Grossberg, S. (2000). How hallucinations may arise from brain mechanisms of learning, attention, and volition. *Journal of the International Neuropsychological Society, 6,* 583–592.

Guido, W., Lu, S., Vaughan, J. W., Godwin, D. W., & Sherman, S. M. (1995). Receiver operating characteristic (ROC) analysis of neurons in the cat's lateral geniculate during tonic and burst response mode. *Visual Neuroscience, 12,* 723–741.

Gur, R. E., Mozley, P. D., Resnick, S. M., Mozley, L. H., Shtasel, D. L., Gallacher, F., et al. (1995). Resting cerebral glucose metabolism in first-episode and previously treated patients with schizophrenia relates to clinical features. *Archives of General Psychiatry, 52,* 57–67.

Hackmann, A. (1997). The transformation of meaning in cognitive therapy. In M. Power & C. R. Brewin (Eds.), *Transformation of meaning in psychological therapies* (pp. 125–140). Chichester, England: Wiley.

Haddock, G., Lobban, F., Hatton, C., & Carson, R. (2004). Cognitive–behavior therapy for people with psychosis and mild intellectual disabilities: A case series. *Clinical Psychology and Psychotherapy, 11,* 282–298.

Haddock, G., McCarron, J., Tarrier, N., & Faragher, E. B. (1999). Scales to measure dimensions of hallucinations and delusions: The Psychotic Symptoms Rating Scale (PSYRATS). *Psychological Medicine, 29,* 879–889.

Haddock, G., Slade, P. D., & Bentall, R. P. (1995). Auditory hallucinations and the verbal transformation effect: The role of suggestions. *Personality and Individual Differences, 19,* 301–306.

Haddock, G., Tarrier, N., Spaulding, W., Yusupoff, L., Kinney, C., & McCarthy, E. (1998). Individual cognitive–behavior therapy in the treatment of hallucinations and delusions: A review. *Clinical Psychology Review, 18,* 821–838.

Hallett, M. (2000, July 13). Transcranial magnetic stimulation and the human brain. *Nature, 406,* 147–150.

Halliday, G. (2005). The emergence of proto-objects in complex visual hallucinations. *Behavioral and Brain Sciences, 28,* 767–768.

Halligan, P. W., & David, A. S. (2001). Cognitive neuropsychiatry: Towards a scientific psychopathology. *Nature Reviews. Neuroscience, 2,* 209–215.

Hammeke, T. A., McQuillen, M. P., & Cohen, B. A. (1983). Musical hallucinations associated with acquired deafness. *Journal of Neurology, Neurosurgery and Psychiatry, 46,* 570–572.

Hammersley, P., Dias, A., Todd, G., Bowen-Jones, K., Reilly, B., & Bentall, R. P. (2003). Childhood trauma and hallucinations in bipolar affective disorder: Preliminary investigation. *British Journal of Psychiatry, 182,* 543–547.

Hamner, M. B., Frueh, B. C., Ulmer, H. G., Huber, M. G., Twomey, T. J., Tyson, C., & Arana, G. W. (2000). Psychotic features in chronic posttraumatic stress disorder and schizophrenia: Comparative severity. *Journal of Nervous and Mental Disease, 188,* 217–219.

Harding, A. J., Broe, G. A., & Halliday, G. M. (2002). Visual hallucinations in Lewy body disease relate to Lewy bodies in the temporal lobe. *Brain, 125,* 391–403.

Hardy, A., Fowler, D., Freeman, D., Smith, B., Steel, C., Evans, J., et al. (2005). Trauma and hallucinatory experience in psychosis. *Journal of Nervous and Mental Disease, 193,* 501–507.

Harris, D., & Batki, S. L. (2000). Stimulant psychosis: Symptom profile and acute clinical course. *American Journal of Addiction, 9,* 28–37.

Havermans, R., Honig, A., Vuurman, E. F., Krabbendam, L., Wilmink, J., Lamers, T., et al. (1999). A controlled study of temporal lobe structure volumes and P300 responses in schizophrenic patients with persistent auditory hallucinations. *Schizophrenia Research, 38,* 151–158.

Haxby, J. V., Horwitz, B., Ungerleider, L. G., Maisog, J. M., Pietrini, P., & Grady, C. L. (1994). The functional organization of human extrastriate cortex: A PET–rCBF study of selective attention to faces and locations. *Journal of Neuroscience, 14,* 6336–6353.

Hayashi, N., Igarashi, Y., Suda, K., & Nakagawa, S. (2004). Phenomenological features of auditory hallucinations and their symptomatological relevance. *Psychiatry and Clinical Neurosciences, 58,* 651–659.

Hayes, S. C., Strosahl, K. D., & Wilson, K. G. (1999). *Acceptance and commitment therapy: An experiential approach to behavior change.* New York: Guilford Press.

Healy, D. (1990). *The suspended revolution: Psychiatry and psychotherapy re-examined.* London: Faber & Faber.

Heilbrun, A. B. (1980). Impaired recognition of self-expressed thoughts in patients with auditory hallucinations. *Journal of Abnormal Psychology, 89,* 728–736.

Heinks-Maldonado, T. H., Mathalon, D. H., Houde, J. F., Gray, M., Faustman, W. O., & Ford, J. M. (2007). Relationship of imprecise corollary discharge in schizophrenia to auditory hallucinations. *Archives of General Psychiatry, 64,* 286–296.

Heinrichs, R. W. (2001). *In search of madness: Schizophrenia and neuroscience.* Oxford, England: Oxford University Press.

Hellerstein, D., Frosch, W., & Koenigsberg, H. W. (1987). The clinical significance of command hallucinations. *American Journal of Psychiatry, 144,* 219–221.

Helmholtz, H. V. (1924). *Treatise on physiological optics* (J. P. C. Southall, Trans.; Vols. 1–3). New York: Dover. (Original work published 1894)

Hemsley, D. R. (1993). A simple (simplistic?) cognitive model for schizophrenia. *Behavioural Research and Therapy, 31,* 633–645.

Henderson, M. J., & Mellers, J. D. C. (2000). Psychosis in Parkinson's disease: "Between a rock and a hard place." *International Review of Psychiatry, 12,* 319–334.

Hermesh, H., Konas, S., Shiloh, R., Reuven, D., Marom, S., Weizman, A., & Gross-Isseroff, R. (2004). Musical hallucinations: Prevalence in psychotic and nonpsychotic outpatients. *Journal of Clinical Psychiatry, 65,* 191–197.

Hibberts, S. (1825). *Sketches of the philosophy of apparitions.* Edinburgh, Scotland: Oliver & Boyd.

Hirono, N., Mori, E., Tanimukai, S., Kazui, H., Hashimoto, M., Hanihara, T., & Imamura, T. (1999). Distinctive neurobehavioural features among neurodegenerative dementias. *Journal of Neuropsychiatry and Clinical Neurosciences, 11,* 498–503.

Hirono, N., Mori, E., Yasuda, M., Ikejiri, Y., Imamura, T., Shimomura, T., et al. (1998). Factors associated with psychotic symptoms in Alzheimer's disease. *Journal of Neurology, Neurosurgery and Psychiatry, 64,* 648–652.

Hoeh, N., Gyulai, L., Weintraub, D., & Streim, J. (2003). Pharmacologic management of psychosis in the elderly: A critical review. *Journal of Geriatric Psychiatry and Neurology, 16,* 213–218.

Hoffman, R. E. (1986). Verbal hallucinations and language production processes in schizophrenia. *Behavioral and Brain Sciences, 9,* 503–548.

Hoffman, R. E., Boutros, N. N., Hu, S., Berman, R. M., Krystal, J. H., & Charney, D. S. (2000). Transcranial magnetic stimulation and auditory hallucinations in schizophrenia. *Lancet, 355,* 1073–1075.

Hoffman, R. E., & Cavus, I. (2002). Slow transcranial magnetic stimulation, long-term depotentiation, and brain hyperexcitability disorders. *American Journal of Psychiatry, 159,* 1093–1102.

Hoffman, R. E., Gueorguieva, R., Hawkins, K. A., Varanko, M., Boutros, N. N., Wu, Y. T., et al. (2005). Temporoparietal transcranial magnetic stimulation for auditory hallucinations: Safety, efficacy and moderators in a fifty patient sample. *Biological Psychiatry, 58,* 97–104.

Hoffman, R. E., Hampson, M., Wu, K., Anderson, A. W., Gore, J. C., Buchanan, R. J., et al. (2007). Probing the pathophysiology of auditory/verbal hallucinations by combining functional magnetic resonance imaging and transcranial magnetic stimulation. *Cerebral Cortex, 17,* 2733–2743.

Hoffman, R. E., Hawkins, K. A., Gueorguieva, R., Boutros, N. N., Rachid, F., Carroll, K., & Krystal, J. H. (2003). Transcranial magnetic stimulation of left temporoparietal cortex and medication-resistant auditory hallucinations. *Archives of General Psychiatry, 60,* 49–56.

Hoffman, R. E., & McGlashan, T. H. (1997). Synaptic elimination, neurodevelopment, and the mechanism of hallucinated "voices" in schizophrenia. *American Journal of Psychiatry, 154,* 1683–1689.

Hoffman, R. E., & McGlashan, T. H. (2006). Using a speech perception neural network computer simulation to contrast neuroanatomic versus neuromodulatory models of auditory hallucinations. *Pharmacopsychiatry, 39*(Suppl. 1), S54–64.

Hoffman, R. E., & Rapaport, J. (1994). A psycholinguistic study of auditory/verbal hallucinations: Preliminary findings. In A. S. David & J. C. Cutting (Eds.), *The neuropsychology of schizophrenia* (pp. 255–267). Hove, England: Erlbaum.

Hoffman, R. E., Rapaport, J., Mazure, C. M., & Quinlan, D. M. (1999). Selective speech perception alterations in schizophrenic patients reporting hallucinated "voices." *American Journal of Psychiatry, 156,* 393–399.

Hoffman, R. E., & Varanko, M. (2006). "Seeing voices": Fused visual/auditory verbal hallucinations reported by three persons with schizophrenia-spectrum disorder. *Acta Psychiatrica Scandinavica, 114,* 290–293.

Holroyd, S. (1998). Hallucinations and delusions in Alzheimer's disease. In B. Vellas, L. J. Fitten, & G. Friston (Eds.), *Research and practice in Alzheimer's disease* (pp. 213–222). New York: Springer Publishing Company.

Honig, A., Romme, M., Ensink, B. J., Escher, A., Pennings, M., & Devries, M. (1998). Auditory hallucinations: A comparison between patients and nonpatients. *Journal of Nervous and Mental Disease, 186,* 646–651.

Hori, H., Terao, T., & Nakamura, J. (2001). Charles Bonnet syndrome with auditory hallucinations: A diagnostic dilemma. *Psychopathology, 34,* 164–166.

Horowitz, M. J. (1975). Hallucinations: An information processing approach. In R. K. Siegel & L. J. West (Eds.), *Hallucinations: Behavior, experience and theory* (pp. 163–195). New York: Wiley.

Hosty, G. (1990). Charles Bonnet syndrome: A description of two cases. *Acta Psychiatrica Scandinavica, 82,* 316–317.

Howanitz, E., Bajulaiye, R., & Losonczy, M. (1995). Magnetic resonance imaging correlates of psychosis in Alzheimer's disease. *Journal of Nervous and Mental Disease, 183,* 548–549.

Howard, R., & Levy, R. (1994). Charles Bonnet syndrome plus: Complex visual hallucinations of Charles Bonnet syndrome type in late paraphrenia. *International Journal of Geriatric Psychiatry, 9,* 399–404.

Howard, R., Williams, S., Bullmore, E., Brammer, M., Mellers, J., Woodruff, P., & David, A. (1995). Cortical response to exogenous visual stimulation during visual hallucinations. *Lancet, 345,* 70.

Hubl, D., Koenig, T., Strik, W., Federspiel, A., Kreis, R., Boesch, C., et al. (2004). Pathways that make voices: White matter changes in auditory hallucinations. *Archives of General Psychiatry, 61,* 658–668.

Hubl, D., Koenig, T., Strik, W. K., Garcia, L. M., & Dierks, T. (2007). Competition for neuronal resources: How hallucinations make themselves heard. *British Journal of Psychiatry, 190,* 57–62.

Hunter, M. D., Griffiths, T. D., Farrow, T. F. D., Zheng, Y., Wilkinson, I. D., Hegde, N., et al. (2003). A neural basis for the perception of voices in external auditory space. *Brain, 126,* 161–169.

Hustig, H. H., & Hafner, R. J. (1990). Persistent auditory hallucinations and their relationship to delusions and mood. *Journal of Nervous and Mental Disease, 178,* 264–267.

Inouye, T., & Shimizu, A. (1970). The electromyographic study of verbal hallucination. *Journal of Nervous and Mental Disease, 151,* 415–422.

Intons-Peterson, M. J. (1992). Components of auditory imagery. In D. Reisberg (Ed.), *Auditory imagery* (pp. 45–72). Hillsdale, NJ: Erlbaum.

Inzelberg, R., Kipervasser, S., & Korczyn, A. D. (1998). Auditory hallucinations in Parkinson's disease. *Journal of Neurology, Neurosurgery and Psychiatry, 64,* 533–535.

Izumi, Y., Terao, T., Ishino, Y., & Nakamura, J. (2002). Differences in regional cerebral blood flow during musical and verbal hallucinations. *Psychiatry Research, 116,* 119–123.

Jackson, J. H. (1931). *Selected writings.* London: Hodder & Stoughton.

Jadri, R., Lucas, B., Delevoye-Turrell, Y., Delmaire, C., Delion, P., Thomas, P., & Goëb, J.-L. (2007). An 11-year-old boy with drug-resistant schizophrenia treated with temporo-parietal rTMS. *Molecular Psychiatry, 12,* 320.

Jakes, S., & Hemsley, D. R. (1987). Personality and reports of hallucination and imagery in a normal population. *Perceptual and Motor Skill, 64,* 765–766.

Jäncke, L., Mirzazade, S., & Shah, N. J. (1999). Attention modulates activity in the primary and the secondary auditory cortex: A functional magnetic resonance imaging study in human subjects. *Neuroscience Letters, 266,* 125–128.

Janssen, I., Krabbendam, L., Bak, M., Vollebergh, W., de Graaf, R., & van Os, J. (2004). Childhood abuse as a risk factor for psychotic experiences. *Acta Psychiatrica Scandinavica, 109,* 38–45.

Jansson, B. (1968). The prognostic significance of various types of hallucinations in young people. *Acta Psychiatrica Scandinavica, 44,* 401–409.

Jaspers, K. (1962). *General psychopathology* (7th ed.). Manchester, England: Manchester University Press. (Original work published 1923)

Javitt, D. C., & Zukin, S. R. (1991). Recent advances in the phencyclidine model of schizophrenia. *American Journal of Psychiatry, 148,* 1301–1308.

Jaynes, J. (1976). *The origin of consciousness in the breakdown of the bicameral mind.* Boston: Houghton Mifflin.

Jenner, J. A. (2002). An integrative treatment for patients with persistent auditory hallucinations. *Psychiatric Services, 53,* 897–898.

Jenner, J. A., Nienhuis, F. J., van de Willige, G., & Wiersma, D. (2006). "Hitting" voices of schizophrenia patients may lastingly reduce persistent auditory hallucinations and their burden: 18-month outcome of a randomized controlled trial. *Canadian Journal of Psychiatry, 51,* 169–177.

Jenner, J. A., Nienhuis, F. J., Wiersma, D., & van de Willige, G. (2004). Hallucination focused integrative treatment: A randomized controlled trial. *Schizophrenia Bulletin, 30,* 133–145.

Jenner, J. A., & van de Willige, G. (2001). HIT, hallucination focused integrative treatment as early intervention in psychotic adolescents with auditory hallucinations: A pilot study. *Acta Psychiatrica Scandinavica, 103,* 148–152.

Jenner, J. A., van de Willige, G., & Wiersma, D. (1998). Effectiveness of cognitive therapy with coping training for persistent auditory hallucinations: A retrospective study of attenders of a psychiatric out-patient department. *Acta Psychiatrica Scandinavica, 98,* 384–389.

Jenner, J. A., van de Willige, G., & Wiersma, D. (2006). Multi-family treatment for patients with persistent auditory hallucinations and their relatives: A pilot study. *Acta Psychiatrica Scandinavica, 113,* 154–158.

Jeste, D. V., & Lacro, J. P. (2000). Characteristics of an ideal drug for behavioral and psychological symptoms of dementia. *International Psychogeriatrics, 12*(Suppl. 1), 213–215.

Jeste, D. V., Wragg, R. E., Salmon, D. P., Harris, M. J., & Thal, L. J. (1992). Cognitive deficits of patients with Alzheimer's disease with and without delusions. *American Journal of Psychiatry, 149,* 184–189.

Johns, L. C. (2005). Hallucinations in the general population. *Current Psychiatry Reports, 7,* 162–167.

Johns, L. C., Cannon, M., Singleton, N., Murray, R. M., Farrell, M., Brugha, T., et al. (2004). Prevalence and correlates of self-reported psychotic symptoms in the British population. *British Journal of Psychiatry, 185,* 298–305.

Johns, L. C., Gregg, L., Allen, P., & McGuire, P. K. (2006). Impaired verbal self-monitoring in psychosis: Effects of state, trait and diagnosis. *Psychological Medicine, 36,* 465–474.

Johns, L. C., Hemsley, D., & Kuipers, E. (2002). A comparison of auditory hallucinations in a psychiatric and non-psychiatric group. *British Journal of Clinical Psychology, 41*, 81–86.

Johns, L. C., & McGuire, P. K. (1999). Verbal self-monitoring and auditory hallucinations in schizophrenia. *Lancet, 353*, 469–470.

Johns, L. C., Nazroo, J. Y., Bebbington, P., & Kuipers, E. (2002). Occurrence of hallucinatory experiences in a community sample and ethnic variations. *British Journal of Psychiatry, 180*, 174–178.

Johns, L. C., Rossel, S., Frith, C., Ahmad, F., Hemsley, D., Kuipers, E., & McGuire, P. K. (2001). Verbal self-monitoring and auditory verbal hallucinations in patients with schizophrenia. *Psychological Medicine, 31*, 705–715.

Johns, L. C., & van Os, J. (2001). The continuity of psychotic experiences in the general population. *Clinical Psychology Review, 21*, 1125–1141.

Johnson, J. H., & McCutcheon, S. M. (1980). Assessing life stress in older children and adolescents: Preliminary findings with the Life Events Checklist. In I. G. Sarason & C. D. Spielberger (Eds.), *Stress and anxiety* (Vol. 7, pp. 111–125). Washington, DC: Hemisphere.

Johnson, M. H., & Magaro, P. A. (1987). Effects of mood and severity on memory processes in depression and mania. *Psychological Bulletin, 101*, 28–40.

Johnson, M. K., Hashtroudi, S., & Lindsay, D. S. (1993). Source monitoring. *Psychological Bulletin, 114*, 3–28.

Johnson, M. K., Nolde, S. F., & Leonardis, D. M. (1996). Emotional focus and source monitoring. *Journal of Memory and Language, 35*, 135–156.

Johnson, M. K., & Raye, C. L. (1981). Reality monitoring. *Psychological Review, 88*, 67–85.

Johnson, M. K., Raye, C. L., Foley, H. J., & Foley, M. A. (1981). Cognitive operations and decision bias in reality monitoring. *American Journal of Psychology, 91*, 37–64.

Johnstone, E. C., Owens. D. G., & Leary, J. (1991). Disabilities and circumstances of schizophrenic patients: A follow-up study—Comparison of the 1975–85 cohort with the 1970–1975 cohort. *British Journal of Psychiatry, 159*(Suppl. 13), 34–36.

Jones, C., Griffiths, R. D., & Humprhis, G. (2000). Disturbed memory and amnesia related to intensive care. *Memory, 8*, 79–94.

Jones, S., Guy, A., & Ormrod, J. A. (2003). A Q-methodological study of hearing voices: A preliminary exploration of voice hearers' understanding of their experiences. *Psychology and Psychotherapy: Theory, Research and Practice, 76*, 189–209.

Jones, S. R., & Fernyhough, C. (2006). The roles of thought suppression and metacognitive beliefs in proneness to auditory verbal hallucinations in a nonclinical sample. *Personality and Individual Differences, 41*, 1421–1432.

Junginger, J., & Frame, C. L. (1985). Self-report of the frequency and phenomenology of verbal hallucinations. *Journal of Nervous and Mental Disease, 173*, 149–155.

Kaplan, H., & Sadock, B. (1981). *Modern synopsis of comprehensive textbook of psychiatry* (3rd ed.). Baltimore: Williams & Wilkins.

Kasai, K., Asada, T., Yumoto, M., Takeya, J., & Matsuda, H. (1999). Evidence for functional abnormality in the right auditory cortex during musical hallucinations. *Lancet, 354,* 1703–1704.

Kastner, S., & Ungerleider, L. G. (2000). Mechanisms of visual attention in the human cortex. *Annual Review of Neuroscience, 23,* 315–341.

Kaufer, D. I., Cummings, J. L., Christine, D., Bray, T., Castellon, S., Masterman, D., et al. (1998). Assessing the impact of neuropsychiatric symptoms in Alzheimer's disease: The Neuropsychiatric Inventory Caregiver Distress Scale. *Journal of the American Geriatrics Society, 46,* 210–215.

Kaufman, J., Birmaher, B., Clayton, S., Retano, A., & Wongchaowart, B. (1997). Case study: Trauma-related hallucinations. *Journal of the American Academy of Child and Adolescent Psychiatry, 36,* 1602–1605.

Kay, S. R., Fiszbein, A., & Opler, L. A. (1987). The Positive and Negative Syndrome Scale (PANSS) for schizophrenia. *Schizophrenia Bulletin, 13,* 261–276.

Kent, G., & Wahass, S. (1996). The content and characteristics of auditory hallucinations in Saudi Arabia and the UK: A cross-cultural comparison. *Acta Psychiatrica Scandinavica, 94,* 433–437.

Kessler, R. C., McGonagle, K. A., Zhao, S., Nelson, C. B., Hughes, M., Eshleman, S., et al. (1994). Lifetime and 12-month prevalence of DSM–III–R psychiatric disorders in the United States: Results from the National Comorbidity Survey. *Archives of General Psychiatry, 51,* 8–19.

Kingdon, D. G., & Turkington, D. (1994). *Cognitive–behavioral therapy of schizophrenia.* London: Guilford Press.

Kingdon, D. G., & Turkington, D. (1996). Using a normalising rationale. In G. Haddock & P. Slade (Eds.), *Cognitive behavioural interventions with psychotic disorders* (pp. 71–85). London: Routledge.

Kingdon, D. G., & Turkington, D. (2005). *Cognitive therapy of schizophrenia.* New York: Guilford Press.

Kirkland, J. (2005). Cognitive–behavior formulation for three men with learning disabilities who experience psychosis: How do we make it make sense? *British Journal of Learning Disabilities, 33,* 160–165.

Klein, C., Koempf, D., Pulkowski, U., Moser, A., & Vieregge, P. (1997). A study of visual hallucinations in patients with Parkinson's disease. *Journal of Neurology, 244,* 371–377.

Kluver, H. (1966). *Mescal and mechanisms of hallucinations.* Chicago: University of Chicago Press.

Kölmel, H. W. (1985). Complex visual hallucinations in the hemianopic field. *Journal of Neurology, Neurosurgery and Psychiatry, 48,* 29–38.

Kosslyn, S. M. (1994). *Image and brain.* Cambridge, MA: MIT Press.

Kosslyn, S. M., Sukel, K. E. & Bly, B. M. (1999). Squinting with the mind's eye: Effects of stimulus resolution on imaginal and perceptual comparisons. *Memory and Cognition, 27,* 276–287.

Kot, T., & Serper, M. (2002). Increased susceptibility to auditory conditioning in hallucinating schizophrenic patients. *Journal of Nervous and Mental Disease*, *190*, 282–288.

Krabbendam, L., Janssen, I., Bak, M., Bijl, R. V., de Graaf, R., & van Os, J. (2002). Neuroticism and low self-esteem as risk factors for psychosis. *Social Psychiatry and Psychiatric Epidemiology*, *37*, 1–6.

Krabbendam, L., Myin-Germeys, I., Bak, M., & van Os, J. (2005). Explaining transitions over the hypothesized psychosis continuum. *Australian and New Zealand Journal of Psychiatry*, *39*, 180–186.

Krabbendam, L., Myin-Germeys, I., Hanssen, M., Bijl, R. V., de Graaf, R., Vollebergh, W., et al. (2004). Hallucinatory experiences and onset of psychotic disorder: Evidence that the risk is mediated by delusion formation. *Acta Psychiatrica Scandinavica*, *110*, 264–272.

Krabbendam, L., Myin-Germeys, I., Hanssen, M., de Graaf, R., Vollebergh, W., Bak, M., & van Os, J. (2005). Development of depressed mood predicts onset of psychotic disorder in individuals who report hallucinatory experiences. *British Journal of Clinical Psychology*, *44*, 113–125.

Krabbendam, L., & van Os, J. (2005). Affective processes in the onset and persistence of psychosis. *European Archives of Psychiatry and Clinical Neuroscience*, *255*, 185–189.

Kraepelin, E. (1971). *Dementia praecox and paraphrenia: With historical introduction*. New York: Robert E. Krieger. (Original work published 1919)

Kraupl Taylor, F. (1981). On pseudo-hallucinations. *Psychological Medicine*, *11*, 265–271.

Kroll, J., & Bachrach, B. (1982). Visions and psychopathology in the Middle Ages. *Journal of Nervous and Mental Disease*, *170*, 41–49.

Krystal, J. H., Karper, L. P., Seibyl, J. P., Freeman, G. K., Delaney, R., Bremner, J. D., et al. (1994). Subanesthetic effects of the noncompetitive NMDA antagonist, ketamine, in humans. Psychotomimetic, perceptual, cognitive, and neuroendocrine responses. *Archives of General Psychiatry*, *51*, 199–214.

Kubany, E. S., Haynes, S. N., Leisen, M. B., Owens, J. A., Kaplan, A. S., Watson, S. B., & Burns, K. (2000). Development and preliminary validation of a brief broad-spectrum measure of traumatic exposure: The Traumatic Life Events Questionnaire. *Psychological Assessment*, *12*, 210–224.

Kuipers, E., Garety, P., Fowler, D., Freeman, D., Dunn, G., & Bebbington, P. (2006). Cognitive, emotional, and social processes in psychosis: Refining cognitive behavioral therapy for persistent positive symptoms. *Schizophrenia Bulletin*, *32*(Suppl. 1), S24–S31.

Kumagai, R., Ohnuma, T., Nagata, T., & Arai, H. (2003). Visual and auditory hallucinations with excessive intake of paroxetine. *Psychiatry and Clinical Neurosciences*, *57*, 548–549.

Lacro, J. P., Dunn, L. B., Dolder, C. R., Leckband, S. G., & Jeste, D. V. (2002). Prevalence of and risk factors for medication nonadherence in patients with schizophrenia: A comprehensive review of the recent literature. *Journal of Clinical Psychiatry, 63*, 892–909.

Lahti, A. C., Weiler, M. A., Holcomb, H. H., Tamminga, C. A., Carpenter, W. T., & McMahon, R. (2006). Correlations between rCBF and symptoms in two independent cohorts of drug-free patients with schizophrenia. *Neuropsychopharmacology, 31*, 221–230.

Langgut, B., Zowe, M., Spiessl, H., & Hajak, G. (2006). Neuronavigated transcranial magnetic stimulation and auditory hallucinations in a schizophrenic patient: Monitoring of neurobiological effects. *Schizophrenia Research, 84*, 185–186.

Larkin, A. R. (1979). The form and content of schizophrenic hallucinations. *American Journal of Psychiatry, 136*, 940–943.

Larkin, W., & Morrison, A. P. (2006). *Trauma and psychosis: New directions for theory and therapy*. New York: Routledge.

Larøi, F. (2006). The phenomenological diversity of hallucinations: Some theoretical and clinical implications. *Psychologica Belgica, 46*, 163–183.

Larøi, F., Collignon, O., & Van der Linden, M. (2005). Source monitoring for actions in hallucination-proneness. *Cognitive Neuropsychiatry, 10*, 105–123.

Larøi, F., DeFruyt, F., van Os, J., Aleman, A., & Van der Linden, M. (2005). Associations between hallucinations and personality structure in a non-clinical sample: Comparison between young and elderly samples. *Personality and Individual Differences, 39*, 189–200.

Larøi, F., Marczewski, P., & Van der Linden, M. (2004). The multi-dimensionality of hallucinatory predisposition: Factor structure of a modified version of the Launay–Slade Hallucinations Scale in a normal sample. *European Psychiatry, 19*, 15–20.

Larøi, F., & Van der Linden, M. (2005a). Metacognition in proneness towards hallucinations and delusions. *Behavioural Research and Therapy, 43*, 1425–1441.

Larøi, F., & Van der Linden, M. (2005b). Normal subjects' reports of hallucinatory experiences. *Canadian Journal of Behavioural Science, 37*, 33–43.

Larøi, F., Van der Linden, M., & Goëb, J.-L. (2006). Hallucinations and delusions in children and adolescents. *Current Psychiatry Reviews, 2*, 473–485.

Larøi, F., Van der Linden, M., & Marczewski, P. (2004). The effects of emotional salience, cognitive effort and meta-cognitive beliefs on a reality monitoring task in hallucination-prone subjects. *British Journal of Clinical Psychology, 43*, 221–233.

Larøi, F., & Woodward, T. (2007). Hallucinations from a cognitive perspective. *Harvard Review of Psychiatry, 15*, 109–117.

Laruelle, M. (2003). Dopamine transmission in the schizophrenic brain. In S. R. Hirsch & D. Weinberger (Eds.), *Schizophrenia* (pp. 365–387). Oxford, England: Blackwell.

Lataster, T., van Os, J., Drukker, M., Henquet, C., Feron, F., Gunther, N., & Myin-Germeys, I. (2006). Childhood victimisation and developmental expression of non-clinical delusional ideation and hallucinatory experiences: Victimisation and non-clinical psychotic experiences. *Social Psychiatry and Psychiatric Epidemiology, 41*, 423–428.

Launay, G., & Slade, P. (1981). The measurement of hallucinatory predisposition in male and female prisoners. *Personality and Individual Differences, 2*, 221–234.

Laurens, K. R., Hodgins, S., Maughan, B., Murray, R. M., Rutter, M. L., & Taylor, E. A. (2007). Community screening for psychotic-like experiences and other putative antecedents of schizophrenia in children aged 9–12 years. *Schizophrenia Research, 90*, 130–146.

Lazarus, R. S., & Folkman, S. (1984). *Stress, appraisal and coping.* New York: Springer Verlag.

Lee, S. H., Kim, W., Chung, Y. C., Jung, K. H., Bahk, W. M., Jun, T. Y., et al. (2005). A double blind study showing that two weeks of daily repetitive TMS over the left or right temporoparietal cortex reduces symptoms in patients with schizophrenia who are having treatment-refractory auditory hallucinations. *Neuroscience Letters, 376*, 177–181.

Lee, S. H., Wynn, J. K., Green, M. F., Kim, H., Lee, K.-J., Nam, M., et al. (2006). Quantitative EEG and low resolution electromagnetic tomography (LORETA) imaging of patients with persistent auditory hallucinations. *Schizophrenia Research, 83*, 111–119.

Legget, J., Hurn, C., & Goodman, W. (1997). Teaching psychological strategies for managing auditory hallucinations. *British Journal of Learning Disabilities, 25*, 158–163.

Lelut, L. F. (1846). *L'Amulette de Pascal pour servir à l'histoire des hallucinations.* Paris: J. B. Baillière.

Lennox, B. R., Park, S. B., Jones, P. B., & Morris, P. G. (1999). Spatial and temporal mapping of neural activity associated with auditory hallucinations. *Lancet, 353*, 644.

Lennox, B. R., Park, S. B., Medley, I., Morris, P. G., & Jones, P. B. (2000). The functional anatomy of auditory hallucinations in schizophrenia. *Psychiatry Research, 100*, 13–20.

Lenz, H. L. (1964). *Vergleichende Psychiatrie: Ein studie über die Beziehung von Kultur, Soziologie und Psychopathologie* [Comparative psychiatry: A study of relationships between culture, sociology and psychopathology]. Vienna: Wilhelkm Mandrich.

Lepore, F. E. (1990). Spontaneous visual phenomena with visual loss: 104 patients with lesions of retinal and neural afferent pathways. *Neurology, 40*, 444–447.

Lesch, K. P. (1998). Hallucinations: Psychopathology meets functional genomics. *Molecular Psychiatry, 3*, 278–281.

Leudar, I., & Thomas, P. (2000). *Voices of reason, voices of insanity: Studies of verbal hallucinations.* London: Routledge.

Leudar, I., Thomas, P., McNally, D., & Glinski, A. (1997). What voices can do with words: Pragmatics of verbal hallucinations. *Psychological Medicine, 27*, 885–898.

Levitan, C., Ward, P. B., & Catts, S. V. (1999). Superior temporal gyral volumes and laterality correlates of auditory hallucinations in schizophrenia. *Biological Psychiatry, 46*, 955–962.

Levitan, C., Ward, P. B., Catts, S. V., & Hemsley, D. R. (1996). Predisposition toward auditory hallucinations: The utility of the Launay–Slade Hallucination Scale in psychiatric patients. *Personality and Individual Differences, 21,* 287–289.

Lewandowski, K. E., Barrantes-Vidal, N., Nelson-Gray, R. O., Clancy, C., Kepley, H. O., & Kwapil, T. R. (2006). Anxiety and depression symptoms in psychometrically identified schizotypy. *Schizophrenia Research, 83,* 225–235.

Li, H.-L. (1974). An archeological and historical account of *Cannabis* in China. *Economic Botany, 28,* 437–448.

Liddle, P. F. (1987). The symptoms of chronic schizophrenia: A re-examination of the positive–negative dichotomy. *British Journal of Psychiatry, 151,* 145–151.

Lindenmayer, J. P. (2000). Treatment refractory schizophrenia. *Psychiatric Quarterly, 71,* 373–384.

Livingston, G., Kitchen, G., Manela, M., Katona, C., & Copeland, J. (2001). Persecutory symptoms and perceptual disturbance in a community sample of older people: The Islington study. *International Journal of Geriatric Psychiatry, 16,* 462–468.

Llinas, R. R., & Pare, D. (1991). Of dreaming and wakefulness. *Neuroscience, 44,* 521–535.

Lobban, F., Haddock, G., Kinderman, P., & Wells, A. (2002). The role of metacognitive beliefs in auditory hallucinations. *Personality and Individual Differences, 32,* 1351–1363.

Løberg, E.-M., Jørgensen, H. A., & Hugdahl, K. (2004). Dichotic listening in schizophrenic patients: Effects of previous vs. ongoing auditory hallucinations. *Psychiatry Research, 128,* 167–174.

Lowe, G. R. (1973). The phenomenology of hallucinations as an aid to differential diagnosis. *British Journal of Psychiatry, 123,* 621–633.

Luria, A. R. (1981). *Language and cognition.* New York: Wiley.

Lyketsos, C. G., Steinberg, M., Tschanz, J. T., Norton, M. C., Steffens, D. C., & Breitner J. C. S. (2000). Mental and behavioural disturbances in dementia: Findings from the Cache County study on memory and aging. *American Journal of Psychiatry, 157,* 708–714.

Lysaker, P. H., Marks, K. A., Picone, J. B., Rollins, A. L., Fastenau, P. S., & Bond, G. R. (2000). Obsessive and compulsive symptoms in schizophrenia: Clinical and neurocognitive correlates. *Journal of Nervous and Mental Disease, 188,* 78–83.

Lyttle, T., Goldstein, D., & Gartz, J. (1996). Bufo toads and bufotenine: Fact and fiction surrounding an alleged psychedelic. *Journal of Psychoactive Drugs, 28,* 267–290.

Mackinnon, A., Copolov, D. L., & Trauer, T. (2004). Factors associated with compliance and resistance to command hallucinations. *Journal of Nervous and Mental Disease, 192,* 357–362.

Malhotra, A. K., Goldman, D., Mazzanti, C., Clifton, A., Breier, A., & Pickar, D. (1998). A functional serotonin transporter (5-HTT) polymorphism is associated with psychosis in neuroleptic-free schizophrenics. *Molecular Psychiatry, 3,* 328–332.

Manford, M., & Andermann, F. (1998). Complex visual hallucinations: Clinical and neurobiological insights. *Brain, 121,* 1819–1840.

Margo, A., Hemsley, D. R., & Slade, P. D. (1981). The effects of varying auditory input on schizophrenic hallucinations. *British Journal of Psychiatry, 139,* 122–127.

Massaro, D. W. (1987). *Speech perception by ear and eye: A paradigm for psychological inquiry.* Hillsdale, NJ: Erlbaum.

Mathew, V. M., Gruzelier, J. H., & Liddle, P. F. (1993). Lateral asymmetries in auditory acuity distinguish hallucinating from nonhallucinating schizophrenic patients. *Psychiatry Research, 46,* 127–138.

Maugière, F. (1999). Scope and presumed mechanisms of hallucinations in partial epileptic seizures. *Epileptic Disorders, 1,* 81–91.

McAlonan, K., Cavanaugh, J., & Wurtz, R. H. (2006). Attentional modulation of thalamic reticular neurons. *Journal of Neuroscience, 26,* 4444–4450.

McGee, R., Williams, S., & Poulton, R. (2000). Hallucinations in nonpsychotic children. *Journal of the American Academy of Child Adolescent Psychiatry, 39,* 12–13.

McGuigan, F. J. (1966). Covert oral behaviour and auditory hallucinations. *Psychophysiology, 3,* 73–80.

McGuigan, F. J. (1978). *Cognitive psychophysiology: Principles of covert behavior.* Englewood Cliffs, NJ: Prentice Hall.

McGuire, P. K., Shah, G. M. S., & Murray, R. M. (1993). Increased blood flow in Broca's area during auditory hallucinations in schizophrenia. *Lancet, 342,* 703–706.

McGuire, P. K., Silbersweig, D. A., Wright, I., Murray, R. M., David, A. S., Frackowiak, R. S., & Frith, C. D. (1995). Abnormal monitoring of inner speech: A physiological basis for auditory hallucinations. *Lancet, 346,* 596–600.

McGuire, P. K., Silbersweig, D. A., Wright, I., Murray, R. M., Frackowiak, R. S., & Frith, C. D. (1996). The neural correlates of inner speech and auditory verbal imagery in schizophrenia: Relationship to auditory verbal hallucinations. *British Journal of Psychiatry, 169,* 148–159.

McIntosh, A. M., Semple, D., Tasker, K., Harrison, L. K., Owens, D. G. C., Johnstone, E. C., & Ebmeier, K. P. (2004). Transcranial magnetic stimulation for auditory hallucinations in schizophrenia. *Psychiatry Research, 127,* 9–17.

McKay, C. M., Headlam, D. M., & Copolov, D. L. (2000). Central auditory processing in patients with auditory hallucinations. *American Journal of Psychiatry, 157,* 759–766.

McKeith, I. G. (1998). Dementia with Lewy bodies: Clinical and pathological diagnosis. *Alzheimer's Reports, 1,* 83–87.

McKeith, I. G., Dickson, D. W., Lowe, J., Emre, M., O'Brien, J. T., Feldman, H., et al. (2005). Diagnosis and management of dementia with Lewy bodies: Third report of the DLB consortium. *Neurology, 65,* 1863–1872.

McKeith, I. G., Galasko, G., Kosaka, K., Perry, E. K., Dickson, D. W., Hansen, L. A., et al. (1996). Consensus guidelines for the clinical and pathologic diagnosis of dementia with Lewy bodies (DLB): Report of the Consortium on DLB International Workshop. *Neurology, 47*, 1113–1124.

McKellar, P. (1968). *Experience and behaviour*. London: Penguin.

McKenna, P. (2003). Is cognitive–behavioural therapy a worthwhile treatment for psychosis? Against. *British Journal of Psychiatry, 182*, 477–479.

McManus, D. (1996). Error, hallucination and the concept of "ontology" in the early work of Heidegger. *Philosophy, 71*, 553–575.

Merckelbach, H., & van de Ven, V. (2001). Another White Christmas: Fantasy proneness and reports of "hallucinatory experiences" in undergraduate students. *Journal of Behaviour Therapy and Experimental Psychiatry, 32*, 137–144.

Milham, A., & Easton, S. (1998). Prevalence of auditory hallucinations in nurses in mental health. *Journal of Psychiatric and Mental Health Nursing, 5*, 95–99.

Miller, L. J. (1996). Qualitative changes in hallucinations. *American Journal of Psychiatry, 153*, 265–267.

Miller, L. J., O'Connor, E., & DePasquale, T. (1993). Patients' attitudes to hallucinations. *American Journal of Psychiatry, 150*, 584–588.

Mintz, S., & Alpert, M. (1972). Imagery vividness, reality testing, and schizophrenic hallucinations. *Journal of Abnormal Psychology, 79*, 310–316.

Mitchell, J., & Vierkant, A. D. (1989). Delusions and hallucinations as a reflection of the subcultural milieu among psychotic patients of the 1930s and 1980s. *Journal of Psychology, 123*, 269–274.

Mlakar, J., Jensterle, J., & Frith, C. D. (1994). Central monitoring deficiency and schizophrenia symptoms. *Psychological Medicine, 24*, 557–564.

Mohanty, A., Herrington, J. D., Koven, N. S., Fisher, J. E., Wenzel, E., Webb, A. G., et al. (2005). Neural mechanisms of affective interference in schizotypy. *Journal of Abnormal Psychology, 114*, 16–27.

Mojtabai, R., & Rieder, R. O. (1998). Limitations of the symptom-oriented approach to psychiatric research. *British Journal of Psychiatry, 173*, 198–202.

Monteiro, I. M., Boksay, I., Auer, S. R., Torossian, C., Ferris, S. H., & Reisberg, B. (2001). Addition of a frequency-weighted score. *European Psychiatry, 16*(Suppl. 1), 5S–24S.

Mori, T., Ikeda, M., Fukuhara, R., Nestor, P. J., & Tanabe, H. (2006). Correlation of visual hallucinations with occipital rCBF changes by donepezil in DLB. *Neurology, 66*, 935–937.

Mori, T., Ikeda, M., Fukuhara, R., Sugawara, Y., Nakata, S., Matsumoto, N., et al. (2006). Regional cerebral blood flow change in a case of Alzheimer's disease with musical hallucinations. *European Archives of Psychiatry and Clinical Neurosciences, 256*, 236–239.

Morrison, A. P. (1998). A cognitive analysis of auditory hallucinations: Are voices to schizophrenia what bodily sensations are to panic? *Behavioural and Cognitive Psychotherapy, 26*, 289–302.

Morrison, A. P. (2001). The interpretation of intrusions in psychosis: An integrative cognitive approach to hallucinations and delusions. *Behavioural and Cognitive Psychotherapy, 29,* 257–276.

Morrison, A. P. (2002). Cognitive therapy for drug-resistant auditory hallucinations: A case example. In A. P. Morrison (Ed.), *A casebook of cognitive therapy for psychosis* (pp 132–147). Hove, England: Brunner-Routledge.

Morrison, A. P. (2004). The use of imagery in cognitive therapy for psychosis: A case example. *Memory, 12,* 517–524.

Morrison, A. P., & Baker, C. A. (2000). Intrusive thoughts and auditory hallucinations: A comparative study of intrusions in psychosis. *Behavioural Research and Therapy, 38,* 1097–1106.

Morrison, A. P., Beck, A. T., Glentworth, D., Dunn, H., Reid, G. S., Larkin, W., & Williams, S. (2002). Imagery and psychotic symptoms: A preliminary investigation. *Behavior Research and Therapy, 40,* 1053–1062.

Morrison, A. P., Frame, L., & Larkin, W. (2003). Relationships between trauma and psychosis: A review and integration. *British Journal of Clinical Psychology, 42,* 331–353.

Morrison, A. P., & Haddock, G. (1997). Cognitive factors in source monitoring and auditory hallucinations. *Psychological Medicine, 27,* 669–679.

Morrison, A. P., Haddock, G., & Tarrier, N. (1995). Intrusive thoughts and auditory hallucinations: A cognitive approach. *Behavioural and Cognitive Psychotherapy, 23,* 265–280.

Morrison, A. P., & Petersen, T. (2003). Trauma, metacognition and predisposition to hallucinations in non-patients. *Behavioural and Cognitive Psychotherapy, 31,* 235–246.

Morrison, A. P., & Wells, A. (2003). A comparison of metacognitions in patients with hallucinations, delusions, panic disorder, and non-patient controls. *Behaviour Research and Therapy, 41,* 251–256.

Morrison, A. P., Wells, A., & Nothard, S. (2000). Cognitive factors in predisposition to auditory and visual hallucinations. *British Journal of Clinical Psychology, 39,* 67–78.

Morrison, A. P., Wells, A., & Nothard, S. (2002). Cognitive and emotional predictors of predisposition to hallucinations in non-patients. *British Journal of Clinical Psychology, 41,* 259–270.

Mortimer, A. M. & McKenna, P. J. (1994). Levels of explanation—Symptoms, neuropsychological deficit and morphological abnormalities in schizophrenia. *Psychological Medicine, 24,* 541–545.

Mosimann, U. P., Rowan, E. N., Partington, C. E., Collerton, D., Littlewood, E., O'Brien, J. T., et al. (2006). Characteristics of visual hallucinations in Parkinson disease dementia and dementia with Lewy bodies. *American Journal of Geriatric Psychiatry, 14,* 153–160.

Muenzenmaier, K., Castille, D. M., Shelley, A. M., Jamison, A., Battaglia, J., Opler, L. A., & Alexander, M. J. (2005). Comorbid PTSD and schizophrenia. *Psychiatric Annals, 35,* 51–56.

Mueser, K. T., Bellack, A. S., & Brady, E. U. (1990). Hallucinations in schizophrenia. *Acta Psychiatrica Scandinavica, 82*, 26–29.

Mueser, K. T., & Butler, R. (1987). Auditory hallucinations in combat-related chronic posttraumatic stress disorder. *American Journal of Psychiatry, 144*, 299–302.

Mueser, K. T., Trumbetta, S. L., Rosenberg, S. D., Vivader, R., Goodman, L. B., Osher, F. C., et al. (1998). Trauma and posttraumatic stress disorder in severe mental illness. *Journal of Consulting and Clinical Psychology, 66*, 493–499.

Murase, S., Honjo, S., Inoko, K., & Ohta, T. (2002). A child who visited the emergency room with stress-related nonpsychotic hallucinations. *General Hospital Psychiatry, 24*, 448–454.

Murase, S., Ochiai, S., & Ohta, T. (2000). Separation anxiety leads to nonpsychotic hallucinations. *Journal of the American Academy of Child & Adolescent Psychiatry, 39*, 1345.

Murphy, H. B. M., Wittkower, E. D., Fried, J., & Ellenberger, H. (1963). A cross-cultural survey of schizophrenic symptomatology. *International Journal of Social Psychiatry, 9*, 237–249.

Myin-Germeys, I., & Myin, E. (2004). Getting real about experience: Commentary on Behrendt and Young. *Behavioral and Brain Sciences, 27*, 801–802.

Naccache, L., Habert, M. O., Malek, Z., Cohen, L., & Willer, J.-C. (2005). Activation of secondary auditory cortex in a deaf patient during song hallucinosis. *Journal of Neurology, 252*, 738–739.

Nayani, T. H., & David, A. S. (1996). The auditory hallucination: A phenomenological survey. *Psychological Medicine, 26*, 177–189.

Ndetei, D. M., & Singh, A. (1983). Hallucinations in Kenyan schizophrenic patients. *Acta Psychiatrica Scandinavica, 67*, 144–147.

Ndetei, D. M., & Vadher, A. (1984). A comparative cross-cultural study of the frequencies of hallucination in schizophrenia. *Acta Psychiatrica Scandinavica, 70*, 545–549.

Nechmad, A., Ratzoni, G., Poyurovsky, M., Meged, S., Avidan, G., Fuchs, C., et al. (2003). Obsessive-compulsive disorder in adolescent schizophrenia patients. *American Journal of Psychiatry, 160*, 1002–1004.

Neckelmann, G., Specht, K., Lund, A., Ersland, L., Smievoll, A. I., Neckelmann, D., & Hugdahl, K. (2006). MR morphometry analysis of grey matter volume reduction in schizophrenia: Association with hallucinations. *International Journal of Neuroscience, 116*, 9–23.

Nelson, H. R. (1982). *The National Adult Reading Test: Test manual*. Windsor, England: NFER.

Niehaus, L., Hoffman, K. T., Grosse, P., Roricht, S., & Meyer, B. U. (2000). MRI study of human brain exposed to high-dose repetitive magnetic simulation of visual cortex. *Neurology, 54*, 256–258.

Nieznański, M. (2005). Reality monitoring failure in schizophrenia: Relation to clinical symptoms and impairment of self-concept. In J. E. Pletson (Ed.), *Progress in schizophrenia research* (pp. 45–76). Hauppauge, NY: Nova Science.

Noda, S., Mizoguchi, M., & Yamamoto, A. (1993). Thalamic experiential hallucinosis. *Journal of Neurology, Neurosurgery and Psychiatry, 56*, 1224–1226.

Nosé, M., Barbui, C., & Tansella, M. (2003). How often do patients with psychosis fail to adhere to treatment programmes? A systematic review. *Psychological Medicine, 33*, 1149–1160.

Oathamshaw, S. C., & Haddock, G. (2006). Do people with intellectual disabilities and psychosis have the cognitive skills required to undertake cognitive behavioural therapy? *Journal of Applied Research in Intellectual Disabilities, 19*, 35–46.

Ohayon, M. (2000). Prevalence of hallucinations and their pathological associations in the general population. *Psychiatry Research, 97*, 153–164.

Ohayon, M. M., Priest, R. G., Caulet, M., & Guilleminault, C. (1996). Hypnagogic and hypnopompic hallucinations: Pathological phenomena? *British Journal of Psychiatry, 169*, 459–467.

Okubo, T., Harada, S., Higuchi, S., & Matsushita, S. (2002). Investigation of quantitative trait loci in the CCKAR gene with susceptibility to alcoholism. *Alcoholism: Clinical and Experimental Research, 26*(Suppl. 8), 2S–5S.

Okulate, G. T., & Jones, O. B. E. (2003). Auditory hallucinations in schizophrenic and affective disorder in Nigerian patients: Phenomenological comparisons. *Transcultural Psychiatry, 40*, 531–541.

O'Leary, D. S., Andreasen, N. C., Hurtig, R. R., Kesler, M. L., Rogers, M., Arndt, S., et al. (1996). Auditory attentional deficits in patients with schizophrenia. A positron emission tomography study. *Archives of General Psychiatry, 53*, 633–641.

Olfson, M., Lewis-Fernandez, R., Weissman, M. M., Feder, A., Gameroff, M. J., Pilowsky, D., & Fuentes, M. (2002). Psychotic symptoms in an urban general medicine practice. *American Journal of Psychiatry, 159*, 1412–1419.

Olin, R. (1999). Auditory hallucinations and the bicameral mind. *Lancet, 353*, 644.

Oliveri, M., & Calvo, G. (2003). Increased visual cortical excitability in ecstasy users: A transcranial magnetic stimulation study. *Journal of Neurology, Neurosurgery, and Psychiatry, 74*, 1136–1138.

Olson, P., Suddeth, J., Peterson, P., & Egelhoff, C. (1985). Hallucinations of widowhood. *Journal of the American Geriatric Society, 33*, 543–547.

Onofrj, M., Bonanni, L., Albani, G., Mauro, A., Bulla, D., & Thomas, A. (2006). Visual hallucinations in Parkinson's disease: Clues to separate origins. *Journal of Neurological Science, 248*, 143–150.

O'Sullivan, K. (1994). Dimensions of coping with auditory hallucinations. *Journal of Mental Health, 3*, 351–361.

Ott, U., Reuter, M., Hennig, J., & Vaitl, D. (2005). Evidence for a common biological basis of the absorption trait, hallucinogen effects, and positive symptoms: Epistasis between 5-HT2a and COMT polymorphisms. *American Journal of Medical Genetics: Part B. Neuropsychiatric Genetics, 137*, 29–32.

Oulis, P. G., Mavreas, V. G., Mamounas, J. M., & Stefanis, C. N. (1995). Clinical characteristics of auditory hallucinations. *Acta Psychiatrica Scandinavica, 92*, 97–102.

Pankow, L., Pliskin, N., & Luchins, D. (1996). An optical intervention for visual hallucinations associated with visual impairment and dementia in elderly patients. *Journal of Neuropsychiatry, 152*, 1470–1475.

Pantelis, C., & Barnes, T. R. E. (1996). Drug strategies and treatment-resistant schizophrenia. *Australian and New Zealand Journal of Psychiatry, 30*, 20–37.

Paulik, G., Badcock, J. C., & Maybery, M. T. (2006). The multifactorial structure of the predisposition to hallucinate and associations with anxiety, depression and stress. *Personality and Individual Differences, 41*, 1067–1076.

Paulik, G., Badcock, J. C., & Maybery, M. T. (2007). Poor intentional inhibition in individuals predisposed to hallucinations. *Cognitive Neuropsychiatry, 12*, 457–470.

Pearlman, L. M., & Hubbard, B. A. (2000). A self-control skills group for persistent auditory hallucinations. *Cognitive and Behavioural Practice, 7*, 17–21.

Penfield, W. (1955). The twenty-ninth Maudsley lecture: The role of the temporal cortex in certain physical phenomena. *Journal of Mental Science, 101*, 451–465.

Penfield, W., & Perot, P. (1963). The brain's record of auditory and visual experience. *Brain, 86*, 595–696.

Perry, E. K., & Perry, R. H. (1995). Acetylcholine and hallucinations: Disease-related compared to drug-induced alterations in human consciousness. *Brain and Cognition, 28*, 240–258.

Persons, J. B. (1986). The advantages of studying psychological phenomena rather than psychiatric diagnoses. *American Psychologist, 41*, 1252–1260.

Phillipson, O. T., & Harris, J. P. (1985). Perceptual changes in schizophrenia: A questionnaire survey. *Psychological Medicine, 15*, 859–866.

Pilling, S., Bebbington, P., Kuipers, E., Garety, P., Geddes, J., Martindale, B., et al. (2002). Psychological treatments in schizophrenia: II. Meta-analyses of randomized controlled trials of social skills training and cognitive remediation. *Psychological Medicine, 32*, 783–791.

Pinfold, V., Toulmin, H., Thorncroft, G., Huxley, P., Farmer, P., & Graham, T. (2003). Reducing psychiatric stigma and discrimination: Evaluation of educational interventions in UK secondary schools. *British Journal of Psychiatry, 182*, 342–346.

Platz, W. E., Oberlaender, F. A., & Seidel, M. L. (1995). The phenomenology of perceptual hallucinations in alcohol-induced delirium tremens. *Psychopathology, 28*, 247–255.

Plaze, M., Bartres-Faz, D., Martinot, J. L., Januel, D., Bellivier, F., De Beaurepaire, R., et al. (2006). Left superior temporal gyrus activation during sentence perception negatively correlates with auditory hallucination severity in schizophrenia patients. *Schizophrenia Research, 87*, 109–115.

Pomarol-Clotet, E., Honey, G. D., Murray, G. K., Corlett, P. R., Absalom, A. R., Lee, M., et al. (2006). Psychological effects of ketamine in healthy volunteers: Phenomenological study. *British Journal of Psychiatry, 189*, 173–179.

Posey, T. B., & Losch, M. E. (1983). Auditory hallucinations of hearing voices in 375 normal subjects. *Imagination, Cognition and Personality, 3*, 99–113.

Poulton, R., Avshalom, C., Moffitt, T. E., Cannon, M., Murray, R., & Harrington, H. (2000). Children's self-reported psychotic symptoms and adult schizophreniform disorder: A 15-year longitudinal study. *Archives of General Psychiatry, 57*, 1053–1058.

Poyurovsky, M., Hramenkov, S., Isakov, V., Rauchverger, B., Modai, I., Schneidman, M., et al. (2001). Obsessive-compulsive disorder in hospitalized patients with chronic schizophrenia. *Psychiatry Research, 102*, 49–57.

Rabins, P. V. (1982). Psychopathology of Parkinson's disease. *Comprehensive Psychiatry, 23*, 421–429.

Rajarethinam, R. P., DeQuardo, J. R., Nalepa, R., & Tandon, R. (2000). Superior temporal gyrus in schizophrenia: A volumetric magnetic resonance imaging study. *Schizophrenia Research, 41*, 303–312.

Rankin, P. M., & O'Carroll, P. J. (1995). Reality discrimination, reality monitoring and disposition towards hallucination. *British Journal of Clinical Psychology, 34*, 517–528.

Rao, V., & Lyketsos, C. G. (1998). Delusions in Alzheimer's disease: A review. *Journal of Neuropsychiatry and Clinical Neuroscience, 10*, 373–382.

Read, J., Agar, K., Argyle, N., & Aderhold, V. (2003). Sexual and physical abuse during childhood and adulthood as predictors of hallucinations, delusions and thought disorder. *Psychology and Psychotherapy: Theory, Research and Practice, 76*, 1–22.

Read, J., & Argyle, N. (1999). Hallucinations, delusions, and thought disorder among psychiatric patients with a history of child abuse. *Psychiatric Services, 50*, 1467–1472.

Read, J., Perry, B. D., Moskowitz, A., & Connolly, J. (2001). The contribution of early traumatic events to schizophrenia in some patients: A traumagenic neurodevelopmental model. *Psychiatry, 64*, 319–345.

Read, J., van Os, J., Morrison, A. P., & Ross, C. A. (2005). Childhood trauma, psychosis and schizophrenia: A literature review with theoretical and clinical implications. *Acta Psychiatrica Scandinavica, 112*, 330–350.

Rector, N. A., & Beck, A. T. (2001). Cognitive behavioral therapy for schizophrenia: An empirical review. *Journal of Nervous and Mental Disease, 189*, 278–287.

Reese, W. D. (1971). The hallucinations of widowhood. *British Medical Journal, 210*, 37–41.

Reisberg, B., Borenstein, J., Salob, S. P., Ferris, S. H., Franssen, E., & Georgotas, A. (1987). Behavioral symptoms in Alzheimer's disease: Phenomenology and treatment. *Journal of Clinical Psychiatry, 48*(Suppl. 5), 9–15.

Reisberg, B., Franssen, E., Sclan, S. G., Kluger, A., & Ferris, S. H. (1989). Stage specific incidence of potentially remediable behavioural symptoms in aging and Alzheimer's disease. *Bulletin of Clinical Neuroscience, 54*, 95–112.

Richardson, J. T. E. (1999). *Imagery*. Hove, England: Psychology Press.

Robins, L. N., Wing, J., Wittchen, H. U., Helzer, J. E., Babor, T. F., Burke, J., et al. (1988). The Composite International Diagnostic Interview: An epidemiological instrument suitable for use in conjunction with different diagnostic systems and in different cultures. *Archives of General Psychiatry, 45*, 1069–1077.

Rockwell, E., Choure, J., Galasko, D., Olichney, J., & Jeste, D. V. (2000). Psychopathology at initial diagnosis in dementia with Lewy bodies versus Alzheimer disease: Comparison of matched groups with autopsy-confirmed diagnoses. *International Journal of Geriatric Psychiatry, 15*, 819–823.

Roman, R., & Landis, C. (1945). Hallucinations and mental imagery. *Journal of Nervous and Mental Disease, 102*, 327–331.

Romme, M. A., & Escher, A. D. (1989). Hearing voices. *Schizophrenia Bulletin, 15*, 209–216.

Romme, M. A., & Escher, A. D. (2000). *Making sense of voices*. London: Mind.

Romme, M. A., Honig, A., Noorthoorn, E., & Escher, A. (1992). Coping with hearing voices: An emancipatory approach. *British Journal of Psychiatry, 161*, 99–103.

Ross, C. A., Anderson, G., & Clark, P. (1994). Childhood abuse and positive symptoms of schizophrenia. *Hospital and Community Psychiatry, 45*, 489–491.

Ross, C. A., & Joshi, S. (1992). Paranormal experiences in the general population. *Journal of Nervous and Mental Disease, 180*, 357–361.

Rossell, S. L., & Boundy, C. L. (2005). Are auditory–verbal hallucinations associated with auditory affective processing deficits? *Schizophrenia Research, 78*, 95–106.

Rossell, S. L., Shapleske, J., Fukuda, R., Woodruff, P. W., Simmons, A., & David, A. S. (2001). Corpus callosum area and functioning in schizophrenic patients with auditory–verbal hallucinations. *Schizophrenia Research, 50*, 9–17.

Rousseaux, M., Debrock, D., Cabaret, M., & Steinling, M. (1994). Visual hallucinations with written words in a case of left parietotemporal lesion. *Journal of Neurology, Neurosurgery and Psychiatry, 57*, 1268–1271.

Rudnick, A. (1999). Relation between command hallucinations and dangerous behavior. *Journal of the American Academy of Psychiatry and the Law, 27*, 253–258.

Rüsch, N., Angermeyer, M. C., & Corrigan, P. W. (2005). Mental illness stigma: Concepts, consequences, and initiatives to reduce stigma. *European Psychiatry, 20*, 529–539.

Saba, G., Verdon, C. M., Kalalou, K., Rocamora, J. F., Dumortier, G., Benadhira, R., et al. (2006). Transcranial magnetic stimulation in the treatment of schizophrenic symptoms: A double blind sham controlled study. *Journal of Psychiatric Research, 40*, 147–152.

Saba, P. R., & Keshavan, M. S. (1997). Musical hallucinations and musical imagery: Prevalence and phenomenology in schizophrenic inpatients. *Psychopathology, 30,* 185–190.

Sack, A. T., van de Ven, V. G., Etschenberg, S., Schatz, D., & Linden, D. E. (2005). Enhanced vividness of mental imagery as a trait marker of schizophrenia? *Schizophrenia Bulletin, 31,* 97–104.

Salanova, V., Andermann, F., Olivier, A., Rasmussen, T., & Quesney, L. F. (1992). Occipital lobe epilepsy: Electroclinical manifestations, electrocorticography, cortical stimulation and outcome in 42 patients treated between 1930 and 1991. Surgery of occipital lobe epilepsy. *Brain, 115,* 1655–1680.

Salkovskis, P. M., & Kirk, J. (1989). Obsessional disorders. In K. Hawton, P. M. Salkovskis, J. Kirk, & D. Clark (Eds.), *Cognitive behavior therapy for psychiatric problems: A practical guide* (pp. 129–168). New York: Oxford University Press.

Sanchez-Ramos, J., Ortoll, R., & Paulson, G. (1996). Visual hallucinations associated with Parkinson's disease. *Archives of Neurology, 53,* 1265–1268.

Sanjuán, J., Gonzalez, J. C., Aguilar, E. J., Leal, C., & van Os, J. (2004). Pleasurable auditory hallucinations. *Acta Psychiatrica Scandinavica, 110,* 273–278.

Sanjuán, J., Lull, J. J., Aguilar, E. J., Marti-Bonmati, L., Moratal, D., Gonzalez, J. C., et al. (2007). Emotional words induce enhanced brain activity in schizophrenic patients with auditory hallucinations. *Psychiatry Research, 154,* 21–29.

Sanjuán, J., Toirac, I., Gonzalez, J. C., Leal, C., Moltó, M. D., Nájera, C., & de Frutos, R. (2004). A possible association between the CCK-AR gene and persistent auditory hallucinations. *European Psychiatry, 19,* 349–353.

Sanjuán, J., Tolosa, A., González, J. C., Aguilar, E. J., Moltó, M. D., Nájera, C., et al. (2006). Association between FOXP2 polymorphisms and schizophrenia with auditory hallucinations. *Psychiatric Genetics, 16,* 67–72.

Santhouse, A. M., Howard, R. J., & ffytche, D. H. (2000). Visual hallucinatory syndromes and the anatomy of the brain. *Brain, 123,* 2055–2064.

Sarbin, T. R., & Juhasz, J. B. (1967). The historical background of the concept of hallucination. *Journal of the History of the Behavioral Sciences, 3,* 339–358.

Sarbin, T. R., & Juhasz, J. B. (1975). The social context of hallucinations. In R. K. Siegel & L. J. West (Eds.), *Hallucinations: Behavior, experience and theory* (pp. 214–227). New York: Wiley.

Sartorius, N., Jablensky, A., Korten, A., Ernberg, G., Anker, M., Cooper, J. E., & Day, R. (1986). Early manifestations and first contact incidence of schizophrenia in different cultures. *Psychological Medicine, 16,* 909–928.

Sartorius, N., Shapiro, R., & Jablensky, A. (1974). The international pilot study of schizophrenia. *Schizophrenia Bulletin, 1,* 21–25.

Sautter, F. J., Brailey, K., Uddo, M. M., Hamilton, M. F., Beard, M. G., & Borges, A. H. (1999). PTSD and comorbid psychotic disorder: Comparison with veterans diagnosed with PTSD or psychotic disorder. *Journal of Traumatic Stress, 12,* 73–88.

Schatzberg, A., & Rothschild, A. (1992). Psychotic (delusional) major depression: Should it be included as a distinct syndrome in *DSM–IV? American Journal of Psychiatry, 149,* 733–745.

Schielke, E., Reuter, U., Hoffmann, O., & Weber, J. R. (2000). Musical hallucinations with dorsal pontine lesions. *Neurology, 55,* 454–455.

Schneider, K. (1957). Primäre und sekundäre Symptomen bei Schizophrenie [Primary and secondary symptoms in schizophrenia]. *Fortschrift für Neurologie und Psychiatrie, 25,* 487–490.

Schneider, L. S., Pollock, V. E., & Lyness, S. A. (1990). A meta-analysis of controlled trials of neuroleptic treatment in dementia. *Journal of the American Geriatric Society, 38,* 553–563.

Schnider, A., & Ptak, R. (1999). Spontaneous confabulators fail to suppress currently irrelevant memory traces. *Nature Neuroscience, 2,* 677–681.

Schreiber, S., Dannon, P. N., Goshen, E., Amiaz, R., Zwas, T. S., & Grunhaus, L. (2002). Right prefrontal rTMS treatment for refractory auditory command hallucinations—A neuroSPECT assisted case study. *Psychiatry Research, 116,* 113–117.

Schreier, H. A., & Libow, J. A. (1986). Acute phobic hallucinations in very young children. *Journal of the American Academy of Child and Adolescence Psychiatry, 25,* 574–578.

Schultes, R. E., Hofmann, A., & Ratsch, C. (1998). *Plants of the gods: Their sacred, healing and hallucinogenic properties.* Rochester, VT: Healing Arts Press.

Schultz, G., & Melzack, R. (1991). The Charles Bonnet syndrome: "Phantom visual images." *Perception, 20,* 809–825.

Schulze, B., Richter-Werling, M., Matschinger, H., & Angermeyer, M. C. (2003). Crazy? So what! Effects of a school project on students' attitudes towards people with schizophrenia. *Acta Psychiatrica Scandinavica, 107,* 142–150.

Seal, M. L., Aleman, A., & McGuire, P. K. (2004). Compelling imagery, unanticipated speech and deceptive memory: Neurocognitive models of auditory verbal hallucinations in schizophrenia. *Cognitive Neuropsychiatry, 9,* 43–72.

Seal, M. L., Crowe, S. F., & Cheung, P. (1997). Deficits in source monitoring in subjects with auditory hallucinations may be due to differences in verbal intelligence and verbal memory. *Cognitive Neuropsychiatry, 2,* 273–290.

Sedikides, C. (1992). Mood as a determinant of attentional focus. *Cognition and Emotion, 6,* 129–148.

Seitz, P. F., & Molholm, H. B. (1947). Relation of mental imagery to hallucinations. *Archives of Neurology and Psychiatry, 57,* 469–480.

Semper, T. F., & McClellan, J. M. (2003). The psychotic child. *Child and Adolescent Psychiatric Clinics of North America, 2,* 679–691.

Semple, D., Smyth, R., Burns, J., Darjee, R., & McIntosh, A. (2005). *Oxford handbook of psychiatry.* New York: Oxford University Press.

Serper, M., Dill, C. A., Chang, N., Kot, T., & Elliot, J. (2005). Factorial structure of the hallucinatory experience: Continuity of experience in psychotic and normal individuals. *Journal of Nervous and Mental Disease, 193,* 265–272.

Shafran, R., & Rachman, S. (2004). Thought-action fusion: A review. *Journal of Behavior Therapy and Experimental Psychiatry, 35,* 87–107.

Shapleske, J., Rossell, S. L., Simmons, A., David, A. S., & Woodruff, P. W. (2001). Are auditory hallucinations the consequence of abnormal cerebral lateralization? A morphometric MRI study of the sylvian fissure and planum temporale. *Biological Psychiatry, 49,* 685–693. (Erratum in *Biological Psychiatry, 50,* 394)

Shawyer, F., Mackinnon, A., Farhall, J., Trauer, T., & Copolov, D. L. (2003). Command hallucinations and violence: Implications for detection and treatment. *Psychiatry, Psychology and Law, 10,* 97–107.

Shedlack, K. J., McDonald, W. M., Laskowitz, D. T. & Krishnan, K. R. (1994). Geniculocalcarine hyperintensities on brain magnetic resonance imaging associated with visual hallucinations in the elderly. *Psychiatry Research, 54,* 283–293.

Sheehan, D. V., Lecrubier, Y., Sheehan, K. H., Amorim, P., Janavs, J., Weiller, E., et al. (1998). The Mini-International Neuropsychiatric Interview (MINI): The development and validation of a structured diagnostic psychiatric interview for DSM–IV and ICD–10. *Journal of Clinical Psychiatry, 59*(Suppl. 20), 22–33.

Shergill, S. S., Brammer, M. J., Fukuda, R., Williams, S. C. R., Murray, R. M., & McGuire, P. K. (2003). Engagement of brain areas implicated in processing inner speech in patients with auditory hallucinations. *British Journal of Psychiatry, 182,* 525–531.

Shergill, S. S., Brammer, M. J., Williams, S. C., Murray, R. M., & McGuire, P. K. (2000). Mapping auditory hallucinations in schizophrenia using functional magnetic resonance imaging. *Archives of General Psychiatry, 57,* 1033–1038.

Shergill, S. S., Cameron, L. A., Brammer, M. J., Williams, S. C., Murray, R. M., & McGuire, P. K. (2001). Modality specific correlates of auditory and somatic hallucinations. *Journal of Neurology, Neurosurgery and Psychiatry, 71,* 688–690.

Shergill, S. S., Murray, R. M., & McGuire, P. K. (1998). Auditory hallucinations: A review of psychological treatments. *Schizophrenia Research, 32,* 137–150.

Sherman, S. L. (2001). A wake-up call from the thalamus. *Nature Neuroscience, 4,* 344–346.

Shevlin, M., Dorahy, M., & Adamson, G. (2007). Childhood traumas and hallucinations: An analysis of the National Comorbidity Survey. *Journal of Psychiatric Research, 41,* 222–228.

Shin, S. E., Lee, J. S., Kang, M. H., Kim, C. E., Bae, J. N., & Jung, G. (2005). Segmented volumes of cerebrum and cerebellum in first episode schizophrenia with auditory hallucinations. *Psychiatry Research, 138,* 33–42.

Shorter, E. (2005). *A historical dictionary of psychiatry.* Oxford, England: Oxford University Press.

Shulman, G. L., Corbetta, M., Buckner, R. L., Raichle, M. E., Fiez, J. A., Miezin, F. M., & Petersen, S. E. (1997). Top-down modulation of early sensory cortex. *Cerebral Cortex, 7,* 193–206.

Sidgewick, H. A. (1894). Report of the census on hallucinations. *Proceedings of the Society for Psychical Research, 26,* 259–394.

Siegel, R. K. (1984). Hostage hallucinations: Visual imagery induced by isolation and life-threatening stress. *Journal of Nervous and Mental Disease, 172,* 264–272.

Silbersweig, D. A., & Stern, E. (1998). Towards a functional neuroanatomy of conscious perception and its modulation by volition: Implications of human auditory neuroimaging studies. *Philosophical Transactions of the Royal Society London B, 353,* 1883–1888.

Silbersweig, D. A., Stern, E., Frith, C., Cahill, C., Holmes, A., Grootoonk, S., et al. (1995, November 9). A functional neuroanatomy of hallucinations in schizophrenia. *Nature, 378,* 176–179.

Slade, P. D. (1976). An investigation of psychological factors involved in the predisposition to auditory hallucinations. *Psychological Medicine, 6,* 123–132.

Slade, P. D., & Bentall, R. P. (1988). *Sensory deception: A scientific analysis of hallucination.* London: Croom-Helm.

Small, I. F., Small, J. G., & Andersen, J. M. (1966). Clinical characteristics of hallucinations of schizophrenia. *Diseases of the Nervous System, 27,* 349–353.

Smeets, R. M. W., & Dingemans, P. M. A. J. (1993). *Composite International Diagnostic System (CIDI), Version 1.1.* Geneva: World Health Organization.

Smith, B., Fowler, D. G., Freeman, D., Bebbington, P., Bashforth, H., Garety, P., et al. (2006). Emotion and psychosis: Links between depression, self-esteem, negative schematic beliefs and delusions and hallucinations. *Schizophrenia Research, 86,* 181–188.

Smith, D. B. (2007). *Muses, madmen, and prophets: Rethinking the history, science, and meaning of auditory hallucination.* New York: Penguin Press.

Sommer, I. E. C., Aleman, A., & Kahn, R. S. (2003). Left with the voices or hearing right? Meta-analysis of lateralization of auditory verbal hallucinations in schizophrenia. *Journal of Psychiatry and Neuroscience, 28,* 217–218.

Sommer, I. E., Ramsey, N. F., & Kahn, R. S. (2001). Language lateralization in schizophrenia: An fMRI study. *Schizophrenia Research, 52,* 57–67.

Sommer, I. E., Slotema, C. W., de Weijer, A. D., Blom, J. D., Daalman, K., Neggers, S. F., et al. (2007). Can fMRI-guidance improve the efficacy of rTMS treatment for auditory verbal hallucinations? *Schizophrenia Research, 93,* 406–408.

Spence, S. A. (2004). Voices in the brain. *Cognitive Neuropsychiatry, 9,* 1–8.

Spitzer, R. L., Williams, J. B., Gibbon, M., & First, M. B. (1992). The Structured Clinical Interview for *DSM-III-R* (SCID): I. History, rationale, and description. *Archives of General Psychiatry, 49,* 624–629.

Sritharan, A., Line, P., Sergejew, A., Silberstein, R., Egan, G., & Copolov, D. (2005). EEG coherence measures during auditory hallucinations in schizophrenia. *Psychiatry Research, 136,* 189–200.

Stant, A. D., TenVergert, E. M., Groen, H., Jenner, J. A., Nienhuis, F. J., van de Willige, G., & Wiersma, D. (2003). Cost-effectiveness of the HIT programme in patients with schizophrenia and persistent auditory hallucinations. *Acta Psychiatrica Scandinavica, 107,* 361–368.

Starker, S., & Jolin, A. (1982). Imagery and hallucination in schizophrenic patients. *Journal of Nervous and Mental Disease, 170*, 448–451.

Startup, M. (1999). Schizotypy, dissociative experiences and childhood abuse: Relationships among self report measures. *British Journal of Clinical Psychology, 38*, 333–344.

Stedman's Medical Dictionary (26th ed.). (1995). Baltimore: Williams & Wilkins.

Stefanis, N., Thewissen, V., Bakoula, C., van Os, J., & Myin-Germeys, I. (2006). Hearing impairment and psychosis: A replication in a cohort of young adults. *Schizophrenia Research, 85*, 266–272.

Stephane, M., Barton, S., & Boutros, N. N. (2001). Auditory verbal hallucinations and dysfunction of the neural substrates of speech. *Schizophrenia Research, 50*, 61–78.

Stephane, M., Thuras, P., Nasrallah, H., & Georgopoulos, A. P. (2003). The internal structure of the phenomenology of auditory verbal hallucinations. *Schizophrenia Research, 61*, 185–193.

Stephens, G. L., & Graham, G. (2000). *When self-consciousness breaks: Alien voices and inserted thoughts.* Cambridge, MA: MIT Press.

Stevens, A. A., Donegan, N. H., Anderson, M., Goldman-Rakic, P. S., & Wexler, B. (2000). Verbal processing deficits in schizophrenia. *Journal of Abnormal Psychology, 109*, 461–471.

Stevens, J. R., & Livermore, A. (1982). Telemetered EEG in schizophrenia: Spectral analysis during abnormal behaviour episodes. *Journal of Neurology, Neurosurgery and Psychiatry, 45*, 385–395.

Stewart, B., & Brennan, D. M. (2005). Auditory hallucinations after right temporal gyri resection. *Journal of Neuropsychiatry and Clinical Neuroscience, 17*, 243–245.

Stip, E. (2000). Novel antipsychotics: Issues and controversies. Typicality of atypical antipsychotics. *Journal of Psychiatry and Neuroscience, 25*, 137–153.

Stirling, J. D., Hellewell, J. S. E., & Ndlovu, D. (2001). Self-monitoring dysfunction and the positive symptoms of schizophrenia. *Psychopathology, 34*, 198–202.

Stirling, J. D., Hellewell, J. S. E., & Quraishi, N. (1998). Self-monitoring and schizophrenia symptoms of alien control. *Psychological Medicine, 28*, 675–683.

Strauss, E. W. (1962). *Phenomenology of hallucinations.* In L. J. West (Ed.), *Hallucinations* (pp. 220–231). Oxford, England: Grune & Stratton.

Strauss, J. S. (1969). Hallucinations and delusions as points on continua function. *Archives of General Psychiatry, 21*, 581–586.

Strauss, J. S. (1989). Subjective experiences of schizophrenia: Toward a new dynamic psychiatry II. *Schizophrenia Bulletin, 15*, 179–187.

Suhail, K., & Cochrane, R. (2002). Effect of culture and environment on the phenomenology of delusions and hallucinations. *International Journal of Social Psychiatry, 48*, 126–138.

Sumich, A., Chitnis, X. A., Fannon, D. G., O'Ceallaigh, S., Doku, V. C., Faldrowicz, A., & Sharma, T. (2005). Unreality symptoms and volumetric measures of

Heschl's gyrus and planum temporal in first-episode psychosis. *Biological Psychiatry, 57*, 947–950.

Suzucki, M., Yuasa, S., Minabe, Y., Murata, M., & Kurachi, M. (1993). Left superior temporal blood flow increases in schizophrenic and schizophreniform patients with auditory hallucinations: A longitudinal case study using ^{123}I-IMP SPET. *European Archives of Psychiatry and Clinical Neuroscience, 242*, 257–261.

Sweet, R. A., Hamilton, R. L., Lopez, O. L., Klunk, W. E., Wisniewski, S. R., Kaufer, D. I., et al. (2000). Psychotic symptoms in Alzheimer's disease are not associated with more severe neuropathologic features. *International Psychogeriatrics, 12*, 547–558.

Szechtman, H., Woody, E., Bowers, K. S., & Nahmias, C. (1998). Where the imaginal appears real: A positron emission tomography study of auditory hallucinations. *Proceedings of the National Academy of Sciences of the USA, 95*, 1956–1960.

Tachikawa, H., Harada, S., Kawanishi, Y., Okubo, T., & Suzuki, T. (2001). Linked polymorphisms (-333G>T and -286A>G) in the promoter region of the CCK-A receptor gene may be associated with schizophrenia. *Psychiatry Research, 103*, 147–155.

Tanriverdi, N., Sayilgan, M. A., & Özçürümez, G. (2001). Musical hallucinations associated with abruptly developed bilateral loss of hearing. *Acta Psychiatrica Scandinavica, 103*, 153–155.

Tanzi, E. (1909). *A textbook of mental diseases* (W. F. Robertson & T. C. Mackenzie, Trans.). New York: Rebman.

Tariot, P. N. (1996). Treatment strategies for agitation and psychosis in dementia. *Journal of Clinical Psychiatry, 57*, 21–29.

Tariot, P. N., Mack, J. L., Patterson, M. B., Edland, S. D., Weiner, M. F., Fillenbaum, G., et al. (1995). The CERAD Behavioral Rating Scale for Dementia. *American Journal of Psychiatry, 152*, 1349–1357.

Tarrier, N. (2002). The use of coping strategies and self-regulation in the treatment of psychosis. In A. P. Morrison (Ed.), *A casebook of cognitive therapy for psychosis* (pp. 132–147). Hove, England: Brunner-Routledge.

Tarrier, N., & Wykes, T. (2004). Is there evidence that cognitive behavior therapy is an effective treatment for schizophrenia? A cautious or cautionary tale? *Behavior Research and Therapy, 42*, 1377–1401.

Taylor, M., & Abrams, R. (1975). Acute mania: Clinical and genetic study of responders and nonresponders to treatments. *Archives of General Psychiatry, 32*, 863–865.

Tellegen, A. (1982). *Content categories: Absorption items (Revised)*. Unpublished manuscript, University of Minnesota, Minneapolis.

Terao, T. (1995). Tricyclic-induced musical hallucinations and states of relative sensory deprivation. *Biological Psychiatry, 38*, 192–193.

Terao, T. (2001). Musical hallucinations in middle age. *Acta Psychiatrica Scandinavica, 104*, 315–316.

Terao, T., & Matsunaga, K. (1999). Musical hallucinations and palinacousis. *Psychopathology, 32,* 57–59.

Terao, T., & Tani, Y. (1998). Carbamazepine treatment in a case of musical hallucinations with temporal lobe abnormalities. *Australian and New Zealand Journal of Psychiatry, 32,* 454–456.

Teri, L., Ferretti, L. E., Gibbons, L. E., Logsdon, R. G., McCurry, S. M., Kukull, W. A., et al. (1999). Anxiety of Alzheimer's disease: Prevalence and comorbidity. *Journals of Gerontology, Series A: Biological Sciences and Medical Sciences, 54,* 348–352.

Tervaniemi, M., & Hugdahl, K. (2003). Lateralization of auditory-cortex functions. *Brain Research Reviews, 43,* 231–246.

Teunisse, R. J., Cruysberg, J. R., Hoefnagels, W. H., Verbeek, A. L., & Zitman, F. G. (1996). Visual hallucinations in psychologically normal people: Charles Bonnet's syndrome. *Lancet, 347,* 794–797.

Teunisse, R. J., Zitman, F. G., & Raes, D. C. M. (1994). Clinical evaluation of 14 patients with Charles Bonnet syndrome (isolated visual hallucinations). *Comprehensive Psychiatry, 35,* 70–75.

Thewissen, V., Myin-Germeys, I., Bentall, R., de Graaf, R., Vollebergh, W., & van Os, J. (2005). Hearing impairment and psychosis revisited. *Schizophrenia Research, 76,* 99–103.

Thomas, P., Bracken, P., & Leudar, I. (2004). Hearing voices: A phenomenological–hermeneutic approach. *Cognitive Neuropsychiatry, 9,* 13–23.

Thomas, P., Mathur, P., Gottesman, I. I., Nagpal, R., Nimgaonkar, V. L., & Deshpande, S. N. (2007). Correlates of hallucinations in schizophrenia: A cross-cultural evaluation. *Schizophrenia Research, 92,* 41–49.

Thompson, J. S., Stuart, G. L., & Holden, C. E. (1992). Command hallucinations and legal insanity. *Forensic Report, 5,* 29–43.

Tien, A. Y. (1991). Distribution of hallucinations in the population. *Social Psychiatry and Psychiatric Epidemiology, 26,* 287–292.

Toone, B. K., Cooke, E., & Lader, M. H. (1981). Electrodermal activity in the affective disorders and schizophrenia. *Psychological Medicine, 11,* 497–508.

Tootell, R. B., Hadjikhani, N., Hall, E. K., Marrett, S., Vanduffel, W., Vaughan, J. T., & Dale, A. M. (1998). The retinotopy of visual spatial attention. *Neuron, 21,* 1409–1422.

Trower, P., Birchwood, M., Meaden, A., Byrne, S., Nelson, A., & Ross, K. (2004). Cognitive therapy for command hallucinations: Randomised controlled trial. *British Journal of Psychiatry, 184,* 312–320.

Trygstad, L., Buccheri, R., Dowling, G., Zind, R., White, K., Griffin, J., et al. (2002). Behavioural management of persistent auditory hallucinations in schizophrenia: Outcomes from a 10-week course. *Journal of the American Psychiatric Nurses Association, 8,* 84–91.

Tsuang, J. W., Irwin, M. R., Smith, T. L., & Schuckit, M. A. (1994). Characteristics of men with alcoholic hallucinosis. *Addiction, 89,* 73–78.

Tucker, G. J., Price, T. R., Johnson, V. B., & McAllister, T. (1986). Phenomenology of temporal lobe dysfunction: A link to atypical psychosis. A series of cases. *Journal of Nervous and Mental Disease, 174,* 348–356.

Tuelth, M. J., Cheong, J. A., & Samander, J. (1995). The Charles Bonnet syndrome: A type of organic visual hallucinosis. *Journal of Geriatric Psychiatry and Neurology, 8,* 1–3.

Turnbull, G., & Bebbington, P. (2001). Anxiety and the schizophrenic process: Clinical and epidemiological evidence. *Social Psychiatry and Psychiatric Epidemiology, 36,* 235–243.

Turvey, C. L., Schultz, S. K., Arndt, S., Ellingrod, V., Wallace, R., & Herzog, R. (2001). Caregiver report of hallucinations and paranoid delusions in elders aged 70 or older. *International Psychogeriatrics, 13,* 241–249.

Valmaggia, L. R., van der Gaag, M., Tarrier, N., Pijnenborg, M., & Sloof, C. J. (2005). Cognitive–behavioural therapy for refractory psychotic symptoms of schizophrenia resistant to atypical antipsychotic medication. *British Journal of Psychiatry, 186,* 324–330.

VandenBos, G. R. (Ed.). (2007). *APA dictionary of psychology.* Washington, DC: American Psychological Association.

van de Ven, V. G., Formisano, E., Roder, C. H., Prvulovic, D., Bittner, R. A., Dietz, M. G., et al. (2005). The spatiotemporal pattern of auditory cortical responses during verbal hallucinations. *Neuroimage, 27,* 644–655.

van der Gaag, M. (2006). A neuropsychiatric model of biological and psychological processes in the remission of delusions and auditory hallucinations. *Schizophrenia Bulletin, 32,* S113–S122.

van der Gaag, M., Hageman, M. C., & Birchwood, M. (2003). Evidence for a cognitive model of auditory hallucinations. *Journal of Nervous and Mental Disease, 191,* 542–545.

van der Werf, M., van Boxtel, M., Verhey, F., Jolles, J., Thewissen, V., & van Os, J. (2007). Mild hearing impairment and psychotic experiences in a normal aging population. *Schizophrenia Research, 94,* 180–186.

van Os, J., Hanssen, M., Bijl, R. V., & Ravelli, A. (2000). Strauss (1969) revisited: A psychosis continuum in the normal population? *Schizophrenia Research, 45,* 11–20.

van Os, J., & Jones, P. B. (2001). Neuroticism as a risk factor for schizophrenia. *Psychological Medicine, 31,* 1129–1134.

van Os, J., Jones, P., Sham, P., Bebbington, P., & Murray, R. M. (1998). Risk factors for onset and persistence of psychosis. *Social Psychiatry and Psychiatric Epidemiology, 33,* 596–605.

van't Wout, M., Aleman, A., Kessels, R. P. C., Larøi, F., & Kahn, R. S. (2004). Emotional processing in a non-clinical psychosis-prone sample. *Schizophrenia Research, 68,* 271–281.

Vercammen, A., de Haan, E. H. F., & Aleman, A. (in press). Hearing a voice in the noise: Auditory hallucinations and speech perception. *Psychological Medicine.*

Verdoux, H., van Os, J., Maurice-Tison, S., Gay, B., Salamon, R., & Bourgeois, M. (1998). Is early adulthood a critical developmental stage for psychosis proneness? A survey of delusional ideation in normal subjects. *Schizophrenia Research, 29,* 247–254.

Versmissen, D., Janssen, I., Johns, L., McGuire, P., Drukker, M., Campo, J. A., et al. (2007). Verbal self-monitoring in psychosis: A non-replication. *Psychological Medicine, 37,* 569–576.

Vignal, J.-P., Maillard, L., McGonigal, A., & Chauvel, P. (2007). The dreamy state: Hallucinations of autobiographic memory evoked by temporal lobe stimulations and seizures. *Brain, 130,* 88–99.

Vollenweider, F. X., Vontobel, P., Oye, I., Hell, D., & Leenders, K. L. (2000). Effects of (S)-ketamine on striatal dopamine: A [11C]raclopride PET study of a model psychosis in humans. *Journal of Psychiatric Research, 34,* 35–43.

Vygotsky, L. S. V. (1962). *Thought and language.* Cambridge, MA: MIT Press.

Wahass, S., & Kent, G. (1997a). A comparison of public attitudes in Britain and Saudi Arabia towards auditory hallucinations. *International Journal of Social Psychiatry, 43,* 175–183.

Wahass, S., & Kent, G. (1997b). Coping with auditory hallucinations: A cross-cultural comparison between Western (British) and non-Western (Saudi Arabian) patients. *Journal of Nervous and Mental Disease, 185,* 664–668.

Wahass, S., & Kent, G. (1997c). The modification of psychological interventions for persistent auditory hallucinations to an Islamic culture. *Behavioural and Cognitive Psychotherapy, 25,* 351–364.

Waters, F. A. V., Badcock, J. C., & Maybery, M. T. (2003). Revision of the factor structure of the Launay–Slade Hallucination Scale (LSHS–R). *Personality and Individual Differences, 35,* 1351–1357.

Waters, F. A. V., Badcock, J. C., & Maybery, M. T. (2006). The 'who' and 'when' of context memory: Different patterns of association with auditory hallucinations. *Schizophrenia Research, 82,* 271–273.

Waters, F. A. V., Badcock, J. C., Maybery, M. T., & Michie, P. T. (2003). Inhibition in schizophrenia: Association with auditory hallucinations. *Schizophrenia Research, 62,* 275–280.

Waters, F. A. V., Badcock, J. C., Michie, P. T., & Maybery, M. T. (2006). Auditory hallucinations in schizophrenia: Intrusive thoughts and forgotten memories. *Cognitive Neuropsychiatry, 11,* 65–83.

Waters, F. A. V., Maybery, M. T., Badcock, J. C., & Michie, P. T. (2004). Context memory and binding in schizophrenia. *Schizophrenia Research, 68,* 119–125.

Watkins, J. (1998). *Hearing voices: A common human experience.* Melbourne: Hill of Content.

Wechsler, D. (1987). *Wechsler Memory Scale—Revised: Manual.* New York: Harcourt, Brace, Jovanovich.

Wei, J., & Hemmings, G. P. (1999). The CCK-A receptor gene possibly associated with auditory hallucinations in schizophrenia. *European Psychiatry, 14,* 67–70.

Weiss, A. P., & Heckers, S. (1999). Neuroimaging of hallucinations: A review of the literature. *Psychiatry Research, 92*, 61–74.

Weiss, E. M., Hofer, A., Golaszewski, S., Siedentopf, C., Felber, S., & Fleischhacker, W. W. (2006). Language lateralization in unmedicated patients during an acute episode of schizophrenia: A functional MRI study. *Psychiatry Research, 146*, 185–190.

Wells, A. (2000). *Emotional disorders and metacognition: Innovative cognitive therapy.* Chichester, England: Wiley.

Wells, A., & Cartwright-Hatton, S. (2004). A short form of the Metacognitions Questionnaire: Properties of the MCQ-30. *Behavioral Research and Therapy, 42*, 385–396.

West, D. J. (1948). A mass observation questionnaire on hallucinations. *Journal of the Society for Psychical Research, 34*, 187–196.

West, L. J. (1975). A clinical and theoretical overview of hallucinatory phenomena. In R. K. Siegel & L. J. West (Eds.), *Hallucinations: Behavior, experience and theory* (p. 292). New York: Wiley.

Wiersma, D., Jenner, J. A., Nienhuis, F. J., & van de Willige, G. (2004). Hallucination focused integrative treatment improves quality of life in schizophrenia patients. *Acta Psychiatrica Scandinavica, 109*, 194–201.

Wiersma, D., Jenner, J. A., van de Willige, G., Spakman, M., & Nienhuis, F. J. (2001). Cognitive behaviour therapy with coping training for persistent auditory hallucinations in schizophrenia: A naturalistic follow-up study of the durability of effects. *Acta Psychiatrica Scandinavica, 103*, 393–399.

Wilcox, J., Briones, D., & Suess, L. (1991). Auditory hallucinations, posttraumatic stress disorder, and ethnicity. *Comprehensive Psychiatry, 32*, 320–323.

Williamson, D. E., Birmaher, B., Ryan, N. D., Shiffrin, T. P., Lusky, J. A., Protopapa, J., et al. (2003). The Stressful Life Events Schedule for children and adolescents: Development and validation. *Psychiatry Research, 119*, 225–241.

Wing, J. K., Birley, J. L. T., Cooper, J. E., Graham, P., & Isaacs, A. D. (1967). Reliability of a procedure for measuring and classifying "present psychiatric state." *British Journal of Psychiatry, 113*, 499–515.

Woldorff, M. G., Gallen, C. G., Hampson, S. A., Hillyard, S. A., Pantev, C., Sobel, D., & Bloom, F. E. (1993). Modulation of early sensory processing in human auditory cortex during auditory selective attention. *Proceedings of the National Academy of Sciences of the USA, 90*, 8722–8726.

Wolters, E. C. (2006). PD-related psychosis: Pathophysiology with therapeutical strategies. *Journal of Neural Transmission, 71*(Suppl.), 31–37.

Wolters, E. C., & Berendse, H. W. (2001). Management of psychosis in Parkinson's disease. *Current Opinion in Neurology, 14*, 499–504.

Wood, S., Cummings, J. L., Hsu, M. A., Barclay, T., Wheatley, M. V., Yarema, K. T., & Schnelle, J. F. (2000). The use of the Neuropsychiatric Inventory in nursing home residents: Characterization and measurement. *American Journal of Geriatric Psychiatry, 8*, 75–83.

Woodruff, P. W. (2004). Auditory hallucinations: Insights and questions from neuroimaging. *Cognitive Neuropsychiatry, 9*, 73–91.

Woodruff, P. W., Wright, I. C., Bullmore, E. T., Brammer, M., Howard, R. J., Williams, S. C., et al. (1997). Auditory hallucinations and the temporal cortical response to speech in schizophrenia: A functional magnetic resonance imaging study. *American Journal of Psychiatry, 154*, 1676–1682.

World Health Organization. (1990). *Composite International Diagnostic Interview (CIDI), Version 1.0.* Geneva: Author.

Writing: Hallucinations. (n.d.). Retrieved October 30, 2007, from http://www.schizophrenia-help-online.com/writing.htm

Wunderlich, G., Suchan, B., Volkmann, J., Herzog, H., Homberg, V., & Seitz, R. J. (2000). Visual hallucinations in recovery from cortical blindness: Imaging correlates. *Archives of Neurology, 57*, 561–565.

Wykes, T. (2004). Psychological treatment for voices in psychosis. *Cognitive Neuropsychiatry, 9*, 25–41.

Wykes, T., Hayward, P., Thomas, N., Green, N., Surguladze, S., Fannon, D., & Landau, S. (2005). What are the effects of group cognitive behavior therapy for voices? A randomized control trial. *Schizophrenia Research, 77*, 201–210.

Wykes, T., Parr, A.-M., & Landau, S. (1999). Group treatment of auditory hallucinations. *British Journal of Psychiatry, 175*, 180–185.

Yamamoto, J., Okonogi, K., Iwasaki, T., & Yosimura, S. (1969). Mourning in Japan. *American Journal of Psychiatry, 125*, 1660–1665.

Yee, L., Korner, A. J., McSwiggan, S., Meares, R. A., & Stevenson, J. (2005). Persistent hallucinosis in borderline personality disorder. *Comprehensive Psychiatry, 46*, 147–154.

Yoshizumi, T., Murase, S., Honjo, S., Kaneko, H., & Murakami, T. (2004). Hallucinatory experiences in a community sample of Japanese children. *Journal of the American Academy of Child and Adolescent Psychiatry, 43*, 1030–1036.

Yoss, R. E., & Daly, D. D. (1960). Criteria for the diagnosis of the narcoleptic syndrome. *Mayo Clinic Proceedings, 32*, 320–328.

Young, H. F., Bentall, R. P., Slade, P. D., & Dewey, M. E. (1987). The role of brief instructions and suggestibility in the elicitation of auditory and visual hallucinations in normal and psychiatric subjects. *Journal of Nervous and Mental Disease, 175*, 41–48.

Zarroug, E. T. A. (1975). The frequency of visual hallucinations in schizophrenia patients in Saudi Arabia. *British Journal of Psychiatry, 127*, 553–555.

Zatorre, R. J., & Halpern, A. R. (2005). Mental concerts: Musical imagery and auditory cortex. *Neuron, 47*, 9–12.

Zhang, X. Y., Zhou, D. F., Zhang, P. Y., & Wei, J. (2000). The CCK-A receptor gene possibly associated with positive symptoms of schizophrenia. *Molecular Psychiatry, 5*, 239–240.

Zikopoulos, B., & Barbas, H. (2006). Prefrontal projections to the thalamic reticular nucleus form a unique circuit for attentional mechanisms. *Journal of Neuroscience, 26*, 7348–7361.

Zimmerman, G., Favrod, J., Trieu, V. H., & Pomini, V. (2005). The effect of cognitive behavioral treatment on the positive symptoms of schizophrenia spectrum disorders: A meta-analysis. *Schizophrenia Research, 77,* 1–9.

Zubin, J., & Spring, B. (1977). Vulnerability: A new view of schizophrenia. *Journal of Abnormal Psychology, 86,* 103–126.

Zuckerman, M. (1999). *Vulnerability to psychopathology: A biosocial model.* Washington, DC: American Psychological Association.

AUTHOR INDEX

Connolly, J., 51, 207
Cooke, E., 42
Cooper, J. E., 80
Cooper, J. K., 206
Copeland, J. R., 75, 76, 227
Copolov, D. L., 25, 32, 33, 35–37, 94, 112,
    166, 168, 189, 210, 220
Corrigan, P. W., 198
Cosoff, S. J., 205
Costa, S. E., 54
Costello, A., 225
Costello, C. G., 6
Cowell, P. E., 156
Cramer, J. A., 184
Crick, F., 173
Critchley, M., 94
Crowe, S. F., 127, 174
Cruysberg, J. R., 43
Cubells, J. F., 224
Cullberg, J., 155
Cummings, L. J., 55, 149, 206, 230
Currie, S., 54
Curson, D. A., 184

d'Alfonso, A. A. L., 186, 187
d'Amato, T., 145
Daly, D. D., 40
Darjee, R., 16
Dary, M., 58
Dattilio, F. N., 202
David, A. S., 6, 7, 15–17, 25, 28, 32, 35, 36,
    43, 47, 53, 57, 58, 60, 66, 94, 101,
    112, 113, 115, 144, 157, 164, 189,
    190, 231, 232
Davies, E., 194
Davies, M. F., 33, 35, 79
Debrock, D., 94
DeFruyt, F., 61, 64, 76, 77, 88, 106, 228
de Haan, E. H. F., 16, 17, 61, 64, 96, 99,
    100, 101, 131, 221
de Lemus, M. L., 30
Delespaul, P., 26, 33, 38, 42, 43, 73, 88, 134,
    191, 193, 226
Della-Sala, S., 57
Del'Osso, L., 205
Dendurkuri, N., 75, 227
Dennett, D., 20
Denukuri, N, 76
DePasquale, T., 25, 212, 233
DeQuardo, J. R., 156
Devanand, D. P., 229
de Vries, M., 26, 88, 134

Dewey, M. E., 61, 102, 221
Dhossche, D., 69–73, 206
Dickerson, F. B., 198, 202
Dickinson, J., 58
Diederich, N. J., 97
Dierks, T., 101, 160, 161, 167, 186
Dill, C. A., 61, 221
Dingemans, P. M. A. J., 81
Dinin, T. G., 111
Ditman, T., 109, 134
Dittmann, J., 191, 193
Dixon, J. J., 67, 207
Dixon, N. F., 103
Dolan, R. J., 92, 158, 174
Dolder, C. B., 184
Dolgov, I., 95
Done, D. J., 117
Donegan, N. H., 94
Dorahy, M., 75
Douglass, M. A., 213
Dowson, L., 75, 76, 227
Drevets, W. C., 57
Duda, J. E., 149
du Feu, M., 48
Dudley, R., 201, 207
Dunn, L. B., 184

Easton, S., 61
Eaton, W. E., 61
Edelbrock, C., 225
Egelhoff, C., 67
Elimalach-Malmilyan, S., 105
Ellason, J., 51
Ellenberger, H., 28
Ellger, T., 26, 40
Elliot, J., 61, 221
Eming-Erdmann, A., 210
Endicott, J., 226
Ensink, B., 51, 64
Ensum, I., 123–125, 134
Eperjesi, F., 58, 216
Erkwoh, R., 210
Errasti, J. M., 138
Escher, A. D., 33, 61, 74, 189, 191, 192, 204,
    205, 207, 211, 226, 234
Escher, S., 43, 73, 74, 193, 226
Esquirol, E., 12
Esquirol, J. E. D., 12, 14, 33
Etheridge, J. B., 45, 61, 64, 87, 99, 222
Etschenberg, S., 99
Eustache, F., 58
Evans, C. L., 101

Evans, J. M., 215
Evers, S., 26, 40
Ey, H., 25

Fallon, I. R. H., 189
Faragher, E. B., 36, 220
Farah, M. J., 103
Farhall, J., 37, 189
Farley, J., 51
Favrod, J., 198, 212
Feinberg, I., 114
Feinstein, A., 53
Feldman, F., 58
Fénelon, G., 39, 55–57, 59, 206, 215
Fenton, G. W., 59
Ferdinand, R., 69, 70, 206
Fernandez, A., 216
Fernyhough, C., 22, 138
Ferris, S. H., 57, 229
Ferroir, J. P., 39, 59
Festinger, L., 137
ffytche, D. H., 58, 101, 160, 164, 223
Fialko, L., 233
Fidalgo, A. M., 142
Finkel, S. I., 54
First, M. B., 82
Fischer, C. E., 40
Fiszbein, A., 220
Fitzgerald, P. B., 186
Flaum, M., 48, 156
Flavell, J. H., 109
Fleming, K. C., 215
Foley, H. J., 121
Foley, M. A., 121
Folkman, S., 189
Ford, J. M., 114, 117, 177
Formisano, E., 167
Forstl, H., 155
Foss, J., 22
Fowler, D., 84, 86, 113, 198
Fowler, I. L., 205
Frame, C. L., 20, 25
Frame, L., 50, 207
Francescani, A., 57
Franssen, E., 57, 229
Freeman, D., 42, 84, 86, 113, 116, 206
French, P., 195
Freud, S., 10, 15
Fried, J., 28
Friston, K. J., 174
Frith, C. D., 92, 110, 113, 114, 117, 122, 158, 161, 167, 172, 177

Frosch, W., 37
Fukuhara, R., 163, 213

Galasko, D., 56
Gallagher, A. G., 111
Galton, F., 14, 19, 97
Garcelàn, S. P., 138, 196
Garcia, L. M., 167
García-Montes, J. M., 30, 138, 139, 142, 196
Garety, P. A., 33, 35, 42, 84, 85n6, 86, 113, 198, 206
Garralda, M. E., 72, 73
Garrett, M., 197
Gartz, J., 150
Gaser, C., 158
Gaudiano, B. A., 198, 201
Gauntlett-Gilbert, J., 26, 36, 38
Gazzaniga, M. S., 8, 162
Gehrbe, M., 189
Geiger-Kabisch, C., 155
Georgopoulos, A. P., 25, 134, 232
Gibbon, M., 82
Gilbert, P., 223
Gilley, D. W., 214
Gledhill, A., 201
Glicksohn, J., 105
Glinski, A., 78, 110
Godwin, D. W., 173
Goëb, J.-L., 70, 72, 74, 185, 206
Goetz, C. G., 55, 97
Goff, D., 198
Goldman-Rakic, P. S., 94
Goldstein, D., 150
Gonzalez, J. C., 35
Good, J., 206
Goodman, W., 201
Goodwin, D. W., 26, 37, 38, 41
Goodwin, F. K., 50
Gorman, J. M., 144
Gottesman, C., 174
Gould, L. N., 110, 112
Gould, R. A., 198
Gouzoulis-Mayfrank, E., 152
Graham, C., 58
Graham, G., 22
Graham, J., 55–57, 60
Graham, P., 80
Grasset, F., 212
Gray, M. J., 207n7
Green, M. F., 95, 110, 111
Green, P., 110
Greenwood, K. M., 189

Husting, H. H., 224

Igarashi, Y., 36
Ikeda, M., 163, 213
Inoko, K., 74
Inouye, T., 110
Intons-Peterson, M. J., 98
Inzelberg, R., 57, 206
Irwin, M. R., 52
Isaacs, A. D., 80
Ishino, Y., 26, 163
Ivry, R. B., 8
Iwasaki, T., 31, 68
Izumi, Y., 26, 163

Jablensky, A., 48
Jackson, H. J., 189
Jackson, J. H., 148
Jacoby, R., 57
Jakes, S., 87
James, I., 213
Jamison, K. R., 50
Jäncke, L., 161
Janssen, I., 65, 74
Jansson, B., 26
Jardi, R., 186
Jaspers, K., 18–20, 33
Javitt, D. C., 152
Jaynes, J., 162
Jenner, J. A., 35, 203, 204
Jensterle, J., 117
Jeste, D. V., 56, 57, 184, 213
Johns, L., 116
Johns, L. C., 3, 15, 29, 33, 35, 47, 61, 63, 64,
    66, 79, 87, 115, 116, 174
Johnson, J. H., 208n7
Johnson, M. K., 100, 118–120, 126, 127, 132,
    134, 176
Johnson, V. B., 54
Johnstone, E. C., 117, 148
Jolin, A., 98
Jones, C., 106
Jones, H. M., 144
Jones, O. B. E., 28
Jones, P., 88
Jones, P. B., 112, 160, 161, 186
Jones, R. B., 88
Jones, S., 34
Jones, S. R., 138, 141
Jørgensen, H. A., 95
Joshi, S., 51, 64
Juhasz, J. B., 12, 40

Junginger, J., 20, 25

Kahn, R. S., 42, 64, 100, 101, 131, 134, 157,
    163, 166, 174, 185
Kalas, R., 225
Kaneko, H., 69, 70, 206
Kaplan, H., 51
Karson, C. N., 26, 38
Kasai, K., 163
Kastner, S., 173
Katona, C., 75, 76, 227
Kaufer, D. I., 230
Kaufman, J., 74
Kawanishi, Y., 154
Kay, S. R., 220
Kent, G., 28, 31, 31n4, 192
Keshavan, M. S., 39
Kessels, R. P. C., 42, 64, 134
Kessler, M., 225
Kessler, R. C., 205
Kinderman, P., 138
Kingdon, D. G., 197, 200, 205
Kinsbourne, M., 110, 111
Kipervasser, S., 57, 206
Kirk, J., 195
Kirkland, J., 201
Kitchen, G., 75, 76, 227
Klaric, S., 225
Klein, C., 55
Kluger, A., 57, 229
Kluver, H., 150
Knight, A., 195
Koempf, D., 55
Koenig, T., 167
Koenigsberg, H. W., 37
Kölmel, H. W., 58, 94
Korczyn, A. D., 57, 206
Korner, A. J., 53
Kosslyn, S. M., 16, 21, 100, 176
Kostianovsky, D. J., 156
Kot, T., 61, 103, 221
Krabbendam, L., 43, 65, 87, 88
Kraepelin, E., 33
Krishnan, K. R., 155
Krol, P., 51
Kroll, J., 29, 30
Krystal, J. H., 151
Kubany, E. S., 208n7
Kuipers, E., 26, 29, 33, 35, 36, 38, 42, 61,
    66, 79, 84, 86, 113, 198
Kumagai, R., 151
Kunert, H. J., 210

SUBJECT INDEX

Avoidant coping style, 192
Awakening, hallucinations on, 40–41
Awake state, 17–18
Axis I disorders, 72, 73

Baillarger, Jules, 13
BAVQ. *See* Beliefs About Voices Questionnaire
BAVQ–R (Revised Beliefs About Voices Questionnaire), 221
BEHAVE–AD (Behavioral Pathology in Alzheimer's Disease Rating Scale), 229
BEHAVE–AD–FW (Behavioral Pathology in Alzheimer's Disease—Frequency-Weighted Severity Scale), 229
Behavioral measures of imagery, 100–102
Behavioral modification, 189
Behavioral Pathology in Alzheimer's Disease—Frequency-Weighted Severity Scale (BEHAVE–AD–FW), 229
Behavioral Pathology in Alzheimer's Disease Rating Scale (BEHAVE–AD), 229
Behavior Rating Scale for Dementia (BRSD), 228–229
Behrendt, R.-P., 21–22
Beliefs
    and command hallucinations, 210
    and imagery, 209–210
    metacognitive, 137–142, 194–196
    and response to hallucinations, 86
    visual hallucinations affecting lasting, 39
Beliefs About Voices Questionnaire (BAVQ), 45, 221, 225, 232
Belladonna, 149
Belshazzar, 10, 11
Benevolence, 33
Benevolent voices, 212
Bentall, Richard P., 16–17, 84n5, 118, 126–127
Bentall's reality monitoring model, 118–136
    culture's role in, 120
    and external stimulation, 120–121
    and reality testing task, 122–125
    source monitoring in, 118–120
    verbal self-monitoring in, 121–122
Bereavement, 67–68
    in children/adolescents, 72
    and coping styles, 192
    and hallucinations, 31
Beriberi, 71

Betts Questionnaire Upon Mental Imagery (QMI), 98–99
Bias
    cognitive, 113
    externalization, 124
    externalizing, 116, 117
    response, 122, 124
The Bible, 11
Bicameral mind, 162
Bilateral basal ganglia, 163
Bilateral lower frontal area, 163
Bilateral parahippocampal gyrus, 160
Bilateral thalamus, 160
Bipolar disorder
    with hallucinations, 50, 60
    and musical hallucinations, 39
    and positive auditory hallucinations, 35
    and visual hallucinations, 38
Blindness, 58
Blood alcohol level, 52
Blood flow, 154
Blood pressure analogy, 87
Blurring, 105
Borderline personality disorder, 38, 53
Bottom-up influences, 176
Bottom-up perceptual processing, 91
Brain, 147–169
    auditory hallucinations and volume of, 157
    and comprehensive model, 172–179
    neuroimaging, 153–168
    neurotransmitters, 148–153
    stimulation studies of, 147–148
Brain activity during hallucinations, 159–168
    activation studies of, 159–164
    cognitive studies of, 164–166
    electroencephalographic studies of, 166–167
Brain diseases, 54
Brain injury, 94
Brain stem hematoma, 54
Brain structure, 154–159
Brain tumors, 54
Brébion, G., 129–130
Brewer, E. Cobham, 14
Brierre de Boismont, Alexandre, 12–14
Broca's area, 156, 158–160, 168
Brodmann's area, 167
BRSD. *See* Behavior Rating Scale for Dementia; CERAD Behavior Rating Scale for Dementia
Bufo alvarius, 150

ABOUT THE AUTHORS

André Aleman, PhD, is a professor of cognitive neuropsychiatry at the University Medical Center, Groningen, the Netherlands. He obtained his MSc (in neuropsychology) and his PhD from the University of Utrecht, the Netherlands. His research foci include the cognitive and neural bases of hallucinations, emotional processing in schizophrenia and depression, and the psychological and neural underpinnings of poor illness awareness in psychosis.

Frank Larøi, PhD, works in the Cognitive Psychopathology Unit at the University of Liège, Belgium. He obtained his BSc from the University of Bath, England; his degree in clinical psychology from the University of Oslo, Norway; and his PhD from the University of Liège. In addition to hallucinations, his research interests include schizophrenia, delusions, cognitive remediation, awareness of illness, and emotional processing in psychopathology.